The
INTIMATE COUPLE

The
INTIMATE COUPLE

Reaching New Levels of Sexual Excitement through Body Awakening and Relationship Renewal

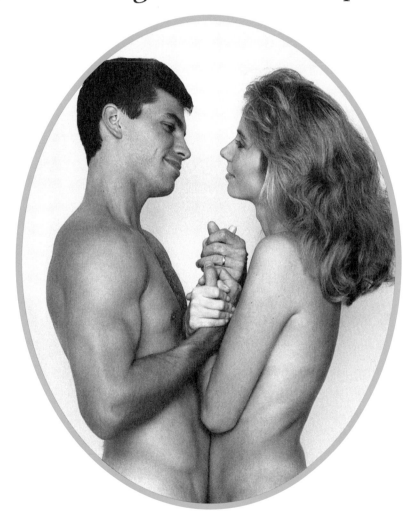

JACK LEE ROSENBERG, PH.D.
BEVERLY KITAEN-MORSE, PH.D.

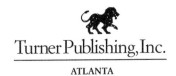

Turner Publishing, Inc.
ATLANTA

To our parents, children, and grandchildren,
the generations who have so enriched our lives

Library of Congress Cataloging-in-Publication Data
Rosenberg, Jack Lee, 1932–
    The intimate couple: reaching new levels of sexual excitement
  through body awakening and relationship renewal/by Jack L. Rosenberg and
  Beverly Kitaen-Morse. —1st ed.
      p. cm.
    Includes bibliographical references (p.   ) and index.
    ISBN 1–57036–222–X (alk. paper)
    1. Sex. 2. Orgasm. 3. Exercise. I. Kitaen-Morse, Beverly.
  II. Title.
  HQ31.R84316 1996
  613.9′6—dc20
                                   95–44191
                                       CIP

Photography—J. Stoll
Illustrations—John Daugherty
Cover design—Michael J. Walsh
Book design and art direction—Karen E. Smith
Photo Editor—Marty Moore
Production Manager—Anne Murdoch

Published by Turner Publishing, Inc.
A Subsidiary of Turner Broadcasting Company, Inc.
1050 Techwood Drive, NW
Atlanta, Georgia 30318

Distributed by Andrews and McMeel
A Universal Press Syndicate Company
4900 Main Street
St. Louis, Missouri 64112

First Edition
10 9 8 7 6 5 4 3 2 1

Printed in the U.S.A.

TABLE OF CONTENTS

A C K N O W L E D G M E N T S

WE WISH TO EXPRESS our gratitude and appreciation to friends, therapists, colleagues, and others who have supported and encouraged us in many ways, including reading our manuscripts and providing introductions to publishers: Vera Dunn, Phyllis Shankman, Jeffrey Trop, Victoria Hamilton, Tracy Kramer, Jane Fonda, Julie LaFond, Linda Graedel, Jonathan Estrin, Michael Rosenfeld, Sr., Michael Rosenfeld, Jr., Loren Miles, Gary LeMel, Lori Steinberg, Harriet Goslins, Nancy Lunney, Loren Basch, Lauree Moss, Leroy Perry, Virginia Barbosa, and Marc LeBel.

A special thank you to Valerie Murphy whose editorial assistance over the years has been invaluable; to our son-in-law and attorney, Charles Fries, for his sound guidance on this project; to our agent Mitchell Hamilburg for his support; and, for clerical assistance, Julie Kawakami, Edith Kitaen Klein, Neal Morse, and Melissa Morse Miles. We wish to acknowledge the Turner Publishing crew for sticking with us through sometimes difficult decisions, and to thank the very cooperative photography models.

To the IBP board members, institute directors, teachers, practitioners, trainees, and clients, we appreciate your enduring enthusiasm for IBP. For providing a milieu in which we could continue to learn and create and for your personal support, we express our gratefulness and continued professional commitment. A special thanks to Marjorie Rand for her contributions to IBP, in particular for helping Jack turn his original professional training groups into a school and coordinating new institutes. She also helped Jack in an early attempt to update the original *Total Orgasm*. Unfortunately, the project was short-lived because the psychological couples work, which was essential to the project, had not yet been developed.

For their love, confidence, support, and patience while our time was so occupied with writing this book, we acknowledge Beverly's mother, Edith Kitaen Klein, her husband, Albert Klein, and our grown children and their children: Neal Morse (Daniella), Andrea Rosenberg Cooper and Vic (Tristan), Melissa Morse Miles (Max and Wyatt), Melissa Rosenberg Spiro and Lev, Jonna Morse Fries and Charles (Roxanne, Charlie, Nicky, Alexandra), Greg Morse and Dorte (Eli and one on the way), K. C. Rosenberg Ramos and Art, Eric Rosenberg, and Mariya MacCuish Rosenberg. Thanks to our former spouses: Sidney Morse, Patricia Connolly, Lynn MacCuish.

Our Story

AFTER WE BECAME A COUPLE, much to our professional chagrin, old struggles familiar to our past marriages began to creep into our idealized romance. To sustain our trust and romance, we turned to the tools of Integrative Body Psychotherapy (IBP). With IBP, Jack had formulated a tremendously effective system of psychotherapy, a mind-body therapy that integrates verbal and cognitive methods with a body orientation and breath work. It draws from many perspectives, including: Object Relations, Self Psychology, Gestalt Therapy, Reichian Therapy, Bioenergetics, Transpersonal Psychotherapy, plus various Eastern disciplines.

IBP helps individuals experience their potential by heightening aliveness and authenticity and through mental-health skills to sustain well-being. Jack first articulated his approach to heightening sexuality in *Total Orgasm,* published in 1972. In 1985 he wrote, with Marjorie Rand and Diane Asay, the psychological applications for IBP in *Body Self and Soul.*

As we used IBP mental-health tools to preserve and deepen our own love and sexuality, we joined forces professionally to develop a new way to do relational and sexual counseling with couples. We have been leading couples workshops together for ten years. By focusing on the body, IBP cuts through the protective facade that perpetuates isolation and the destruction of intimacy. The secret is to reawaken authenticity and aliveness in the body.

One of the struggles in writing this book was in collaborating and finding a voice that spoke for both of us. Initially, we wrote every word together, but this proved slow and cumbersome. Eventually, each piece was written by one, with the other editing, the manuscript moving between us until we could no longer tell whose words were whose. Our challenge was to develop a language and style to describe an experience to a reader who may not have had the experience, and, in addition, talk about what can only be known through a body experience. Therefore, there may be many facets of our work that you will not fully understand *unless you do the exercises.*

We have a committed, equal, and reciprocal relationship. We keep it vital and exciting by using the principles we write about, our understanding for resolving struggles, and building a bond for love and sexuality throughout life. We wish to pass on these precious discoveries so that others will not have to say, "If only we had known."

A Map for the Journey

THE INTIMATE COUPLE is written in the spirit of adventure and discovery, with abounding hope for monogamous relationships and sexuality; for couples who are rediscovering the treasure of sexual fidelity and are ready to work toward its full potential. It has been written both to enhance lovemaking in the best of relationships and to reignite the spark of loving, erotic sexuality for those who find themselves in troubled waters. *The Intimate Couple* will help you heighten your orgastic experience and enable you and your partner to be more open and emotionally available to each other during sexual lovemaking.

Couples of today hold higher levels of expectation for a relationship, and with this comes a new challenge: to build and sustain the excitement and passion of sexual lovemaking within a sexually exclusive, loving, and reciprocal relationship. Most couples want the feeling of equality and reciprocity in all aspects of their relationship, including sexuality, and they want to retain the desire and passions that characterized their first sexual experiences together. *The Intimate Couple* provides these lovers with a way to regain their early passion and increase the level of intimacy in their relationship, as well as the quality of erotic sexual excitement, and it provides the secrets for sustaining a deep sense of union.

It is rare that we find individuals or couples who actually have a sexual problem based on a physical limitation. Most sexual problems stem from other problems in a relationship. Every issue that is troubling a relationship is bound to be acted out in lovemaking. We each bring to the relationship a set of unconscious psychological patterns that alter our perspective and influence our behavior that we need to remain consistently aware of. These personal patterns have an ongoing effect on the state of our intimacy, sexuality, and the relationship itself.

The Intimate Couple will provide you with the means to achieve heightened sexuality in several ways:

- The energetic model of sexuality presented will enhance your potential by showing you a new way of thinking about sexual lovemaking and orgasm.
- Psychological guides will help you resolve your barriers to intimacy and find a renewed and elevated capacity for love, trust, well-being, mutuality, and sexuality.
- The many mental health tools you will find can help you put yourself and the relationship back together again when necessary.
- The exercises, through breathing and movement, will help you open your body for love and sexuality while establishing the potential for total orgasm

in your body. The first set of exercises are done alone, without the distractions that come with intimacy. They provide the opportunity for you to learn how to build your own charge and spread it through your body as you develop a comfort with higher levels of excitement. The next series of exercises, done with your partner, create an atmosphere of mutuality, of being seen and touched and known, of being in tune with each other. Then you and your partner assist each other in opening your bodies to your most natural and alive states.

• The final chapters provide illustrations and guides for making sex better. We show a variety of sexual positions and how you can improve your favorites. You will discover how to bring to lovemaking all that you learned in the earlier chapters.

If you only read this book but don't do the exercises, you will gain valuable insights, but you will not achieve a different experience in your body. In order to change, you need the internal body experience as well as the mental insight. As in learning a sport or a dance, you need specific information, time, and kinesthetic experience to become proficient. Your body has its own wisdom. After a few repetitions it will remember the natural, open feelings and movement you are teaching it. You will be able to discover for yourself what is interfering psychologically and physically with your lovemaking. This will set you free to experience your natural inborn capacity for aliveness and sexual fulfillment. This feeling in your body of optimal functioning is often the missing link in your sexual experience. Once felt, you will have a body memory that will allow for consistency in your lovemaking.

The Intimate Couple *will not so much teach you something new as help you unlearn something old: outmoded, automatic, restrictive body-mind patterns.*

Many people look toward others, rather than within themselves, for the source of their sexual excitement. "You just don't turn me on anymore," is an implied demand. The notion that sexual charge should be generated by somebody else is a fib we love to believe. We can, of course, be stimulated by others at times. But if we come to believe that our excitement must come from our partner, we are left without the empowering sense of self necessary for heightened sexuality. In long-term relationships we each must learn how to keep love and sexuality alive within us and be able to arouse erotic excitement within our own bodies.

We describe an approach to an awakening, a mutual joining in love and sexual intimacy, a union grounded in an environment that often embraces a sacred dimension. Without our habitual barriers to self and intimacy we can choose to appear from behind our protective masks and truly know one another. This awakening is a necessary component for heightened sexuality or what we call the total orgasm.

A total orgasm results when sexual energy is built to a high level and spread throughout the entire body so that the sensation of release into orgasm is profoundly heightened, intensified, and felt not merely in the genitals but throughout the body. This orgasm can involve your whole being. A total orgasm results in a heightened experience of aliveness that can reawaken a body experience of self. There are no words to explain this experience. This inner awareness of self speaks from the core of our being through the confusion of our protective and learned themes. It is an experience felt in the body of well-being, of "I am," one that is sustaining through both the existential and everyday experiences of life.

Perhaps no other experience can come closer to a profound emotional and physical union between two people and give rise to an inner awakening than sexual lovemaking. The orgasm is the culmination of sexual excitement and is one of our most pleasurable, satisfying, and intense natural gifts. Yet it is transitory.

There is no one right way to make love. You only need a willingness to understand yourself and to take responsibility for your feelings and behavior, a positive intention toward your partner, and, most importantly, a willingness to be fully alive.

Most people who seek sexual counseling need only basic but specific information and guidelines, minimal psychotherapy, and effective body opening–enlivening techniques to relieve physical, psychological, relational, and sexual limitations. Because the psychological principles, mental health tools, and energetic movement and breathing exercises employed in *The Intimate Couple* are based on human nature, they have been proven to work cross-culturally. In addition, it makes no difference whether a couple is made up of a man and woman or two people of the same gender.

It seems rather presumptuous to tell others how they should make love. It's like telling someone how they should live or die. Men and women have been making love for some time. Making love with the same partner over and over again, and keeping lovemaking not only enticing and exciting, but also an enduring means for deepening the bond between you, is difficult, but it is an achievable reality. Good sex is not difficult to establish, but there is much more. The essence of love, as expressed in erotic sexual lovemaking, goes beyond: It nurtures the soul and sustains excitement and aliveness within a monogamous relationship.

BEGINNING
the
JOURNEY

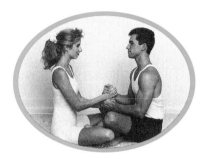

C H A P T E R   O N E

Erotic Sexual Lovemaking

NEITHER LOVE NOR SEXUALITY has to diminish over time. When you can risk being emotionally vulnerable during sexual lovemaking in a committed relationship, it will not be newness or novelty, but the familiarity and trust you have developed within yourself and between you and your partner, that will allow you to open your mind and body. This is a journey of discovery to fulfill your capacities individually and as a couple.

THE JOURNEY

FOR REALLY CONSISTENT and satisfying sexual lovemaking you must be able to develop your ability to love and trust; to become comfortable with intense and authentic experiences; to build, contain, spread, and release larger and larger amounts of energy in your body; and to show up fully as a lover for a mutually pleasuring experience. These are the capacities that you will learn to develop throughout this book.

When you come face to face with intense and profound experiences of intimacy, sexuality, and spirituality, the most important and challenging aspect is the ability to sustain your sense of self. You must have a strong enough sense of yourself that you can be vulnerable and fully available and giving, and not lose your inner stability. This balance is inherently difficult and is part of the ongoing struggle of relationships.

As you realize how sexual energy, or energy in general, builds in your body, you will understand beyond a doubt how love, which is an opening of the heart, can exponentially expand and deepen your sexual experience. You will also recognize why sex without love eventually leads to boredom, no matter how many partners you have, sex tools you use, sexual positions you master, or dangerous risks you take. For when two people are emotionally close they can generate a powerful synergy of sexual excitement.

Love and trust can melt the emotional barriers you build in mind and body to defend yourself against life's pain and disappointments. Emotional fears and injuries can cause your body to contract and tense, limiting your ability to feel love, trust, security, and sexual desire.

When love is just a memory rather than an energetic charge sparked between lovers, sexual potential is limited. Without time, experience, and emotional availability, love and trust cannot grow. Though we usually associate the feelings of love and sexual excitement with someone or something outside of ourselves, these feelings originate within us. Once you identify your internal source of erotic excitement, you can increase your aliveness and share it with another. To participate in the adventure of heightened lovemaking, you must know more about your body and its language and how this affects your sexuality.

How you think about something affects how your body functions. Your physical state affects how you think. Both mind and body influence and are affected by your emotions. This intertwined system can be altered from any one of the three component sources: mind, emotions, or body. The methods in *The Intimate Couple* allow profound sexual change because they incorporate all three simultaneously.

Most people are unaware of how stress or emotional and physical inundation can numb their feelings and cause their bodies to tighten. People often believe the deadness in their bodies indicates that they no longer feel love or erotic sexual desire toward their partner. "I don't feel sexual desire; therefore, I must not be in love anymore," is an all too common refrain.

This emotional and physical shutting down does not indicate sexual incompatibility or a lack of love. Lifelessness can creep into the most loving relationships. Love and sexuality are more than thoughts; they are different experiences felt in the body. Sex, love, trust, hope, erotic feelings, jealousy— such emotions are all experiences that cannot be known by the intellect alone. In addition, each feels differently in the body. You may love someone and not trust them. You can have trust but not feel love or sexual arousal. Or you may feel sexual without any of the other emotions.

Loving

In long-term relationships without intimacy, there is no support for heightened sexuality. With sex, the trick is to allow surrender to emotional openness without losing sexuality and passion. If you focus on the sexuality and passion, you may miss the intimacy. If you overemphasize the intimacy, you may miss out on the erotic passion. The way to total sexuality is by the opening of your whole being, through the loving of your heart and not through the sexuality of the pelvis alone.

Love sometimes feels like a deep familiarity: "Somehow I've always known you, and here we meet again." It is in a committed relationship that this depth of knowing one another can provide a window through which you can glimpse the joy and radiance at your core. And as you open more deeply into love, a commitment to loving in all forms will grow. The more you involve your whole body and mind in lovemaking, the more emotionally "present" you can remain with yourself and your partner, and the deeper, more exciting, and passionate you and your relationship can become.

Many people have a romantic, wishful belief that if they really love someone, they should feel this love all the time. Unfortunately love, like other emotions, tends to come and go. "I'm loving you right now," is a good self-reminder of this ebb and flow. You may know you love someone and at the very same time feel anger, frustration, even hate. As you learn to manage these feelings and keep your body open, you will be able to feel love more consistently. "I know I love you even if I can't feel it right now," is also a good reminder to oneself. Love, like any living entity, must be consistently nurtured.

Love is an emotional body feeling, and certain behaviors and considerations emanate from this feeling. Love is not an excuse for hurtful, insensitive neglectful behavior. "If you really loved me you would..." is one of the most destructive forms of emotional blackmail in which a couple can participate.

There is no way to prove that you love someone.

Eve couldn't believe that Matt loved her. No matter what he would say, she felt unloved, not cared for. When she left him, Matt wrote this poem:
>And then my broken heart shattered
>into a thousand pieces,
>and I lay flat on the boards for weeks
>staring at no-heaven.

Even though Matt adored Eve, she did not feel loved by him. And Harry, Tom, and George could not make her feel loved either. No matter how much you love someone, if they cannot love themselves first, they won't feel loved by you. It's like telling someone who does not feel beautiful that they are beautiful. Most likely they not only will disregard what you have said but will feel discouraged or just plain unseen. Eve does not experience a self-validating inner voice, one she can feel in her body; therefore she cannot feel the tremendous love that Matt had for her.

TRUSTING   AN INTIMATE RELATIONSHIP should be a sanctuary with trust as its foundation. Fortunately, we usually choose a mate because we feel, "This one I can trust." Although there are people who are not trustworthy, if mistrust is a recurring theme in your life, it probably has something to do with you. It is often difficult to trust because of the hurts you received early in your life: Your body, if not your mind, retains a memory of these hurts and predisposes you for mistrust. When your body opens for love and sexuality it also opens to all the warnings you have accumulated over your lifetime. These warnings, or memories, color how you see and treat your partner.

All that we experience affects our psyches and our bodies. When you are anxious at home or at work, your body tightens; when you witness violence in the media, your body harbors a feeling of caution, a reminder to be careful. We carry reminders of our daily experiences in our bodies and bring the messages home with us: "Be careful." "Someone could take advantage of me, hurt me." "Don't trust."

Positive Intention, Good Will

Being in an intimate relationship is like dancing in a small closet: You are bound to step on each other's toes once in a while. When this happens, if you carry a body experience of mistrust, you are liable to misjudge your partner. It is imperative to remember that even though your body may feel mistrust, your partner may not be doing what you think he or she is doing. Positive intention means that when your toes are stepped on, you can sustain a belief that your partner didn't do it on purpose, until you ask them of their intention.

When you lose trust, you lose intimacy. A relationship without trust is neither safe nor intimate. Sustaining heightened sexuality is not possible without the intimacy of trust. Therefore, trust is not to be taken for granted or to be thrown about carelessly in the heat of an argument. It has to be protected, nurtured, honored, and, if injured, brought back to health.

Trusting means approaching a relationship with a positive intention, the intention to solve problems and misunderstandings, not to hurt or blame. Trusting means remembering that your partner also intends well toward you and your relationship, and is worthy of trust. If at any time you believe your partner has a negative intention toward you, ask. If your feelings are hurt, it implies doubt. Ask your partner what his or her intention toward you is:

body-mind awakening

"Was it your intention to make me feel foolish and abandoned?" If you are holding a thought of *negative intention*, then when you feel stepped on, you may try to get even or prove that your partner is bad, defective, stupid, or trying to control you. If you have a *positive intention*, you will assume that your partner was not out to hurt you on purpose. You must remember that no matter how bad things look in the moment, if you have worked out differences and emotional injuries before, you can once again sort out your own and your partner's intentions each time doubt arises. But you must remain focused on solving the problem rather than reacting to it.

If you believe that your partner is truly out to demean, punish, hurt, or use you in some way, this is not a loving relationship. Change it or get out. It is not a healthy place to be. *If you believe your partner does not have a negative intent toward you, don't treat your partner as if she or he does, even in humor.* It only creates emotional injury, mistrust, and distance. If you are trying to suppress your partner in any way so that you will feel bigger or better, stop. It is abusive. It is far better to empower your partner and to empower yourself. The ability for you and your partner to work together within an intimate environment depends on each of you maintaining a positive intention toward the other, particularly when you are making love.

In order to trust you must, on a regular basis, take time to assess whether the inner warning light you carry in your body has much to do with your partner. Your body experience of trust may be dim. Trust needs consciousness and nurturing to be sustained.

EROTIC SEXUALITY

THOUGH COUPLES HAVE THE CAPACITY for erotic sexuality, many just do not always have the ability to find and sustain an erotic sensibility in themselves or in their sexual interactions. So they settle for mediocrity, sex without much excitement. They do not allow their inner erotic pleasures to flourish because they are afraid of or embarrassed by their core erotic nature, or they conceal its existence, even from themselves.

Eroticism is not the same as feeling sexual or engaging in sexual behavior. It is about an internal experience of sexual energy felt in concert with the five senses. Erotic energy makes everything feel more sensually pleasurable and satisfying. When sexual energy arising from the pelvis blends with the energy circulating throughout the entire body—intensifying all your senses—it is called erotic energy. Erotic energy is felt as undulating sensations. It is more about the movement of free-flowing sexual excitement arousing sensations throughout the body and less about the genitals, sexual behavior, or sexual release. Many couples engage in sex that is devoid of eroticism because their senses are not fully engaged.

When eroticised energy is present it radiates from the body as light does from a lamp. Erotic energy brings added delight to whatever you do, no matter how mundane: taking a bath, drinking a glass of lemonade, or asking for a cup of tea. Merely allowing yourself to feel fully the erotic energy in your body can easily arouse erotic sensations and sexual desire in others.

Eroticism can be aroused by taking full pleasure through all of your senses. Eating a nectarine can delight your erotic senses if you allow yourself to indulge in experiencing the sweet-tart flavor, the abundant dripping juices, the slippery smooth textures, and tantalizing aroma. Listening to music or reading poetry can arouse the deepest of erotic body experiences if you allow yourself to join fully with the sounds, rhythms, feelings, and sensations these activities invite in your body. Bringing full attention to your senses, together with intensifying your sensations and spreading them through your body (as you will be learning to do with *The Intimate Couple* exercises) can awaken all the sensibilities of the body including sexuality and love. When love and sexuality flow in concert with the heightened erotic senses, pleasure is greatly heightened.

Two basic elements of eroticism are sexual energy from an awakened pelvis and a heightened awareness of the senses. Your senses help the erotic energy to spread through the body. A third element is interiority, the ability to feel your internal experience as it is occurring. Thoughts can interfere

"Eroticism and passion are the missing ingredients for the vast masses of sexually functional people who never experience the full impact of their sexual potential."

SCHNARCH,
*CONSTRUCTING THE
SEXUAL CRUCIBLE,* 1991

with the ability to reach heightened sensory awareness. When the mind ceases to be in control, an interior experience is aroused. Therefore, all interruptive thoughts must be put aside. When you dance or make love you must "get out of your head." Or as Fritz Pearls said, "Lose your mind and come to your senses." This helps your body to soften, making way for emotions and sensations, and for trusting the rhythmic, undulating movements of the body as a guide.

Erotic sensations feel differently depending on which parts of your body are sensually stimulated. The simplest way to describe this is through the Kundalini Yoga system, which affirms that, depending on which sites in the body are awakened, one's energy is in the service of security, sexuality, power, loving, or more spiritual levels of consciousness. For example, when erotic energy is in the service of power it is more aggressive than when it is in the service of love, but as these two energies blend you have passionate love. As you add erotic energy, you have passionate sensual energy that is both sexual and loving. The nature of eroticism always depends on what part or how much of the body is engaged through the senses. The more the body is enlivened, the more its sensibilities—or centers of energy—participate. Your joining becomes more powerful with loving and even more so as you reach higher centers of consciousness.

Eroticism is an interior experience. It involves pleasure and movement throughout the body more than thoughts limited to the mind. The belly dancer is very erotic, implying sexuality as she circulates energy through her body in undulating movements. Wherever erotic energy is found it hints of sexuality and the passions of the night. Most pornographic movies are prime examples of sex without eroticism and heart. Consequently, they become boring after the initial novelty wears off. True eroticism never omits the heart, nor does it become boring.

Some people fear that erotic energy is so powerful that, if allowed into their sensory awareness, it will control them and lead them into inappropriate sexual behavior; or they feel that the embodiment of this energy will arouse undesired sexual attention from others. It is true that this energy is powerful, but these fears are not actually due to erotic sexuality. The underlying fear is of being fully alive with a sense of well-being.

Whenever Sylvia felt a flush of erotic energy creep through her body she turned to Frank, whom she adored. Wanting him to match her passion she would whisper, "Let's pull off all our clothes and have sex right here on the stairs." She hoped that the immediacy would break through his mental control and allow his erotic excitement to surge. But Frank was always practical. He loved that Sylvia had an erotic spark to her, but it also made him feel uncomfortable. More than anything else, her eroticism made him more conscious of his lack of interior erotic sensibilities. It was easier to feel criticized by her than face his own feelings of inadequacy. The erotic energy Sylvia brought to her approach was enough to trigger his internal fear that he was not enough as a man. He not only believed, erroneously, that he was supposed to supply the

The Loss of Eros

Human beings have long tried to explain this feeling in our loins and in the depths of our being that is the expression of our aroused sexuality. Perhaps no other culture has so systematically expressed in metaphysical abstractions the timeless essence that underlies our sexuality than the ancient mythologies of the Greeks. Eros, the winged god of love, son of Aphrodite, the goddess of beauty, personifies the meaning and form of human sexuality.

> To the Greeks, Eros was seen as a complex multidimensional archetype which, at the physical levels, impelled the philosopher's passion for intellect, beauty, and wisdom, culminating in the mystical vision of the eternal, the ultimate source of all beauty.
>
> Plato suggested that the highest philosophical vision is possible only to one with the temperament of a lover. The philosopher must permit himself to grasp the most sublime form of Eros—that universal passion to restore a former unity, to overcome the separation from the divine and become one with it. (Richard Tarnas, *The Passion of the Western Mind*, 1991)

When Eros, this energetic life force, is redefined as something bad and suppressed it affects the aliveness and joy we allow ourselves to feel in our bodies and relationships. This loss is evident as we listen to couples struggling to find their inner spark of sexual desire and vitality.

It is easier to understand the erotic energy of Eros if we think of sexuality as expressed in Eastern Tantric texts and traditions, that is, sexuality is neither good nor bad. The erotic is just one way the Kundalini, the basic energy of life, can be expressed.

body-mind awakening

As children our erotic energy often frightens our parents because it reminds them of what they have given up. And to protect their comfort, we thwart our ability to feel it in our bodies. But, since Eros is an important, indispensable part of our being, it later rises again in the privacy of the bedroom. The excitement and wonder of sexuality remains alive within us.

In youth, pleasure comes from the rush of hormonal urgency and the release of this tension. At the height of virginal adventure there is scarcely time for learning to be a lover. With release as the goal, sex is supreme, and it is easy to mistake surging hormones for erotic sensation and expression. Because of this confusion, as hormonal urgency diminishes with maturity and experience, people often believe their eroticism has died. In an attempt to resuscitate their erotic feelings, many couples turn to emotional or physical tension, which creates crises not eroticism.

Erotic experience is not exclusive to the young. As we age we can grow closer to our partners. Life's tensions subside, or we can deal more effectively with them, and our capacity for eroticism and loving increases. We cannot go back to the urgency of youth, but we can go forward into heightened sexuality and love and deeper expression of our erotic being.

Sharing erotic thoughts, fantasies, and desires with one another is not a good idea because our erotic symbols often mean little to others. Rather than arousing desire, this sharing often causes emotional injury. Bringing forth erotic energy to make contact with your partner is preferable to sharing internal images. Reviving the lost feeling of Eros in your body to heighten the expression of your life force, your being, is one of the purposes of this book.

erotic energy for the two of them, he also feared that by shifting from thinking to feeling he would lose control. So he just answered, "What do you want from me? You're never satisfied."

Helen turned away from Carl every time she caught a glimpse of his erotic spark. She loved but couldn't tolerate the intensity in his eyes and felt embarrassed, as if she were seeing him truly naked to the core. He interpreted her turning away as a sign of disapproval and felt like a chastised child. What was once a flame quickly turned to ash.

It is very clear when a couple is not inhibited in their erotic expression. The aliveness and excitement surrounding them is almost palpable.

Some people confuse eroticism with lewd thoughts, feelings, and behavior. When sexual behavior is separated from our compassion and respect for others, or when we use others to satisfy our desires, it is offensive and dehumanizing. This cannot happen with true eroticism that arouses all the centers of the body, including love and a higher consciousness. With sexuality, it is imperative that other centers in the body are functioning so that we bring compassion to our erotic lovemaking. The lover who seduces a chosen mate through an eroticism that is alive and well, will be met with delight and enthusiasm.

SPEED LIMITS FOR EROTIC SEXUAL LOVEMAKING

YOUR PRESENT COMFORT LEVEL with sexuality and eroticism was set when you were a child, almost like a speed limit, which you were taught not to exceed. This limit was formed by the attitudes of your family and social environment long before you could decide for yourself. It is now mostly unconscious and is thoroughly embodied and incorporated in your being.

The function of *The Intimate Couple* is to help extend your erotic sexuality beyond these internalized speed limits that have the power to sabotage your best intentions and efforts. Speed limits surface as discomforts—uncomfortable sensations or emotions in your body—or as a memory, usually of a problem, particularly one with your partner. If you wish to extend your limits for erotic sexual lovemaking, it is important to identify the speed limits set for you long ago in childhood.

Think back to your family environment, more in terms of feelings and tone than actual words or behavior. What was the general attitude about sexuality? Did anyone embody erotic energy? Can you imagine your parents enjoying loving, erotic sexuality? Were you supported in sustaining your erotic curiosity and experimentation?

On a scale of one to ten, with one being the least, rate your family's speed limit. Even though you probably have never thought about it before, venture a guess. Most people rate the level of erotic sexuality allowed in their family at about three. Some assign a minus number, and a few guess above six or seven. Those who rate their families above seven usually find, under closer scrutiny, that what was said and what was actually allowed were different.

> Before they were married Muriel and Joseph made love at the drop of a zipper. But her ardor and enthusiasm began to wane when they moved in together. A year later they were married, adopted two dogs, and became a family. Her sexual passion came to a screeching halt, replaced by, "I've got a headache," or a thousand other substitutes for no. Joseph can't understand why the traffic signal is always red in their bedroom, but he doesn't seem to mind much any more. Sometimes Muriel is turned on and masturbates for relief and wonders, "I don't know why I don't want Joseph any more. It just feels too uncomfortable in my body."
>
> As Joseph and Muriel settled into feeling like a family, they unconsciously responded to old rules learned in their families during childhood and remembered silently in their bodies. They have both unconsciously returned to the comfort of their old family speed limits.

If your internal limit for sexually erotic excitement is low, as you become a family you may hope that your partner will provide the missing erotic sexual spark, even while you hasten to extinguish it. The limitations and the spark are both within you, and, like most people, you have probably chosen a partner with a speed limit similar to your own. Therefore, blaming your mate or expecting your mate to resolve your dilemma will not work.

To raise your speed limit, you will need to give yourself permission to do so. And remember, when doing the exercises in this book or when making love, if your good feelings suddenly disappear, it probably means that your old limitations are being challenged, even surpassed. This is not a crisis; on the contrary, it is a sign of success.

To heighten sexual excitement you must become comfortable with the intensity of sensations and emotions in your body. For the fullest lovemaking experience, it is essential that you learn to tolerate the intensity of intimacy, sexuality, eroticism, and heightened aliveness.

All the body-mind practices provided in this book are designed to help you tolerate new levels of aliveness, particularly sexual aliveness. You will learn how to change the energetic limitations you bring to sexual lovemaking, individually and as a couple.

SENSUAL BODY CONTACT

TO BEGIN THIS JOURNEY we suggest you start by building a body-to-body, nonverbal relationship with your partner. Bypass the walls of words, explanations, demands, and daily scuffles. Move through the emotional distance and, in nonsexual ways, find each other again. You will be surprised how nondemand body contact can calm, soothe, comfort, and establish a feel-

Three Ways to Look at Sexuality

- **The physical-sexual-energetic level.** This is the actual, practical, mechanical, physiological, energetic way of improving sexuality and excitation for yourself and your partner. This level includes opening the body for tolerating, charging, containing, and releasing excitement to heighten orgastic response and sensual pleasure. The exercises in this book systematically teach this level.

- **The interpersonal or relationship level.** Because sexuality is an expression of your relationship, you must look at anything that persistently interrupts the intimacy of the relationship: any problems that undermine the closeness or bond between you and your partner—such as struggling and fighting, creating an atmosphere of crisis, or even being overly nice and careful. Ignoring problems is just as deadening to sexuality as hostility.

Any lies or destructive patterns experienced in your relationship will be expressed in sexuality. You can't bypass these issues and still have good sex—not in a long-term, monogamous relationship. When there is a struggle and two people clear their way to a resolution, the repair deepens trust and strengthens the bond of the relationship.

- **The intrapsychic or personal level.** This category includes all of who you are. You bring all the patterns (body-mind habits) you learned as a child plus everything you are today to every aspect of your life. Sex is no exception. Emotionally, many adults still act out behaviors born in the nursery, which are now self-perpetuating and largely undermining to one's self and intimate relationship. Sexuality, by its nature, is self-exposing and an opening to the core of our being. It is impossible to fully join with another and, at the same time, keep aspects of one's core self hidden.

All three of these levels are going on at the same time all the time, and they are all an expression of your sense of self. Heightened, deepened sexuality requires the meeting of two people at this level of authenticity and a mutual savoring of eroticism.

Building additional skills as a lover is just the icing on the cake. Once you have opened to love, developed a comfort with heightened excitement, and know how to build, contain, and release energy from within the core of your being, the rest will come easily and naturally.

ing of communion and deepen your bond. By "nondemand" we mean all you have to do is show up and be physically close. Nothing more is expected. Two ways to initiate and sustain a deeper intimacy are through Hug Time and Skin Time.

Hug Time. Every culture has a way of touching as a form of greeting. Some kiss on either cheek, hug, or shake hands. Many couples have given up their body-to-body connection for a perfunctory peck on the cheek or a shout down the hall over the heads of their kids. Maintaining a calming, sensory bond of recognition and attunement need only take a few moments if both people are emotionally present. If you don't keep the physical bond alive and well throughout your day, you can't make up for it with sex at night.

Each time you and your partner meet or take leave of each other for a period of time, instead of just an inattentive, mechanical "hello" and "goodbye," stop to give each other a whole-body hug. It's nice if you also kiss or touch cheek to cheek, but that is not necessary. If you do kiss, a quick peck is more discounting than affirming. Emphasize the feeling of the energy and warmth between and within you with a full body-to-body hug.

For those brief moments, focus all your attention on your embrace and the sensations brought about as your bodies touch. You may notice that you bring thoughts and emotions, negative or positive, that have nothing to do with the body-to-body contact. Let the intruding thoughts and emotions go, stay with the body-to-body sensations. When both people make true physical, sensory, body-to-body contact, many struggles and anxieties fade away. After body contact, the time you spend apart is more comfortable, and the transition is easier when you rejoin.

If you consistently hug in this way each time you say hello and good-bye, you won't have to construct an intimate relationship from scratch every time you are ready to make love.

Skin Time. All human beings need a certain amount of physical touching and closeness when they are infants or they will become emotionally injured or die. The need to be touched doesn't disappear when we become adults. But the need for this sensory physical closeness and the need for sexuality can become confused. When sex is used to satisfy a need for physical closeness, the person is left with a feeling of dissatisfaction, and the cause of the dissatisfaction is often blamed on sex or the relationship.

Couples do best when they plan for skin time. We recommend that couples enjoy skin time at least three to five times a week, for just five to ten minutes. Skin time is time without clothing, lying together, holding each other, bare skin to bare skin. The best time is just before falling asleep or when awakening. This time must be separate from sex, sexual stimulation, or the promise of sex. It doesn't work if you combine skin time with sex because couples need a time just to feel close without distractions or demands. Without skin time a basic lack of attunement can be perpetuated or even exaggerated.

Skin time creates a bond that serves as a foundation for love and sexuality by allowing each partner to feel the body experience of trust and safety. This is a time of joining with your partner by focusing on positive feelings of physical closeness and enjoying the sensual experience. This means allowing your body to feel your partner's energy, contours, temperatures. If you show up with your body but keep a sensual-emotional distance and don't really let yourself feel the love and closeness, it won't work. No talking, no TV, no massaging. Just lie together and breathe slowly and fully. Don't let your attention stray. Focus on the physical sensations as your body is skin-to-skin with another. Stay awake. Keep the lights on. Learn to tolerate the intensity.

AND THERE IS MORE . . .

In former times, if people wanted to explore the deeper mysteries of life, they would often enter a monastery or hermitage far away from conventional family ties. For many of us today, however, intimate relationship has become the new wilderness that brings us face to face with our gods and demons. It is calling on us to free ourselves from old habits and blind spots, to develop a full range of our powers, sensitivities, and depths as human beings—right in the middle of everyday life.

JOHN WELWOOD,
LOVE AND AWAKENING, 1996

THERE ARE MOMENTS in each intimate relationship that awaken the core of our soul, moments that allow us to experience the closeness, the wonder of life's secrets—to feel transcendent. There are moments, however brief, that let us know without any doubt that we are not alone in our personal journey through time. In the ecstasy of these moments, we know that our relationship is bountiful. An intimate relationship is a teacher, not an interference or disruption, but a guide, a path to our innermost relationship to our self.

The transcendent quality of sex is not a thought. It is a feeling in your body. Spirituality deepens the intensity of the excitement, joining, and openness with another being. Deep feelings often unconsciously trigger the procreative soul. To create life is a natural desire that emanates from our deepest being. It is not necessarily the same as wanting to have a child, although many people experience profound joy in consciously creating new life with a partner they cherish.

It is this ongoing presence of spirituality and its themes played out in our lives that affords depth to our experience of aliveness. Therefore, to foster great depth of feeling in our intimate relationships, it is essential to acknowledge our interior spiritual life. A relationship without spirituality is like sex without love. Both are enjoyable, but leave one feeling unfinished and incomplete, haunted by the question, "Is that all there is?" Sex without spirituality is like a relationship without love. Eventually it becomes boring.

CHAPTER TWO

A Psychological Overview: The Four Arenas

IT IS DIFFICULT TO UNDERSTAND the transitory nature of sexuality if you only think in terms of sex and orgastic release. For sustaining and heightening sexuality in a long-term relationship, each partner's well-being and how they are relating to each other is as important to acknowledge as what they do together sexually.

To experience heightened sexuality with any consistency, you must be able to meet your partner unadorned, *without a facade or pretense.* To do this, you must know yourself, beyond the confusing, masking themes of your interior world—psychological, emotional, and physiological. Identifying these themes and seeing that *they are not who you are* holds the secret for sustaining your authentic core sense of self, for maintaining the integrity of your relationship, and for reaching ecstatic states.

LIFE IS A SOMATIC EXPERIENCE

"Much of what passes for 'culture' and 'personality' in our society tends to fall into this substitute category, and is in fact the result of running from silence, and from genuine somatic experience."
BERMAN,
COMING TO OUR SENSES, 1989

FOR MANY PEOPLE a sense of self is an elusive concept, because it is based on how others see us, how we look, what we own, what we do, and how we act in the world. In an attempt to become self-validating, we may define ourselves by our intellectual assumptions, ideas, and beliefs, tending to favor perceptions received through the mind rather than felt in the body—a somatic experience. Again, this is elusive. In general, most people have been taught to ignore the deeper, more authentic experiences of self that can only be felt in the body, thereby missing out on a rich and amazing inner life.

This body, or somatic, awareness of self, is the most fundamental experience in life. At this level we are able to witness the messages of our inner voice and experience a deep internal feeling of stability, consistency, the wonder of being alive, and a nonverbal body experience of truth and authenticity. Somatic experience allows us to acquire a sense of self that can be sustained no matter what we are faced with in life. But when our sense of self is not grounded in our body, we do not know where to look for the missing experience. Without somatic awareness, to avoid the feeling of emptiness and instability, we are compelled to try to find a substitute for the experience of self through "doing" behaviors.

There are moments between lovers when something breaks through and we feel who we are beyond our masquerade. Feeling emotionally vulnerable, we may become momentarily frightened by our authenticity, our suddenly naked selves. If we can't tolerate this exposure, we may do or say something to shield us from our discovery and create a comfortable distance. Yet this experience of truly being seen, of being unmasked, is what we strive for again and again.

When our bodies are awakened we are more aware of our emotions and sensations. We have a deeper and fuller experience of self. There are certain experiences that we can not have unless our bodies are awakened and our attention is focused inside our being. We call these *body experiences*. Trust, love, eroticism, and an experience of self are all examples of experiences in which a feeling in your body is essential for validation. Typically, when people have a body experience they say, "I kind of knew that, but now it feels different, like I really know."

Unfortunately for many people, their body has gone to sleep, so to speak, and their own body experiences are absent. To compensate, they may often mistakenly look to others for what can only be found in an interior experience: for the validation of their own feelings of how to be and who they are, for their erotic spark, and for their own capacity for love, trust, and spirituality. As a result of this lack of interiority, they do not build a stable internal experience of self.

By constantly looking outside ourselves to know our internal states, we miss the opportunity to build self-trust and an inner knowing at our core, and we are left with the feeling that our sense of self is fragile. Only with an awareness of our somatic core can we feel experiences of high intensity, act with true volition, and feel our life is our own.

We have divided into four "arenas" the recurring psychological themes that mask core self-experience. What happens in these arenas—when they remain outside of your awareness—causes most of the problems experienced in your intimate-sexual relationship. The arenas are Primary Scenario, Character Style, Agency, and Existential-Transpersonal. The themes of each arena form unconscious, repetitive ways of being, that become all too familiar patterns.

When you explore these arenas you will be working with underlying universal aspects of human nature. Each arena represents a fundamental part of our underlying nature. By working on such a broad scope you will find that you don't have to solve every wrinkle in your past or in your relationship. Couples who understand and take charge of these arenas are better able to stabilize their sense of self and sustain heightened intimacy.

For a deeper, more direct experience of self you must be able to identify your patterns within each arena separate from who you are. The arenas are a disruptive part of your emotional life and a stimulus for interior and relationship upsets and ensuing behaviors. *But they are not who you are.* If you confuse these arena patterns with who you are instead of seeing them as an internal voice that merely echoes the past, they remain automatic and they imprison you.

When you no longer identify these old patterns as self, your facade fades and your true self can shine through. This allows you to experience the radiance at your core, the fourth arena, which is the spiritual realm. With this, the existential-transpersonal experiences of life within and beyond the self are felt and known. It bestows a deeper, spiritual truth, a special internal knowing that you are not alone and there is so much more.

The Intimate Couple will help you identify these self-destructive, defensive behavioral and emotional patterns. The exercises in this book will help you differentiate reactions that arise from early childhood influences from those triggered by present experience. The body exercises will help you feel more open and alive, and they will also help you establish a focal point in your body for self and well-being that is internally sustainable.

For your sense of self to be authentic and stable, you must be able to witness who you actually are as well as your protective cover. You must know yourself undivided, not only the parts you like to admit but that which you avoid and conceal from yourself. You must also learn to live with the paradoxes of being human. For example, you must feel in your body that you are separate from others, while at the same time feel that we are one, intrinsically related. For an experience of self, you must take charge of the unfolding of your life.

Unscrambling Your Body-Voice

body-mind awakening

Unfortunately for most people, their inner voice is not always trustworthy. Messages come through like scrambled radio signals. It is often difficult to sort the messages of the authentic core self, what Gandhi called "the still small voice," from distorting, repetitive arena patterns and longings held in the body. Identifying your arena patterns will help you unscramble the messages. Differentiating your core body-voice messages from the arena's damaging cycles of self-destructive thoughts and resulting behaviors can free you. Tapping into this rich voice of authenticity and consciousness requires taking a route directly to where these nonintellectual experiences lie— in the body.

The most common complaint we hear from couples is that they are unable to communicate effectively. In our experience, communication is not the problem. The problem is what they communicate. They communicate their longings, upsets, frustrations, and arena responses. This is our "craziness," our protective facade, and more often than not, leads to emotional distance, injury, and confusion. It is difficult to feel understood when what you express is not who you are. Separately and together, these arenas play out in your life creating your everyday reality.

THE FOUR ARENAS PRIMARY SCENARIO

THE HISTORY OF YOUR CHILDHOOD is explored in this arena. This includes the relationship patterns and the sense of yourself and others that you formed as you were growing up. Your blueprint for later patterns of intimacy and limits for erotic sexuality were designed and established during this time. To sustain a core sense of self in intimacy, you must identify these relationship patterns you learned in childhood.

The uniqueness of our being begins very early in life. A newborn will understand its parents' caring attitudes, moods, desires, and needs, and these will be energetically imparted in important "parent messages," not through words or tasks but through presence, emotions, and touch. These messages from a good mother and father will be integrated into the core of the child's being. Once received, they provide the inner supports that allow a child to grow up with confidence, a sense of self-worth, and the ability to form close relationships. A parent who as a child received these messages (beginning with "I love you; I want you; you are special to me.") easily, naturally, and automatically passes them on. A parent who didn't receive them finds this more of a challenge.

The good parent messages are supported by words and deeds but, without the full energetic quality that comes from openness, authenticity, and presence in the givers, the messages are empty. If parents can't express love, if they are depressed or merely following "rules," their words will be false promises and will not foster a positive sense of self in the child. If parents are split off or cut off from their own bodies, not emotionally and energetically "present" (see chapter 3, The Energetic Model), the messages are not sufficiently passed. When children who missed these messages are adults, even though they may love their partner, they may not be transmitting these messages energetically. And/or they may not feel loved no matter how kindly treated. This pattern can be changed with an understanding of the arenas and body exercises.

No one has ever received all the messages perfectly. What we have not received we must fulfill for ourselves as part of our own self-development. If we don't, we will exist in an emotional void, hungering for these messages, but no longer from our parents. As adults, until we can give these messages to ourselves, the barrier we erect does not allow us to take them into our core selves when given by others.

We have translated these good parent messages into "feeling tones," which parents impart to their children by consistent gestures, smiles, body contact, warmth, attitude, and behavior, as well as words. To have your own body experience of these messages, write them into your journal. The ones that you are uncomfortable with in some way are probably the ones you didn't get enough of as a child and are now trying to get from your partner. Each message will promote a different body feeling.

The first fifteen in our list we call Good Mother Messages simply because, as they are the earliest messages that can be given by parents, they have traditionally been given by the mother. The Good Father Messages come later. Optimally, all messages should be given by both parents.

Each message elicits a distinct body experience, that can be identified in a different part of your body. "I love you" feels different from "I want you," or, "You are special to me," and so on. Allow yourself to experience the feelings. Learn to listen to your body, not just your mind.

Good Mother Messages (earliest childhood messages)   mental health aid

1. I love you.
2. I want you.
3. You are special to me.
4. I see you and I hear you.
5. It is not what you do but who you are that I love.
6. I love you, and I give you permission to be different from me.
7. I'll take care of you.
8. I'll be there for you; I will be there even when you die.
9. You don't have to be alone anymore.
10. You can trust me.
11. You can trust your inner voice.
12. Sometimes I will tell you "no," and that's because I love you.
13. You don't have to be afraid anymore.
14. My love will make you well.
15. I welcome and cherish your love.

Good Father Messages ("out in the world" messages)   mental health aid

1. I can set limits, and I am willing to enforce them.
2. If you fall down I will pick you up.
3. I am proud of you.
4. I have confidence in you, I am sure you will succeed.
5. I give you permission to be the same as I, to be more or less.
6. You are beautiful (handsome).
7. I give you permission to love and enjoy your erotic sexuality with a partner of your choice and not lose me.

Imagine how different your life would be if you already had received these messages and were no longer compelled to seek them from outside of yourself.

There is only a brief period of time or "window" in childhood during which each of these messages can be provided by your parents. When that time passes, the window closes. Even if your own parent belatedly recognizes your need and strives to fill it, it is too late. Your basic needs can no longer be completely satisfied from outside yourself. You may find yourself fruitlessly trying to obtain these messages from your partner and children.

To begin the process of "giving" these messages to yourself, memorize the first fifteen. Write those you can remember into your journal; then read the messages again and fill in the ones you missed. If you do this each day, you will discover that the few you keep forgetting are the ones you probably did not sufficiently receive in childhood and, consequently, are still seeking.

As you write the messages, you might want to imagine that you are saying them to different aspects of your self: the child; the sexual, competent, alive man or woman you are; the wise old person you are becoming. Some people feel best when imagining that the messages are being sent from God, or the sun. Ultimately what matters is finding a way to trust and allow them in. What you are not prepared to believe rarely feels authentic when expressed by others in words or through deeds.

The Good Father Messages are also very important. However, their "window of receptivity" is wider because these messages are meant to be received later in childhood, at a time when you can more easily provide for yourself. Some people who missed these messages try to seek them through an older lover. Whether these messages are fulfilled or not, they usually have to leave the relationship eventually because they have treated their partner as parent, which will cause the erotic nature of sexuality to fade.

Although we now dry our own tears and no longer throw tantrums, our bodies know when something is still incomplete. This knowing brings forth a driving force we call longings. They are like embers that kindle romantic fantasies and make us vulnerable and human. If you try to sexualize your longings, you set yourself up for disappointment—in yourself, your lover, and in sex itself.

If your attraction to another is based on the hope of fulfilling good parent messages, your sexual approach will be childlike. As one woman so poignantly lamented, "When I first started having sex with my husband I always felt turned on. Now when he approaches me I feel sucked on."

Two things that people unsuccessfully try to satisfy from the outside are longings and sexuality. Together they are sure-fire sexual turn-offs for both partners. For heightened sexuality, it is necessary that both partners have a sense of self that is self-sustainable.

You can discover issues most likely to cause problems in intimacy and sexual lovemaking by charting your own psychological history. These surveys in the appendix guide you to the most relevant questions you must ask yourself for an understanding of your interior and intimacy patterns. The story you tell yourself is often a fantasy (overly negative, idealized, or incomplete) and therefore does not serve as a supportive foundation. By clarifying the history of your first intimate relationships you can form a new narrative of your life, one that is more adult, comprehensive, and authentic. The sexual history exercise helps you understand how your past sexual experiences affect your sexual satisfaction.

There are many themes left over from childhood that couples act out in their relationship. Perhaps the most destructive one is gender prejudice. The rest of the themes that we feel are important for you to look at are found in chapter 11, Primary Scenario.

<table>
<tr><td>

GENDER PREJUDICE
THEME

</td><td>

THIS IS THE MOST IMPORTANT THEME for a couple to confront. If it is not resolved, working on other problems is futile. Gender prejudice is an inherited, recurring bias, discomfort, devaluation, fear of, or anger against one gender or the other. It is the most prevalent and insidious of all themes, having the power to destroy intimacy and sexuality. Although mostly unconscious, when present this infuses every interaction with resentment and mistrust. Prejudice does not allow you to feel the body experience of trust. Therefore, it can provide you with a reason never to feel loving or sexual.

Prejudice is hard to acknowledge when it is clearly opposite to your conscious beliefs. But, if you are attracted to men but think them insensitive and not worthy of your trust, or if you like women but think them controlling or not too bright, then you are probably prejudiced. Friends don't count, since you choose them as exceptions to the rule.

This prejudgment devalues people by seeing them as "too much" (controlling, manipulative, abusive, narcissistic) or "too little" (stupid, wimpy, shallow, unstable, incompetent, insensitive). You can "just not trust" them, or you use their character-style traits (chapter 12) to justify your prejudice.

Prejudice against your own gender profoundly disturbs your sexuality by causing you to dislike, become distant from, or deaden your own body, making it impossible for you to feel a sense of gender-specific erotic sexuality. Hidden prejudice against your own gender can undermine your sense of self and impair your ability to express yourself fully as a man or a woman.

Your parents may have been prejudiced against your gender, even though you were exactly the gender they wanted, if they also assumed that under their influence you would become "better" than others. "You'll never grow up to be that kind of man (woman). We're going to raise you differently." This form of prejudice is learned from the child's earliest caretakers, from their subtle, nonverbal attitudes as well as their not-too-subtle overt actions. Once you absorb it, you go through life finding evidence to reinforce it. When later you chart your primary scenario, try to recall whether men or women were devalued to you in one way or another.

</td></tr>
</table>

Gender prejudice was usually inherited through the mother, because she was usually more involved with the children at the very young age when this prejudice was instilled. Fortunately this seems to be changing as men become a more integral part of the family. But gender prejudice certainly can be compounded by the father, particularly since couples who marry generally have the same prejudices.

Gender Prejudice Identification Exercise

The unfortunate nature of prejudice is that we don't easily recognize it in ourselves. Yet, it is easy to recognize when we are the brunt of it. The following exercise will expose the nature of your gender prejudice. Uncovering this theme is vitally important to intimacy and sexuality and for the stability of your relationship, particularly when the prejudice is against your own gender.

Use this same exercise whether you are a man or woman. In your journal divide a page into four columns. Using one column for each, write down the names of *your maternal grandmother, your mother, and yourself.* Leave the fourth column for insights. Now, pretend that you are your grandmother being interviewed: "Tell me about men in general, what are they like?" (For example, are they bright, trustworthy, kind, faithful, sensitive? If not, what are they good for? Are they placed in groups of bad and exceptions to the rule?)

Answer the question from her viewpoint. Write down whatever comes to mind. It's all right to exaggerate; it helps identify her perspective. Just guess when you do not know the answer.

Now, as your mother, answer the same question, then as yourself. Look at the answers you have written down. Are there themes that repeat from grandmother to mother to you? What is the general feeling and tone?

Do the exercise again, this time asking the same people: "Tell me about women in general, what are they like?"

Once you have identified your prejudice, for the best results work on resolving the one against your own gender first. Any prejudice you have against your own gender will surely affect how you see members of the opposite sex.

To further identify your themes of judgment, run this little survey for yourself. When you see a stranger of your gender, note your attitude and your first thoughts about that person. If you have the opportunity, start a brief conversation. You can choose either to look for evidence to back up your prejudice or you can consciously set your identified prejudice aside and see who the person really is. Do this at a party, a restaurant, or anywhere there are crowds of people. Experiment with about twenty people and note your judgments and insights in your journal. You can learn to see yourself and others beyond your prejudice.

Although there are exceptions as to how this theme is passed on, it usually works in the following ways. If the mother has a prejudice against women, the father—if he is not discounted and has no prejudice against women—can counter it. He can tell the children, for example, "Those are your mother's beliefs about women, but I know women are just as bright and capable as men." If the mother has a strong prejudice against men, the father is powerless to dispel it because the family prejudice against men invalidates his opinion. Nor, for the same reason, can he dispel any prejudice the mother may have against women. But she can counter his prejudice against men if she is not herself disqualified by prejudice.

If a parent is trustworthy, successful, kind, gentle, and supportive, seen through prejudice he or she is apt to be discounted as weak. You will often hear people say, "I don't trust men (or women)." Every once in a while, a person is idealized and seen as an exception to the rule, "My father was wonderful, unlike most men." If the father is bad, he just proves the point. If there is no gender prejudice in the family but ample reason to regard the father or mother as really "bad," this feeling will remain specific to the parent and won't be generalized.

These days we have considerable freedom and autonomy and fewer gender-specific roles in our lives, so one doesn't have to be a victim of gender prejudice. Rather than feel enraged and controlled if you suspect that your partner holds a prejudice against your gender, check to see if you, yourself, have a parallel prejudice. Are you trying to be an exception to the rule for your gender? This implies prejudice. Trying not to be like your same sex parent is a prejudice. In addition, trying not to be like someone else does not allow the unfolding of one's own potential. (See Masturbation in chapter 8 for the effect gender prejudice has on the body.)

Understanding the Primary Scenario arena is relatively simple. It is just a matter of repeating family themes and having to carry the pain of childhood emotional injuries around in your body, sometimes mistaking these feelings as statements about you or your current life.

The next two arenas, character style and agency, are more complex as they are the ways we compensate for our lost somatic core self-experience. These arenas are so much a part of our way of being that we rarely recognize how consistently they now cause injury to the core self they were meant to protect. Forged in childhood, the protective and defensive patterns you developed in relationship to your parents are now yours, and only serve to carry childhood themes and injuries into your adult relationships.

CHARACTER STYLE

YOUR CHARACTER STYLE was formed as a protection, a way to defend yourself against real or imagined dangers to your true nature, your core self. In the formative years, our core sense of self is tentative, fragile, and vulnerable to our need for closeness and to the sometimes overwhelming feelings when it is not available. We are vulnerable to our parents and their ideas and assumptions about who we are and how we should be. To please them we may adapt to their needs, silently compensating by developing a protective cover to preserve our essential nature. But, unfortunately, after a while our core self becomes so concealed by its cover that its existence is hardly recognizable.

When as an adult you turn inward for your experience of self-identity for guidance, you are liable to mistake your defensive cover, or character style, for the true self-identity it was formed to protect.

Each person acts out his or her style in the form of personal characteristics. In your relationship, you may have caught glimpses of these traits and called them idiosyncrasies or personality quirks. They are most often seen as isolated incidents, flaws or irritations in yourself and people you are otherwise fond of. Yet, most of us don't see these ways of being as whole, consistent, definable styles for protecting one's self in intimacy.

Your style keeps you acutely alert, searching for possible dangers that are similar to those you encountered in childhood. If your spouse says, "Let's make love," and you always had to be constantly on guard to not be controlled, you may hear this as parallel and therefore a command. If so, you may feel, "Don't tell me what to do," and communicate "no," not necessarily with words, but by your body expression and attitude. Character style responses are more of an echo of the past than a realistic assessment of the present and can cause you to feel childlike and as if old injuries were happening now.

The traits of character style dwell in what C. G. Jung so astutely called the "shadow" aspects of our being. They are parts of ourselves that we wish to deny. The more you try to hide these traits, the more obvious they are to others. If you try to hide what others see so clearly, you seem like a phony, and engender mistrust.

EMOTIONAL PIE

LOVE IS A STATE OF CONSCIOUSNESS that is difficult to sustain because it triggers the underlying fears of character style. Like waves on the beach, love may surge through your body only to fade away into an ocean of uncomfortable feelings—just when you feel wonderfully loving, character style rises as a warning that danger is near. Yet, most often the warning is misplaced and greatly exaggerated.

These interruptions to loving are triggered by love's special power to open our body and arouse old emotional injuries. When we were children what happened to us during our first experiences of loving and being loved, aroused emotions within us. These old emotions inevitably arise each time we now feel love. The emotional joys and fears of early childhood are forever bound to future states of loving. As adults, when we feel love, it often takes only moments for the childhood association to be felt. Then the love seems to fade. With the experiment on the next page, discover how you interrupt love.

The most dramatic example of the emotional love pie happened to us in the early months of our sexual lovemaking. One evening we were at Jack's house. We were not living together yet. There was a fire in the fireplace, candlelight, the music was just right. We were in love. It was one of those moments when life and loving move in a mystical spiritual realm.

Beverly: I was so happy being with Jack. He was so caring, present, attentive, exciting, and a good cook. Everything was perfect. We were at the height of sensual, sexual erotic loving, energetically flowing and connected, our hearts and bodies joined in rhythm.

Suddenly I felt Jack's energy shift. Instead of closeness there seemed to be a terrible distance between us. I felt abandoned and didn't know what had happened. I thought I had done something wrong to turn him off. When I

Your Emotional Pie Experiment

To find out what causes love to fade for you, try the following experiment. On a piece of paper draw a pie with one wedge marked "love."

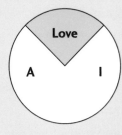

Heighten your body experience by sitting up straight and taking ten full breaths. After you have read the instructions, close your eyes and place the palms of your hands on your chest.

Think of a time when you loved someone—a lover, a child, a friend, a pet. Focus on the feeling of love for a few minutes. Let the feeling expand in your body. Notice that as you feel the love, other feelings and thoughts begin to appear. As you stay with the loving feelings, you will soon feel something else. When you recognize the interrupting feeling or thought, open your eyes. *Make sure you have done the experiment before reading on.*

When you felt love, what were the interrupting feelings, thoughts, or fears that arose in your body?

Many people feel warm, tender, joyful, caring, protective. These are all extensions of the feeling of love. When some people feel love, they also feel fear. "What if something happens to my lover, my dog, my child? What if they go away and leave me, or what if they die? What if the loving stops? What if I die?" In some way, for them, their loving triggers the body experience of *abandonment.*

When other people feel love, the fear of being told what to do takes over and they feel flooded, invaded, smothered, or controlled. Something or everything is too much. Generally, they feel overwhelmed or trapped. Loving, for them, triggers the body experience of *inundation.*

Still others experience the feelings of abandonment and inundation equally when they feel love. They may alternate between the two or feel both anxieties at the same time. Because this is more confusing, their answers are usually not as clear. "I don't know what I feel. I don't feel anything. I can't feel on command. I can't put my feelings in a box."

Of the multitude of thoughts and emotions you could have had with love, the one you unconsciously chose to experience is your self-perpetuated theme. Even though your feeling may have been about your partner, you are the one who gives meaning to your experiences through choice. You can listen to the voice of your defensive cover, or listen beyond to the core self that it protects.

Draw your emotional love pie using the diagrams below as a guide. Indicate how much abandonment (A) and inundation (I) is part of your inner world.

Equal Abandonment and Inundation	Higher Abandonment	Higher Inundation
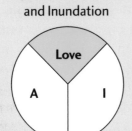	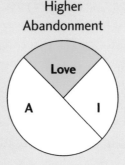	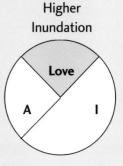

asked him what had happened, he came out of his emotional pie "trance" and reconstructed his thoughts.

Jack: I could not have felt more caring nor have been closer to Beverly. I was so in love and finally had everything I ever wanted. Suddenly, an inner voice started nagging at me, "Jack, remember that later Beverly will be driving home. She will be in her little convertible. It's not safe for her to be out late and alone. She could get hit by a bus." Within a millisecond, the vision of the bus crashing into her car and crushing her head into the steering wheel had an immediate impact on my body. "She could die and I would lose her forever." It closed my heart and chest, collapsing my emotions from love and excitement to abandonment, mourning, and pain.

I then realized that a catastrophic thought follows whenever I have feelings of love—feelings I so dearly want in my life. I had never recognized my destructive, speedy, transition from love to abandonment before that night.

Unconsciously Jack had invited a "bus" into bed with us. When an interruption (a bus) drives into bed with us now, we both know we are just feeling more love than we can tolerate at the moment. Our options are clear. We can choose to climb on the bus and ride off into the problem. Or we can see that our upset is due to old, outgrown fears and longings. Because we realize that the only function the bus—our character style—has is to interrupt our loving, and maintain old speed limits, we dismiss the bus and go back to our loving.

The abandonment or inundation anxieties carried by your character style may just fade away if, with a sense of humor, you remind yourself, "This is not a crisis. I am probably just feeling loving."

THE BALANCING ACT

A PARENT AND CHILD together need to accomplish three tasks for a child to grow up emotionally healthy and stable: 1) form a bond, 2) develop an empathic attunement, and 3) maintain enough breathing room for the child to develop a secure sense of self. In a successful loving relationship there must be a continual balancing of these same three tasks. In childhood, these tasks fulfilled furnish a secure sense of self felt in the body. When not fulfilled, the emotional injury forms an *anxiety that remains in the body*. Protecting one's self against this anxiety forms character styles.

The Bond: Abandonment Anxiety
The first task, forming a strong bond with a primary caretaker, allows a child to feel secure, cared for, and loved in a consistent way. Without enough of this trusting, nurturing bond, infants can die. If a child is separated for too long from the primary parent or a parent is emotionally depressed or distant, the natural longing for a physical and emotional union becomes exaggerated. Any injury in this stage of development leaves the child constantly trying to secure that bond in intimate relationships throughout their adult life.

Even when two people clearly have a loving alliance, a fear of abandonment generated in childhood can ignite the old terror of loss in the present situation. When this childhood insecurity is acted out as character style, as if it were a present reality, the bond of the relationship is liable to be pestered to the breaking point. This is guaranteed to stress a relationship and cause real abandonments to occur.

Breathing Room: Inundation Anxiety

All children need freedom and autonomy to test out their core self, to have their own thoughts, to make their own decisions and their own mistakes. Without breathing room, the child can't individuate, can't develop a healthy sense of a separate self, a sense of personal volition, confidence, curiosity, achievement, or safety in the outer world.

A child with controlling, inundating parents is likely, as an adult, to have feelings of claustrophobia, suffocation, or panic in an intimate relationship. Adults with this history may continually break the bonds of trust and hope in order to fend off the threat of control and gain the feeling of room to breathe. They often do this by insinuating a love or sexual interest in another person or by actually having affairs. This will usually create more distance than they bargained for, even if the affairs remain unacknowledged by both parties. Any desire on the part of another to be close, helpful, loving, or sexual may be interpreted as controlling behavior and seen as a threat.

Attunement: Both Abandonment and Inundation Anxieties

Attunement is necessary for mutuality. It is the most spiritually uplifting aspect of intimacy, a feeling you can't quite grasp, but you know when you have it and when you don't. Attunement is impossible to attain when abandonment and inundation anxieties are acted out. There are three basic aspects of attunement:

1) To be seen and heard: We all want to understand and be understood by the one we love. You must be able to see your partner's essence beyond what they speak and act out through their character style and beyond what you "need" them to be. You must also allow yourself to be seen unadorned by a character style facade.

2) Mutuality or shared experience: Mutuality is the body experience of looking across a room and feeling that you both understand the meaning of what has happened without speaking. Shared experience is engaging in things together, having most of the same, hopes, visions, desires, and commitments. Watching television together, for example, leads to familiarity and comfort, but it does not promote mutuality, the spirit of attunement, getting to know your partner on a deeper level, heightened intimacy, and functioning as a team.

3) Communion versus communication: Communication means "to exchange

or transmit information with the attempt to alter another's belief or action system." Communion means, "to share another's experience with no attempt to alter or change what that person is doing or believing." (Stern, *Interpersonal World of the Infant,* 1985) Communion, not communication, is the lack most couples feel. This sorrow causes people to feel alone no matter what is communicated.

When an abandonment character style is acted out, there is a clinging to the bond. When an inundation character style is acted out, the bond is broken. When there is a struggle between these two anxieties, attunement—the experience of mutuality, reciprocity, and shared experience—is impossible.

An adult who did not experience this attunement as a child may be most comfortable and familiar with more superficial aspects of relationship. Without attunement, they and those with whom they are the closest will find themselves yearning for some missed essence of the human spirit. We all want to be known and understood in a deeper way, to share meaning, to feel the attunement of intimacy. Those who did not receive attunement in childhood have difficulty tuning in to others. They may not know when their partner is upset or how to emotionally comfort or soothe anyone. They don't know how to create a feeling of mutuality.

With the character style profile surveys in chapter 12, you can identify your style so that as you do the exercises you will be able to recognize more clearly the difference between core self and character style experiences. Because the combination of living with both abandonment and inundation acts upon us and our relationships so profoundly, the chapter will help you understand this dilemma and its six traits more thoroughly. In the appendix, you will find a helpful guide for living with abandonment and inundation anxieties. There are many things that you can change, but your character style is relatively unchangeable so it is best to learn how to live with it. If you can acknowledge your defensive patterns and learn how to attenuate the traits of your profile, you can reduce their potentially negative effect on your life.

AGENCY

IT IS THE LACK OF SEXUAL DESIRE and boredom, not the loss of love, that is the most common complaint in long-term monogamous relationships. When we hear such a cry for help we suspect that at least one of the partners has taken responsibility as an agent for the well-being of the other. An agent is a helper who feels an obligation to fulfill the needs of other people, to fix, help, please, or otherwise stabilize them. They do this so intently that a sense of who they are and what they want at a core level, dims or becomes inaccessible.

Agency is developed in childhood, often in infancy. Infants are born with the capacity for self-agency, the ability to feel, know, and, later, act in their own behalf. But, if a child comes to believe its survival depends on its ability to attend to the parent, to be or do what the parent wants, to please and calm the parent, self-agency psychologically takes a back seat.

Daniel N. Stern, in his 1985 groundbreaking book *The Interpersonal World of the Infant,* described self-agency as one "of the experiences available to the infant, and needed to form an organized sense of core self." He defined self-agency as "the sense of authorship of one's own actions and the nonauthorship of the actions of others: having volition, having control over self-generated action...."

The agent's hyper-vigilance toward others severely limits the body experience of self-volition, and the trust, satisfaction, and heightened energy felt when acting in one's own behalf. Taking on responsibility for the life, actions, and well-being of others establishes a lifetime pattern of core self-abandonment. Because of this, even while surrounded by those that love them and appreciate their goodness, they often feel empty and alone. These children fear that if they can't fix their parent they will not be cared for and will die. In hope of finding their inner feeling of self, stability, and worth, they mistakenly try to fix others to attain self-validation, rather than turning inward to their own core body voice.

As an agent, a young child takes on an impossible task trying to make a parent feel fulfilled, happy, stable, and content. This is not something any person can provide for another, much less a child for a parent. Therefore the child is doomed to have nothing more than temporary victories. Even the small victories are a lie that just perpetuates the agency stance. The parent's momentary "fixes" can cause the child to feel omnipotent, but because it never lasts for long, the child ultimately feels bad about himself or herself. They feel that they have done something wrong, failed at this job that is so vital to their survival and well-being. As an adult, they are haunted by the irrational feeling that they are bad and have done something wrong. To compensate for this gnawing emotional feeling in their body, they spend their whole lives trying to be the best they can.

Agency is driven by an inner desperation; yet, from outside appearances, an agent can look the epitome of strength, competence, and wisdom . . . until they collapse . . . often with a physical illness. Their body screams, "Pay attention to your inner voice. If you don't, I will speak louder in the only voice I know, the voice of pain and illness." Over time, the more consistent the agency, the more somatic distress is accumulated.

The problem for the agent is not the helping behaviors. It is the loss of self. As a child, because of the fear of death the agent learned to relinquish any true self-awareness and expression to attune to the needs of others. In childhood, the family rules prevented acting directly in his or her own behalf.

Now, even when they no longer wish to live life as an agent for others, they have a difficult time making any significant change because of the fears associated with breaking this rule. Each time they are successful in doing something for themselves, the core self-experience produced causes an anxiety in their body that something horrible will happen. In this case the anxiety is a healthy sign of success, a sign that they have broken the dysfunctional rule and are doing something that is self-affirming.

Sexual desire, which is highly dependent on feeling good about one's self and knowing that you can trust yourself to act in your own behalf, is lost when time after time a lover chooses to act as an agent for their partner's satisfaction and well-being while their own core self remains neglected.

When this way of being is carried into intimate adult relationships, it is often mistaken for love. Yet, it is more a way of trying to earn love than real loving and caring. Trying to earn love implies that you are not inherently lovable. A loving relationship imparts a genuine reciprocity and respect for each other's capacities, the ability to restabilize when thrown emotionally off balance, to problem-solve, to be empathetic and humane. Agency, on the other hand, implies that one's partner is inadequate, inept, or immature and is more like overextended parenting than a mature love shared between adults. Because agency is more like parenting than sexually provocative, both partners' excitement dwindles and vanishes. Taking on another's problems and issues as one's own eventually causes the recipient of the agent's "generosity" to feel incompetent and unworthy, the opposite of the agent's intention. This way of over-giving undermines the most loving of relationships. It deadens sexuality and the body, creates bewildering anger, and surprisingly, puts distance between people.

Because agency creates a "one up, one down" relationship, it is not equal and reciprocal. Some couples, in an attempt to be fair, form "agencies" rather than relationships. They sign up to insure the well-being of one another, not really knowing the consequences of this contract. With the best of intentions they end up "niceing" their relationship to death and wondering what happened to their excitement and erotic passion. This does not allow for people to be authentic, for partners to accurately reflect one another. Nor does it create an environment for mutuality in which each person has the support, respect, and breathing room for solving his or her own problems.

If agency is treated as a behavioral problem—doing things for others—it neglects to address the real problem, which lies in the body, the denial of core self-experience in the body. It can also heighten somatic symptoms and destroy the relationship. No matter how much a person focuses on doing or *not doing* for others, the core self remains inaccessible, hidden out of awareness in the body. Stopping the behavior without reestablishing a somatic experience of self-guidance does not produce the needed feeling of inner stability or well-being.

Most people with a propensity for agency believe that if their mates would change or just "stay fixed," the pressure would be gone and they could take better care of themselves. But this is not true. The habit, motivating beliefs, desperation, and somatic loss of self are all felt and maintained in the body and psyche of the agent. Agency began in the primary relationship in childhood and is acted out in the relationships of today, but it is not a relationship issue, nor can it be resolved by working on the relationship. Because an agent is always acting in response to someone else, and even when alone they are usually thinking in terms of someone else, agency looks like a relationship issue. *It is not.* Agency is an internal, self-perpetuated process.

Agency is the psychic glue that can keep old scenario patterns and character style firmly entrenched forever, no matter how much you are working on yourself. It keeps you looking into the eyes of others to see who you are. The agent, generous to a fault, gives so much away that he or she feels, to some extent, like a nonentity valued only for his or her successful acts of agency. When a problem arises, an agent does the only thing an agent knows how to do, give more and try harder.

NOTHING LIKE A GOOD OLD "FIXER UPPER"

SOME PEOPLE CHOOSE A MATE who is like an old car or house—great potential, but needs a lot of work. To feel loved and wanted, the agent needs someone to fix or help. An agent doesn't know another way to be in a relationship or to be loved. If a partner gets "fixed," the agent feels at a loss and fears abandonment. If one partner won't stay "defective," another will be found. Agents need their disabled to remain disabled.

Agency is a system made up of an agent and an agency target. A good target consistently comes up with another problem just at the time their agent needs a boost and says the magic words, "You are the only one who can save me and make me feel good about myself." This assurance of being special keeps the agent feeling loved and safe, but only for the brief time that the target stays "fixed" and grateful. Alcoholics and addicts are perfect targets.

If you are an agent, the slightest call for help from a loved one, your "target," will, even if you do nothing, trigger a tightening in your body and the resulting loss of self-volition. If you simply deal with your behavior and not your body reaction, your body will continue to stay closed, responding to the old body fear—If I don't do what you need I will die.

As a representative of others, your pay-off for soothing, fixing, and satisfying them will be different depending on your character style. Someone with a high fear of abandonment will use agency to avoid disaffection and a breach in the relationship. "I'll do anything, just don't leave me." Those with both abandonment and inundation will use agency to gain validation for his or her professed identity. A person with just high inundation will not be in agency.

Interestingly, these two roles of agent and target may be filled by either partner, as people often switch roles.

Both of Marion's parents worked. By the time she was ten years old she took full charge of her sister and disabled brother and had dinner ready for her parents when they came home. She was in agency to the whole family. She was a mother before her time.

To escape, Marion got married. But she then took on the role of agent to her husband, taking care of all his needs and feelings about himself. Then, far too quickly, she got pregnant and soon had another little person around that she automatically became an agent for. Then two more. Marion never had a choice as she didn't know how to be in relationship, only how to be in agency.

Her children grew up and her husband died. She thought she wouldn't have to be in agency anymore to anyone. Mind you, she didn't know she was in agency, but she did know that she now had a chance to live her own life. But when she started to date other men she automatically advertised herself to them as a good agent. She would say, in effect, "I'm a good cook and a good caretaker—love me." It didn't take very long to find a man who said, "This is great," and offered marriage.

After the wedding, Marion, once again, required to be an agent to be loved, was very sad. This increased when her ailing father moved in and she took care of him. Meanwhile, of course, she acts as an agent to her grown children and takes care of them whenever they have an upset.

Marion is now seventy years old and continues to wait for a time when she can focus on her core self. If she can't do it now, when? Agency is not going to go away. It is like an addiction. The alcoholic wants another drink, the smoker always wants another cigarette, and the agent will always find someone to take care of.

AGENCY MANTRAS

AGENCY IS PERPETUATED by both mind and body. Your beliefs cause your physical holding patterns, and your holding patterns perpetuate your beliefs. No matter how many times you release physical blocks, they will return if you don't work with the psychological causes. And all the insight in the world won't unhook the body component.

The following mantras deal with erroneous beliefs that cause and perpetuate agency. You will know what is causing the pain in your life when you identify which mantras you cannot say and believe intellectually and feel as a truth in your body. Take your time and feel each of the twelve statements. If they do not ring true like a clear-sounding bell, figure out why you can't bestow this basic kindness on yourself.

The first statement is the most important. Make sure that you can say it without a doubt before you move on. If you think you are bad, figure out what your "crime" is and how long you have been serving your sentence. Is your crime a thought crime in which you do not have pure thoughts? Is your crime that you haven't been perfect (i.e., you have been human like the rest of us)?

With the second mantra, define first what it meant to "fix" your mother and other members of your family. Then identify your current targets. Identify your primary target of the moment. Then make sure you say the whole sentence together: "I'm not bad because I couldn't fix my mother, and I am not bad because I can't fix…" It is important to keep repeating the sentence until you can feel the connection between the childhood agency hook (mother) at the same time as you feel the current one.

Use your journal to work on any of the statements you can't easily say with emotional confidence. Take your time with each statement. Say them aloud, then notice what you feel in your body. It is the feeling in your body that will let you know if you truly believe each statement on a deeper, more meaningful level. If you read a statement quickly and move on, suspect that it has an important meaning to you that you are avoiding. Go back and read it again slowly and pause to feel you body response.

Agency Mantras

If one of these is a truth you need to hear, adopt it, repeating it to yourself again and again. Sometimes it will take a while for the body experience to penetrate to your core.

1. I am not bad. I haven't done anything wrong. I am worthy of love.

2. I am not bad because I couldn't fix my mother (father, sister, brother, etc.). And I am not bad because I can't fix… (current agency target).

3. I am not selfish when I think of myself or act in my own behalf. I have a right to my own body-voice, my own body, my own toothbrush, to know what I think and want, and to speak up and ask for it.

4. I don't have the power over, control of, or responsibility for other people's lives. I was taught that I had these powers. This is a lie I now tell myself.

5. When I make the well-being of others my responsibility, when I try to change how they feel, no matter how pos-

itive my intention, it's invasive and cripples them. With agency, I undermine those I try to fix as well as myself.

6. I will not abandon myself when I most need my own support.

7. I don't have to depend on someone else or wait for them so that I can live my own life.

8. This is not a crisis; only my agency habit makes me think it is. Agency is a habit I do not have to continue.

9. I have a right to my own interior life, my own thoughts, hopes, and dreams; and I'm not bad if I don't tell anyone about them.

10. I have a right to feel good about myself without feeling swollen-headed, narcissistic, or grandiose.

11. I have a right to my own soul, my own destiny, my own personal communication with God, even if others don't agree.

12. Only in my body can I know the difference between an act of caring and an act of agency. The end of agency is not the end of love. It is the beginning.

Using the following agency mantras is an important step toward maintaining your core sense of self within a monogamous intimate relationship. It is only in your body that you can feel the difference between an act of agency and an act of love. You must pay attention to your body signals, the ones that speak on your behalf—exactly what the agent avoids.

In chapter 13 you will find more help with your agency and find out how your relationship can be healing.

EXISTENTIAL-TRANSPERSONAL

"But have a real relationship with a person that goes on for years—well, that's completely unpredictable. Then, you've cut off all your ties to the land, and you're sailing into the unknown, uncharted seas. And I mean, people hang on to these images of father, mother, husband, wife, again, for the same reason, because they seem to provide some firm ground. But there's no wife there. What does that mean? A wife? A husband. A son. A baby holds your hands, and then suddenly there's this huge man lifting you off the ground, and then he's gone. Where's that son? You know?"

SHAWN AND GREGORY,
MY DINNER WITH ANDRE,
1981

THIS ARENA OF SPIRITUAL AWAKENING involves the most basic issues of human existence, those that touch our soul. It powerfully affects you and your intimate relationship. When you truly make love, not just have sex, you invite a spiritual consciousness into your life.

The transpersonal experience is one in which a person gains an awareness of self as something extending beyond his or her limits as an individual. We use the term "transpersonal" more or less synonymously with "spirituality." The spirituality we speak of is grounded in the body and in the realities of everyday life. This experience usually involves a realization, an insight, or an understanding that touches the core essence of self and is perceived by the body as undeniably true. These truths come from within the individual and are verified intuitively. There is a feeling of knowing linked with a reassessment of life's priorities. And this journey of spiritual consciousness is a somatic one—that is, it is revealed in the body where we feel the passions and zest for life.

The scientist who finds a universal truth in his lab may have a transpersonal experience, just as a mystic in a mountain cave may, or two lovers in a heightened erotic union. Creating a life and becoming a parent can, perhaps, be the most transpersonal experience of all. There is nothing like participating as a parent in the creation, birth, care, growth, and discoveries of a child to move you past and expand all previous self-limits of awareness and consciousness.

The personal growth of our being—the journey of the soul—can not be entirely fulfilled by any relationship, no matter how perfect. A relationship can be an exquisite vehicle to the transpersonal and can deepen your bond, but this journey is ultimately carried out alone, and yet you are not alone. Whether you are in a relationship or not, you must develop a healthy somatic sense of self before you can move to a more fulfilling, higher consciousness. In addition, you have to have lived long enough and had enough life experience to know in your body that there is more to life than sexuality and to be ready for it.

There is no better mirror in which to see yourself than the one presented in an intimate relationship. And there is more reflected than just the flat images of a regular mirror. You no longer look with your eyes but with your heart. You know there is something deeper in life, something more profound and it is at this level that all the truly important discoveries and battles are made.

FRAGMENTATION

WHEN ONE OR MORE of the arena patterns destabilizes your feeling of emotional well-being, you may experience a state of emotional and physical fragmentation. Fragmentation is like a period of insanity that intermittently disrupts your state of mind, causing you to see life in a distorted fashion.

Like most people, there are periods in your life when things are good and life just flows along, and then there are periods when it all seems to fall apart, when you feel "off" and your emotions and responses are exaggerated, distorted, and fragile. At these times your thought process may seem a little bizarre to you and to others, this is why we sometimes refer to this state as intermittent insanity. Your judgments become black or white, and thoughts turn negative and hopeless—a jumble of "You always…You never…What's the use? I'm too fat, too dumb, too ugly…" Your eyes blur and stop seeing in vivid color. Your mind dulls. You can't find your keys, your wallet, your sense of self, or sense of humor. You either don't want to have sex or think you can't live without it. You stumble and trip over words and thoughts. You feel smothered by loved ones or abandoned by them or both at the same time, and all your defensive patterns become exaggerated. We call this state fragmentation.

When you are fragmented it does no good to pretend to yourself or others that you are perfectly fine. It is not a time to make important decisions or wage an argument, and having sex is, at best, only a temporary bandage. This condition of being fragmented is not an idea that you can talk yourself out of; it is a confusing and disconcerting body experience.

Fragmentation makes relationships much more difficult than they need to be. Surprisingly, most couples have a positive intention and a strong bond and can adapt to bumps, bruises, and differences. But when either partner is fragmented, no matter how sincerely each tries to work out their differences, problems seem to magnify. The struggle feels unending, and results are less than satisfying. The fact that one or both partners is not in a state of interior well-being brings an underlying irritability, fragility, and lack of trust and hope to the couple's interactions.

Most couples find that once their fragmentation is dealt with, the undercurrent (caused by the arenas) subsides and differences are once again relatively easy to resolve. Strangely, it doesn't seem to matter where or with whom the fragmentation occurs.

When fragmented, some people emotionally fall apart while others become physically ill, or tight and rigid in their bodies. Others grab on to something or someone. They try to feel whole by turning to addictive work, food, love, alcohol, drugs, or sex. If your partner habitually turns to you for a sexual "fix" to resolve his or her fragmentation, your own sexual excitement will surely vanish.

Sometimes a person is not aware that they are fragmented. They find themselves feeling irritable, angry, depressed, horny, hungry, or split off. These feelings don't seem associated with anything specific. This shift in body and mood is not random or without reason. Something has caused the upset. But dealing only with the current, obvious, external, or superficial symptoms and not the underlying arena patterns allows "the blues" to hang on.

Fragmentation is brought about by the themes of your primary scenario, character style, agency, or transpersonal issues. If you have an upset today and nothing about it triggers these four arenas, the upset will be just an upset. It won't cause the deeper, more debilitating symptoms of fragmentation—the "crazy," rigid, unrealistic, incompetent behavior that can wreak havoc upon your body and life, especially your intimate relationship.

Some people get sick, and this causes them to fragment. Others become so fragmented that it affects their immune system and they become ill. While every physical illness has its psychological component, illness, if it arouses an underlying psychological theme can cause a fragmentation. People who know how to work with their fragmentations can manage to sustain their sense of well-being when they become ill.

You can't maintain yourself or a relationship in a constant state of well-

The Windsurfing Story

A few years ago we were in Hawaii, watching a group of young men windsurfing. It was wonderful to see how they attacked the huge waves, jumping or crashing through them for a thrilling ride.

They seemed to fly, hitting the waves, apparently without ever falling down. This amazed us. Most of the windsurfers we had ever seen spent the majority of their time falling down, struggling to get back onto their boards, then fighting to stay upright.

It seemed impossible that these young men never fell, so we watched them more closely. What we saw at first seemed like magic, because their movements were so swift and smooth. They did, indeed, fall. In fact, because they weren't afraid of falling they moved freely, ventured more risk, and fell a lot. Their falls, we saw, were a graceful part of the ride. As they hit the water they swung their big sails

body-mind awakening

toward the sky, and their bodies and boards lifted as if by magic onto the next big wave without missing a beat.

So it seems, the secret in windsurfing is not how to stay up, but mastering the art of *getting back up* when you are down.

What a great metaphor for mental health! In windsurfing, as in good mental health, no one can stay up all the time. We all have times when we get fragmented or knocked into the water, so to speak.

But the secret in mental health, as in windsurfing, is in knowing how to get up again rapidly. Many people expend most of their energy trying to stay up and that is impossible. Relationships are the same way. Working on them constantly is exhausting; learning how to get back up is much more exciting. With a little practice, you can learn to "surf" your own well-being and that of your relationship.

being. We all fall into self- and relationship fragmentation. The trick is not to spend all your time trying not to fall apart, but to focus instead on getting yourself together again as quickly as possible.

The simplest, most basic type of fragmentation is when something happens in the present that is similar to an emotional injury or theme in your childhood. This apparent reenactment of a past injury can make you feel as if you are catapulted back to the time in your childhood when the original injury occurred. The childlike emotions that emerge can feel overwhelming. Then you not only have the current injury to deal with, but you must also contend with the emotional weight and intensity of the childhood injury.

For example, if as a young child you didn't receive one of the good parent messages such as, "I see you and hear you," then you as an adult will be hyper-sensitive to not being seen and heard. Claire has difficulty feeling as though Pete sees or hears her. When he doesn't say good-bye in the morning she can be fragmented all day. When he forgot their anniversary she became so fragmented that she felt she had to get a divorce.

Sam, growing up in the middle of seven brothers and sisters, never felt the message, "You are special to me." When he was passed over for a promotion he interpreted it to mean that, in his office "family," once again, he wasn't special. He fragmented so badly that he quit his job on the spot. Later he was horrified by what he had done. This hasty action was an exaggeration of other symptoms of his ongoing fragmentations caused by his perpetual body feeling of being excluded.

Character style and agency can cause further fragmentations. Although these arenas are part of your primary scenario, having developed in response to your childhood relationships, they have a life of their own, and each needs different treatment. When your character style or your tendency to agency works against your best interests, you can, and will, fragment.

When it rained the day of her wedding, Rita became immobilized in fragmentation. Her rigid idea of how her wedding should be, in the garden, made it impossible for her to smoothly shift her idea with the weather change and move the wedding into the sanctuary of the church. She was devastatingly fragmented by her own character style.

Raymond made an agency, unilateral contract with Sara, "I'll be nice to your mother during her visit, then when she leaves you'll have sex with me." When Sara just wanted to be left alone after her mother left, he was shocked, fragmented, and started an argument. "How dare you ignore me after how nice I was to your mother. You're unloving, frigid, and never consider my feelings," he thought. It never occurred to him that he had made his contract with himself, not Sara. If he had thought about it, he would have realized that Sara always becomes inundated by her mother's visits and then needs a short period of being alone before she is ready to be intimate and sexual.

Existential-Transpersonal fragmentation occurs when you come face to face with life, death, and impermanence and this shatters your reality of existence. Reaching back in time, this awakens archetypal struggles. Reaching forward it opens uncertainty and the questions of personal survival.

Gary's life was going along exceptionally well. New job, new wife, and finally his previous wife was remarried so he no longer had to pay alimony. But then, the big earthquake came along to shake up his smug reality. He saw the structure where he parked his car collapse. Deep in his body he realized that everything he unconsciously counted on, could change in a moment. "If I had been in my car I would have been crushed," he thought. The reality of the nearness of death and the body experience of not being able to count on anything, not even the earth being stable shook his complacent belief in his reality. Fragmented, he called everything into question, his new marriage, his career, his life, and his sense of self.

If you are in an intimate relationship and don't clear up your own fragmentation, your negativity and distorted feelings can cause your partner and then the relationship itself to fragment and fall apart. You can strain the bond of the best of relationships until it breaks.

In the morning June spoke to her father on the phone. She fragmented when, in his usual way, he began to tell her she wasn't doing a good job raising her children. Instead of realizing that she was fragmented and working it out in her journal, she walked around all day feeling like a chastised, powerless child again under her father's control. When her husband, Hank, asked her to type part of his manuscript, because she was fragmented, June felt that Hank was also trying to control and demean her, trying to "tell her what to do." Her desire to be nice and have him think well of her overrode her rage. So she said she would do it. But she procrastinated, forgot, and became irritable and withdrawn. Hank fragmented in turn because he felt that once again he was dealing with his irresponsible, angry mother who he could never trust. The bond of trust now severed—fragmented—they both began to think of divorce, how to divide up the money, the house and the kids.

This basic theme in their relationship, *their perennial argument,* caused one fragmentation after the other. Now, they each had to resolve their own individual fragmentations, and they also had to find a way to mend the bond of the relationship.

You will find the steps for guiding you out of this debilitating state and a guide for prevention in chapter 15. The section on existential fragmentations will help keep you from making unnecessary crises in your life.

Pandora's Box

To sustain and heighten the excitement of sexuality in a long-term relationship, it is important to understand how certain psychological themes can sabotage sexual excitement and manifest themselves in your body.

When people first join in an intimacy of love and sexuality, the body, which is our storehouse of feelings and emotions, can open up like Pandora's box. If you are only having sex, or if you are only loving without becoming sexual, this does not seem to happen. It is the combination of love and sexuality that fully opens your body, revealing the hidden contents of your psyche.

What actually surfaces can be a surprising collection of old wounds, a disconcerting mixture of unconscious fears linked to psychic scars and faulty relationship patterns of childhood. Even though these disturbing memories come from within you, you are most apt to experience them as current abuses by whomever is closest. These old injuries arouse a need to protect yourself and can lead you to blame your chosen mate. Instead, it is more productive to attend to your aroused interior feelings.

With the storehouse of injustices from your past laid bare, the fallout can become evidence that your worst fears have come to pass. When this happens, the perfectly logical, rational, sane ways of being together, of understanding, communicating, and loving can just fall apart.

Even a subtle injustice today that parallels a trauma from the past can become greatly exaggerated causing deep misunderstandings between two people. Over time, making love works like a key, unlocking in our bodies deep-rooted childhood experiences, releasing the pains as well as the unrealized potential for joy. Throughout The Intimate Couple we will show you how to recognize and address the old pains so they don't stand in the way of your potential for joy.

Your emotional health is not determined by what happened to you as a child or what "comes at you" in life. What you do with what happens to you now makes the difference. The distortions you perpetuate will undermine your emotional stability.

SUSTAINING A SENSE OF SELF IN MUTUALITY

"Though oneness is the essence of love, the vitality of love comes from the partnership of two whole, in-the-flesh human beings who respect each other's separateness. Ultimately every facet of human existence is reflected in the reconciliations of oneness and separateness."

KAPLAN, *ONENESS & SEPARATENESS: FROM INFANT TO INDIVIDUAL*, 1978

THE FOUNDATION AND SUPPORT for heightened sexuality is the ability to establish and sustain a sense of self and at the same time join in a mutual union with another. For many people, a separate self and mutuality sound like direct opposites. Such a lack of understanding causes struggle, pain, and hopelessness within an intimate relationship.

Some people try to resolve this through compromise, others through surrender. In either case, both people lead one life, his or hers. Then it doesn't matter who compromises or surrenders, both lose out. Others try to solve this paradox by leading parallel lives without much mutuality. Still others break the bond of the relationship every time a sense of self is desired. The bond can be broken with intimidation, hurt, anger, indifference, righteous indignation, doing the one thing your partner can't tolerate (like having an affair), or threatening to leave the relationship. None of these tactics works well for long because no one really gets what they want, and self and mutuality both suffer.

A separate sense of self and intimate mutuality can exist side by side if you learn to understand the nature of your internal longings and can fulfill them or put them to rest from within. You also need to establish a different base for your sense of self, one that is somatic. (See chapter 7.)

THE EMOTIONAL PAIN originating from childhood injuries and unfulfilled longings will never completely go away. You will need to identify, understand, and learn to tolerate these sometimes painful interior body messages when they arise and learn how to manage their impact on you and your relationship.

As you join with a lover and your heart and body open to feelings of joy, the openness can cause you to feel other emotions as well. You may feel the emotions of all the times it wasn't safe to be so open and alive, when it was not possible to be so perfectly attuned to another. You may feel the disappointments all the way back to your first intimate relationships with your parents and those throughout your life, from childhood to the present. There can be pain associated with closeness and pain associated with the lack of it. Is it any wonder that we often hesitate to enter profound states of intimacy with another?

It is not as difficult to tolerate these emerging emotions from the past if you are able to recognize them for what they are. Your emotions may turn to self-questioning: "Why didn't I ever do it this way before?" "Will it ever happen again?" "Will I lose myself in my longings and give myself away to love or sex?" It is most important to recognize that the emotions these thoughts are based on are about the past, not the present, and they are about

Keep in Mind

New psychological information can be destructive to your relationship if you use it as a weapon to hurt, demean, or intimidate your partner, as psychological or spiritual blackmail, or "one-upsmanship." Use this information to work on yourself—for your own benefit. Please remember that the psychological issues we present here are within the general range of healthy human experience.

You can obstruct your success in accomplishing the aim of *The Intimate Couple* by not clearing up the destructive psychological patterns in your relationship. Yet, working with psychological-relationship issues alone is not enough to greatly heighten your sexual excitement and orgasmic response. Insight alone—psychological, spiritual, or otherwise—can't appreciably change your body's energetic patterns. The mind and body work

body-mind awakening

together. For every physical response pattern, for every distortion of your energetic process, there is a psychological component. In an ongoing intimate relationship your mental and emotional states affect your body, your sexuality, and your sexual relationship. To maintain physical, mental, and emotional health takes awareness, authenticity, and accountability.

The way we participate in an intimate relationship is with both mind and body. For many, the opening of sexual desire is the first expression of the body's participation in the relationship. For some, closeness and excitement start with the heart and loving. For others it is intellectual stimulation. Whether one leads with the heart, the head, or the genitals, moving experiences of impact affecting the relationship will always be felt in the core of the body.

you, not your partner. If you focus on these distracting emotions and thoughts, it will cloud your sense of satisfaction just as you attain exactly what you have been searching for. Here and now holds the possibilities for satisfaction. Don't let these distracting interruptions unnecessarily deprive you of love and loving.

THE GOOD-ENOUGH PARTNER

Fundamentally, constancy is our emotional acceptance of the idea that we are neither saints nor demons but whole persons who are capable of ordinary human love and ordinary human hatred. By uniting our loving emotions with our emotions of anger and hatred, constancy confirms our sense of personal wholeness. We all strive to protect and uphold the good images of self. When constancy is weak, the only way to protect the cherished parts is to split them apart and to keep them fenced off. When the good and the bad are split apart, the wholeness of the self fragments and disintegrates. And then it becomes impossible to appreciate and respect the wholeness of others.

KAPLAN,
ONENESS & SEPARATENESS: FROM INFANT TO INDIVIDUAL, 1978

THE GOOD-ENOUGH PARENT, as described by D. W. Winnicot, is not just a compromise but is the best parent. The good-enough parent allows a child room for self-experience. A child with an all-giving parent does not have room to build his or her own sense of self through experimentation and accomplishment. In the same way, the best partner is one who is present, interested, supportive, and caring, but neither takes on responsibility to resolve the other's frustrations nor hands his or her own frustrations to his or her partner. Too many people spend their whole life looking for the perfect partner who will take care of, soothe, calm and comfort, see and hear them perfectly, gratify all their longings—believing that only then can they be happy and able to feel a sense of self. As with the overprotected child, this doesn't work because it undermines the ongoing development of self.

Remember, a sense of self, by its nature, must come from one's own interior. It doesn't mean that you can't take in and enjoy with great satisfaction what you receive from others; it simply means that what you receive from the outside is not self-actualizing. If a great deal of your needs are satisfied from the outside instead of through your own volition, you will have little opportunity for an experience of self. Self-volition is a stimulant for heightened life experiences, including erotic sexual excitement.

We need to have enough self-experience to feel our own volition and desires, to take care of our own inner life, our bodies' needs and interests. If you receive an abundance of soothing and comforting, you miss the opportunity for self-soothing. Self-trust requires experience. To trust yourself you must have experiences of picking yourself up when you have fallen down. Experiences that lead to trust in one's self are important prerequisites for desire and erotic feelings. If, in an intimate relationship, all of your longings are fulfilled by your partner, sex goes dead because your inner volition is not being exercised. Dependency is not self-empowering and therefore not a "turn-on."

Some people see others as either "good" or "bad." This is a simplistic and unrealistic approach. It also has a backlash effect as it causes you to see others, including yourself, in a compensatory distortion. "If I am good, you must be bad," or vice versa. A child is often subtly encouraged to see one parent as good and the other bad. When our illusions keep us seeing a parent as bad, we can't enjoy the part within us that is like them, or the healthy parts of the parenting we received. Once learned in childhood, this same splitting is apt to be repeated with your partner: "If I am good, then you must be bad," or vice versa.

In a long-term intimate relationship, little injuries and insecurities can, over time, dampen your spirits and cool your love. To sustain hope and keep an expansive, ever-growing aliveness, undiminished by time, takes a little consciousness, goodwill, and some psychological sophistication. The emotional complexities of a relationship can dull your body's erotic sexual aliveness. A little time and effort in this area promises the greatest rewards.

Battlegrounds of Intimacy

Most couples find that any struggles that occur between them eventually intrude on their sexual relationship. When relationship problems affect sex, it looks as if sexuality is the problem. Then sex becomes a battleground upon which these unresolved personal or interpersonal issues are waged. For some couples, sex and intimacy disappear in the fray. Others continue to have sex, believing that this will resolve everything else. But when the real problem is not sex but arena issues, you can't expect that by having sex, the underlying problem will be resolved or just go away. No matter how much you work on your sexuality, underlying problems remain.

Sexuality is only one of the favorite battlegrounds in which the struggles of the arenas show up. Fighting in any battleground affects sexuality. Some of the favorite battle-grounds are: the Bank (money), Baby (children), Broom (cleanliness and order), Bottle (drugs and alcohol), Belief (religion and politics), Blemish (flaws and imperfections), Business (work), Body (illness, sleep, food, weight), the Blonde (fidelity), Being (sense of core self), and the favorite, of course, the Bedroom (sexuality).

Because sex is a physical manifestation of the bond between partners and is integrally linked to the body and emotions, making sexuality a battleground can become lethal to the relationship. Sustaining a core sense of self is the foundation for building and sustaining the bond, and sexual battles undermine both. Without the closeness of sex to nourish the love, hope, trust, and support that make a relationship worth mending, the relationship often becomes dead or falls apart.

WRITING IN YOUR JOURNAL

THERE IS NO GREATER TOOL than writing in a journal to help you become a witness of your own life. A journal is not necessarily a record of events and experiences. It is also an opportunity for an inner journey. It can be an honest mirror, a friend, and an intimate companion that can help you gain a deeper sense of yourself. To take a profound journey to the core of your being, you must accept and face yourself with all your humanness. To become a witness of your life, you must allow yourself to see who you are beyond your defenses, your protective facade.

Have you ever noticed that often it's easier to see and understand another person's problem than your own? You can usually tell when someone else's way of thinking is off. Just thinking about your own problems doesn't give you enough perspective. Habitual ways of thinking take over, creating blind spots. Writing in a journal involves your body with your mind and provides a perspective that allows you to witness and examine your interior life. It is the best way to take charge of mind-body patterns that are so close to your being that they have become automatic and outside the realm of your awareness. Habitual ways of looking at and resolving problems will most likely always bring you to the same conclusions, whether they work or not.

The body-mind exercises in this book and the information for making sex better will, we hope, bring your life issues to the foreground and provide a means for many new and insightful realizations. Take this opportunity to take charge and witness who you are and how you function. As you read and do the exercises, write down your insights and feelings, otherwise in a short time you will lose these precious awakenings.

The best kind of journal to use is one that is bound so that you can't tear out or lose the pages. A journal with blank pages instead of lines is best so that you can write freely and even draw pictures. If you can, use a special pen that you feel comfortable with and keep it with your journal. If you are concerned about privacy, use a journal that you can lock. We strongly suggest that couples learn to turn to their journals when a disagreement is not easily resolved. Arguing rarely will help you get to the heart of the problem, whereas using the steps out of fragmentation will (chapter 15).

The journal is best used as a companion for:

- **Collecting your insights.** The insights you gain as you read and practice—the ones you most think you will never forget—are the ones most apt to vanish. They are difficult to retain over time because they challenge your habitual way of being.

- **Clearing up issues that are cloudy.** The journal is the best place to sort out and clarify your feelings. Throughout this book we will show you ways in which you can reestablish your inner sense of well-being, whether you are feeling a little "off-track" or completely "down and out."

- **Storing ruminating thoughts and emotions.** When interruptive thoughts plague you during your exercises or lovemaking, write them down and you will be more able to stay present for yourself and your experience. When you know that the emotions you are feeling are more than a situation warrants, your journal is your best friend and confidant. Journal writing is excellent for emptying out your mind before you go to sleep or when your sleep is interrupted. (See the emptying out exercise chapter 15.) As you do the exercises, if your interruptions are repeating or are keeping you from being present, stop and write the distracting thoughts down. Once you have written out the problem you will probably no longer be distracted. You can work on your upset at another time. What is unfinished will tend to plague you. Writing it down creates a completion.

- **Collecting your dreams.** Most often your dreams speak to you from your unconscious body-mind. They carry important guiding messages from a deeper source of knowing. It is not as important that you work on your dreams as it is that you write them down. The writing introduces your unconsciousness intuitive process into your waking hours. Learning to live with your dreams is a means to heightened intuition, creativity, and consciousness.

- **Becoming a witness to your life.** In a sense the witness is the soul, that part of us that remains constant throughout life, or perhaps even death. The first step on the journey of awakening consciousness is the acknowledgment of a soul. As Ken Wilber has said in *Grace and Grit,* "The witness is the soul shining through."

It is from your core self that your private journey must be chronicled so that you can see yourself more objectively, as clearly as you can see others. Being human is not easy.

The constant presence of the witness shines a light on life's path reminding us we are not alone in this precarious existence. The art of witnessing is the art of exploration. The art of understanding is the gift of compassion. The witness is indispensable to compassion.

THE WONDROUS FABRIC OF RELATIONSHIP

A SUCCESSFUL, LOVING RELATIONSHIP must be consciously woven like an intricate fabric. The arenas are the threads that give this wondrous fabric its color and texture. They weave through a relationship, creating its distinctive and unique qualities. Some couples want a lot of togetherness, others weave loosely for more breathing room. No one couple's "fabric" is inherently better or worse than another's. The only test for worth, satisfaction, and durability is whether the fabric suits the two people and is sufficiently flexible for comfort and growth. A relationship based on an idea of how a relationship "should be" is rigid and never comfortable.

To all relationships you bring your unique blend of the four arenas that forms your personality. In an intimate relationship, not only are your arena issues intensified, but you must deal with the complexity of two human beings functioning together. If a couple weaves their fabric without awareness of each person's primary scenario (arena 1), it will be thin and without substance; with its secret themes, it will become riddled with holes and eventually fall apart. Character style (arena 2) gives the fabric its color, texture, and, most importantly, its fit. Woven with too much agency (arena 3) it will be a smothering blanket. The existential-transpersonal (arena 4) provides vision, hope, endurance, the wonder of life, and the feeling of meeting as soul mates. It provides the graciousness to endure the inevitable passages of life. The fabric of your relationship provides warmth, vitality, trust, love, constancy, and hope for you as a couple.

The arenas hold the potential for the deepest love and caring as well as for the deepest pain.

BASIC BODY-MIND PRACTICES
for the
INTIMATE COUPLE

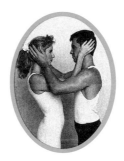

C H A P T E R   T H R E E

The Energetic Model

MOST PEOPLE THINK OF SEXUALITY, including orgasm, as beginning and ending with genital stimulation, but there is so much more. If you can expand your perspective by seeing that sexuality is a process of building and releasing energy in your body, you will have a deeper understanding of your sexuality and a greater potential for change and variation. You will also realize that your capacity for heightened sexuality is the same as your capacity for a heightened aliveness in general.

BUILDING A CHARGE OF
ENERGY IN YOUR BODY

WE NOW KNOW that if we examine the body with an electron microscope, we will find that we are not solid matter but waves and particles of energy. We can alter this energy in our bodies and influence the level of aliveness and excitement we feel.

Besides feeling the energy in our own bodies, we can also feel the energetic presence of others. Sometimes we can sense by their energy that someone is in the room without seeing, smelling, or hearing them. Sometimes a person's energy is magnetic—when they walk into a room people are attracted to them. This energetic charisma is called *presence*.

An infant, sucking at its mother's breast, feels the mother's energetic presence—or lack of it. If the mother withdraws her attention, the infant can sense the loss as a void or disconnection. If the mother is attentive, but her body is closed, the child will not feel her energetic warmth shine through. Energetically, the infant, without language, is aware of and will respond to its mother's anger, delight, depression, or any other emotional state.

As adults, dependent as we are on words for communicating, we sometimes forget we also communicate nonverbally, not only through bodily expression and other nonverbal behaviors, but through energetic expressions of who we are and what we feel. This information that a person transmits energetically—his or her "spark" or level of aliveness—is often the basis of a first attraction to a lover. You may not, however, be aware that you can directly take charge of this level of aliveness and excitement in your own body. You can learn how to boost this energy, or "charge," and move and spread it to different parts of your body, such as to your heart to increase loving or to your pelvis to increase sexuality. The greater the energy that you build in your body, the more enjoyable the sexual experience and the more energy you have available to release during orgasm.

Consider this example of building and releasing a charge of energy. If you

Genital Stimulation

Stimulating the genitals arouses very intense sensations, which can be enjoyable when a charge is high. Yet, as any lover knows, if your genitals are aroused intensely while the level of charge is still low, it can be quite uncomfortable or even painful. As sexual lovemaking begins, the genitals are the last place to touch. When stimulating genitals, begin slowly and gently for both men and women. If you intermittently shift your touch to different areas of the genitals, to the surrounding region of the body, then to other parts of the body, and then back to the genitals, you help to spread the energy throughout the body. If only the genitals are stimulated, the charge remains localized in the pelvis, and the resulting orgasm is small in nature.

That's why when Harry asked Beth to slow down, he didn't mean "go away." He meant, "ease off until I catch up with you."

But Melanie *did* mean "go away." She was afraid of her sexuality, so she kept her charge very low. When Carl tried oral sex, her body was too shut down to let the increasing intensity spread out to a tolerable

level. Had he listened to her and kissed her elsewhere on her body, or even gently around her genitals instead of directly on her clitoris, he could have kept the stimulation apace with her slowly building charge. The spreading sexual energy might have warmed her and helped to melt her fears.

Before they make love, Julia always says to Tom, "Be gentle with me. Don't go so fast." But what she is thinking is, "When you touch my nipples I feel like you're turning the dials on an old radio, but you can't find the right station, volume, or tone."

Too much too soon can set up a pattern of avoiding sex in order to escape discomfort the next time. It can make one's body close down rather than open. The feeling of "that's too much" can become associated with a particular sexual activity or even being asked for sex at all. In addition to physical discomfort, you may feel disregarded as a person or treated like an object, as if your partner is trying to *make* you feel something rather than respecting and tuning into your feelings and physical responses during stimulation.

wish a pistol to shoot farther you must load the bullet or cartridge with more powder, which is the charge. The pistol will not shoot any farther or "produce a bigger bang" if you just pull the trigger harder. During sex, the genitals and nipples are triggers for orgasm. People often fail in their attempts to heighten their sexual experience—produce a bigger bang—because, rather than focusing on building a higher charge, they stimulate the trigger more and harder. Pulling the trigger too soon results in less pleasure for sexuality and a less intense orgasm.

In addition to orgasm, the charge elevates and expands, or minimizes, the sensations of pleasure, excitement, and sexual enjoyment during lovemaking. If you wish to heighten your sexual experience appreciably, you will have to learn how to build a high charge without triggering an orgasm until the charge is built sufficiently high for a total orgasm.

Stimulating genitals can, of course, cause some charge to build. But, because the genitals also function as a trigger for the release of energy, or orgasm, the orgasm is often triggered prematurely. The higher the charge, the more you feel and the more pleasurable it can become.

To build higher charges for a more intense sexual experience and orgasm, you must also learn how to contain the energy as you build it and to spread the charge throughout your body. The further unfolding of the energetic model begins with an understanding of the containment process and the energetic *holding patterns,* which inhibit the expansion and spread of energy in the body.

CONTAINMENT OF ENERGY IN YOUR BODY

ANY TIME YOU GENERATE EXCITEMENT, your body must serve as a container to hold the energy you build. It must be flexible enough to expand as the energy builds and able to retain the energy so that it doesn't "leak out" as fast as you build it. People who have trouble with energetic containment manifest this in a number of ways in their everyday life. Often they can't hold on to money, secrets, and good feelings or maintain limits with work, food, alcohol, or sex.

Although we speak of the body as a container, our energy is not limited only to our physical bodies. What we mean by "body" does include our physical being, but it expands beyond and is much more than our corporeal self. It is an integrated self composed of body, mind, emotions, and spirit—a total energetic system.

To avoid the loss of energy you must be able to stay energetically present and maintain self-boundaries. The following will help you first understand *presence* and how it affects sexuality.

Energetic Presence

The first step in improving your sexual relationship is found in a very simple message: You have to show up! You would think that if a person were going to show up anywhere it would be for sex. But, surprisingly, this is exactly when many people aren't fully present. They bring their physical bodies, but they are simply "not at home" energetically and emotionally. A lack of presence directly lowers the charge of energy and aliveness in the body. As you will see in later exercises, if you "space out," out goes your energy. Avoiding presence is a way some people find relief from the sometimes overwhelming emotions and sensations of sex. This flight from interiority is an attempt at self-protection. But it actually lowers your sexual excitement and orgastic potential, denying you access to your core internal source of energy and volition. To have a high charge during sexual lovemaking, you must be able to remain keenly aware, not only of your immediate surroundings, but also of your interior sensations, thoughts, and emotions. Only when you are completely present with yourself can you be truly in contact with another. Two of the most common ways of not being present are to be energetically or emotionally split off or cut off.

Split Off: If your physical awareness is blurred or focused elsewhere, if it is covered over by thinking or distracted by problem solving, you are not present, you are "split off" from your body and your energetic charge. If your charge builds at all, it will quickly dissipate.

People split off during sex for many reasons. Sometimes it's performance anxiety, and sometimes it's a defensive reaction to having an emotion or to being in close physical proximity with another. Most of all it comes from the reluctance to feel emotional longings—especially those aroused by heightened sexual excitement. Whatever the cause, without presence, all the techniques for increasing excitement and making sexual lovemaking better are futile.

When you are not in the "here and now"—present, but "gone" into the past, future, or just out in space—you are not able to be or do your best. Not only are you not able to build and contain your aliveness or sexual charge, but your partner knows you "aren't there" and feels lonely and abandoned.

Exercise for Presence When Energetically Split Off   exercise one

There are many ways to get present. One of the easiest is to use your senses.

Begin: To bring yourself back to your senses, use your eyes.

Step 1: Aloud, quickly list the colors and objects you see around you, e.g., blue shirt, green pants, brown chair, red fire, etc. The faster you do this exercise the better. Going slowly just helps maintain your split-off stance.

Step 2: Notice if you get into a repetitive rut, where you're not really paying keen attention (red pillow, black pillow, yellow pillow). Make sure you say both color and object for each thing you see (red pillow, gold lamp, white sheet). Look closely, focus on what you are looking at, and get present.

There is no energy for you to share and no one with whom you can join.

Burt lives his life in a state of "when-then." Life is never in the moment. Whether in the office or in bed making love, he is always thinking, planning, problem solving, or fretting about which move should come next. Sara, his wife, says, "I don't know what's the matter with me. I feel so hopelessly lonely when I'm with Burt."

Cut Off: While you can usually identify a person who is split off by the vague or distant look in their eyes, a person who is "cut off" can look you directly in the eye. They do something in their body to impair their ability to feel sensations and emotions. They do this by "muscling" their feelings out, "fatting" them out, or "thinning" them out. Any extreme produces a protective shield of rigid muscular patterns in the body that can inhibit the flow of energy and deaden an awareness of internal feelings. Unfortunately, cutting off forms a barrier to a deeper sense of self, and this loss of interiority undermines a feeling of connection to others.

The rigid muscular patterns that cut off emotions and body sensations restrict your energy so that it is in a tight container unable to expand. If you are cut off from inner feelings, it is easier to treat yourself as a thing or object and pay little attention to pain or discomfort. This lack of presence leads to feeling isolated from oneself and one's partner, and the rigid patterns can cause difficulty in releasing energy during orgasm.

Unaware of emotions and feedback sensations in his body, Stan would insensitively push his way through difficult situations with little consideration for himself or for others. During sex, his fiancée, Mary Lou, thought she might as well have been a plastic Barbie doll for all he noticed. Lack of presence leads to low energy, no way to join, and great loneliness, especially for the partner who *is* present.

Exercise for Presence When Energetically Cut Off   exercise two

Begin: To bring yourself back to your senses, become keenly aware of your body.

Step 1: Start at your toes. Say, "Now I am aware of my toes." Move your toes. Tighten your toes as much as you can, and let go. "Now I am aware of the bottom of my foot."

Flex your foot. Tighten and release. "Now I am aware of my ankle." Now rotate your ankle. Tighten and release.

Step 2: Continue heightening your awareness by tightening and releasing each area as you travel up through your body, paying attention to the sensations and emotions this activity creates.

Boundaries help to establish a separate sense of self. Once we have an energetic sense of our boundaries we can feel when our comfort is being

Experiencing Energetic Boundaries

So that your experience will not be influenced by our explanations, you can try the following boundary exercise before you read the explanations that follow each set of steps.

One person will be called Partner 1 and the other Partner A. Each person will need a piece of chalk.

Begin: Sit on the floor facing each other.

Step 1: Simultaneously, take a piece of chalk and draw a space on the floor around yourself. *Do this before reading further.*

Step 2: Notice if it makes any difference to have a defined space—a boundary—around you.

Some people feel very limited and confined and do not like to have a defined boundary. Others feel safer and more together and solid, as though the boundary accentuates their sense of self. Some feel trapped, enclosed, isolated, or limited by the circle. Some people draw their circle right through their partner's circle; others have difficulty even drawing the circle. For some people a boundary makes no difference whatsoever, but most people are naturally territorial.

Step 3: To exaggerate your body experience of this space, Partner A, use your hand to trace the perimeter you have drawn and say to your partner, "This is my space." Now allow your energy to extend out to the edge of the boundary you've drawn. Don't let your energy go any farther than your own boundary.

Step 4: Partner 1, try the same experiment. In turn, tell your partner what it feels like to define your space. Is the space you have drawn too small or too large or just right? How do you know this? Where in your body do you feel the sensation? Do you feel a right to have a separate boundary? One at a time, try erasing your boundary in front of your partner. What do you feel in your body with and without this boundary? What do you feel like in your body when your partner does and doesn't have a boundary? Have you or your partner overlapped each other's boundaries? If so, discuss how this feels and then experiment by drawing the spaces again so that each person has a separate circle. Are you telling your truth?

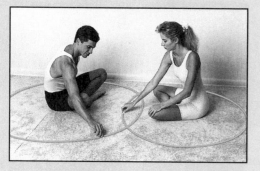
Step 1.

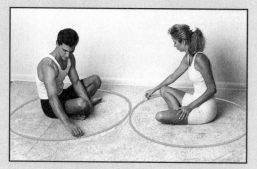
Step 1.

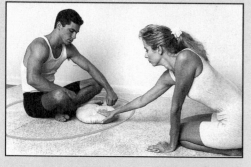
Step 6.

Step 5: Partner 1, have your partner put a small pillow just outside the boundary you have drawn. Pretend for a moment that the pillow is your mother. Now, out loud, tell your mother, "This is my space, and I don't want you to come into it unless I ask you."

Step 6: Partner A, slowly push the pillow into Partner 1's space until it touches his or her body. Partner 1, what emotions and physical sensations are stimulated for you? Partner A, what physical (energetic) reactions do you notice in your partner when you move the pillow into his or her circle?

Note: Notice how easy it is to have a body response by just allowing a pillow to enter your space (or your partner drawing into your circle). This shows how deeply imbedded the early patterns are. These automatic responses are active in our bodies, unconsciously influencing our emotions. These boundary emotions are the same ones that we, as adults in present time, consistently respond to on an unconscious level with our intimate partners. The reason we suggest you refer to the pillow as "mother" is that in most cultures the mother is the primary caretaker of the infant, during the early years when these responses were established in our body-mind. With this exercise it is most important to see that these patterns were formed because of early childhood experiences, not because of what your intimate partner, who is pushing the pillow into your circle, does or does not do.

Common reactions to boundary invasion include a constricted feeling in the chest, severely limited breathing, a loss or flush of skin color, abdominal tightening or nausea, a blank or spacey sensation, anger, fear, a contraction in the body. These body responses are what we call symptoms of inundation anxiety. Some people will have these symptoms even though they are inviting the pillow to come closer and saying how good it feels.

Step 7: Partner A, now pull the pillow slowly out of Partner 1's space. Partner 1, tell Partner A when you first feel comfortable again and to stop if a new discomfort begins as the pillow continues to be withdrawn. What emotions and physical sensations are stimulated this time?

Note: Common reactions to the new discomfort are a flooding of emotions, especially longings or a fear of loss, a reaching out with the eyes, a leaning forward with the body, or hyper-vigilance. Again, the person may turn pale or flush. The reactions to the pillow being too far away are what we call symptoms of abandonment anxiety. Once triggered, some people can't let go of the inundation feeling (step 6), which prevents the anxiety of abandonment from surfacing (step 7). Others focus on the abandonment so fiercely that they forget about their inundation anxiety.

Remember, the body responses you learned in childhood are the same you experience in your present intimate relationship. Notice just how much closeness and how much distance is comfortable for you.

impinged upon psychologically and energetically through words, behaviors, and physical proximity. This awareness, and the right and responsibility to take care of what is inside your boundary, allows you to sustain your sense of self. Without a somatic sense of boundaries, two lovers tend to lose a sense of themselves and energetically merge into one. This causes a distancing from a somatic experience of self, affecting sexuality in two ways. First, the loss of boundaries can cause a person to be afraid of a loss of self to another. With a feeling of safety gone, the lover is apt to limit any further letting go into deeper realms of sexuality. Second, without boundaries, the energy of the body will dissipate. When two lovers meet with their self boundaries intact, the potential for deepening the experience and heightening the charge is greatly expanded.

Boundaries provide the possibility for interiority—knowing yourself from the inside—the right to an internal private world, and knowing, from feeling rather than thinking, a sense of what you need to do to take care of yourself. Boundaries also nonverbally communicate your limits to others. They are necessary for a presence with yourself and to be able to feel in emotional contact with others. To expand the container so it can hold more energy, your body must be free of holding patterns.

HOLDING PATTERNS THAT BLOCK THE SPREAD OF ENERGY

TOTAL ORGASM OCCURS when energy is free to build throughout your whole body and is contained until you are ready for a full release. When your entire body is reasonably limber, toned, and sexually alive, the potential amount of energy it can contain is greatly expanded. Unfortunately, most people have places in their body that chronically inhibit the expansion of energy. These blocks are called *fixed holding patterns*. They prevent energy from spreading from one part of the body to another, which limits the amount of charge that can be built. The pelvis can fill with sexual energy rather rapidly, but it isn't a very big space, and a small amount of contained energy will lead to a small orgasm. Your entire body must be open. Many body holding patterns were formed early in childhood, and the remnants of these injuries show up in sexuality.

Energetic holding patterns are caused and effectively perpetuated jointly by body, mind, and emotions. Rigid beliefs and a rigid body stance play off each other. Emotions can cause our body to pad, muscle, or thin our feelings away. Tight muscle patterns will be held together by the rigidity of the muscles and by the beliefs and fears that were the original cause of the tension. As holding patterns are most often a result of how we view the world, the blocks hold and perpetuate that view on a body level. Therefore, insight is not enough to bring about any depth of change; the body pattern that supports it must also be worked with. And the psychological and emotional beliefs and fears must be addressed. In sexual lovemaking, body patterns tend to soften and release as they do with massage, yoga, and other body practices. As holding patterns release, you may notice thoughts or emotions that seem to come out of nowhere. These are apt to be the psychological aspects of the patterns coming to the surface.

Mike, who was four when his parents divorced, went to stay with his aunt. At this time he began to wet his bed. His aunt severely punished and shamed him. He desperately tried to stay awake so that he wouldn't lose control. He wouldn't touch his penis for fear it would make him have to urinate. He learned, too well, which muscles to tighten to insure safety.

Sherry's pelvic holding patterns were formed by her mother's compulsion to have her toilet trained by the time she was a year old. For each mistake, Sherry received a spanking, and then her mother wouldn't speak to her for the rest of the day.

Both Mike and Sherry were emotionally and physically punished for natural developmental struggles of childhood. Now when they make love and charge begins to build, body-mind holding patterns that they've carried for years release feelings of anxiety, which remind their muscles to tighten as excitement builds, preventing the physical expansion that their bodies need to increase the charge.

These blocks develop over the years as a natural attempt to protect oneself from hurtful situations. Some come from physical injuries such as surgery, accidents, or other trauma; others come from psychological injuries such as abandonment, invasion, or other betrayals. To heighten sexual enjoyment and increase intimacy, you must be able to loosen the physical holds that your mental, physical, and emotional injuries have on you. The breathing and movement exercises throughout this book will help you to relieve holding patterns.

THE ORGASTIC RELEASE OF ENERGY

ORGASM IS A SUBJECTIVE EXPERIENCE that is impossible to measure and definitely describe. There is no standard orgasm; each depends on an individual's physiological and psychological health, belief system, and capacity for pleasure and excitement. An orgasm is a powerful release of sexual energy—or charge—and is usually accompanied by an intense emotional and physical sense of exquisite satisfaction. It can bring forth feelings of love and intimate closeness.

For men, orgasm is usually accompanied by an ejaculation of seminal fluid, though this is not always the case. An orgasm is not an ejaculation. The sensations are different. Men sometimes have ejaculations without an orgasm, which is less satisfying than with the energetic high of an orgasm. This occurs when they ejaculate before building enough charge for an orgasm. (See chapters 4 and 8.)

It has been found that some women have ejaculations, a release of fluid, even though they don't have semen. Grafenberg reported in the early 1950s that, "the same structure that becomes paraurethral glands in the female during fetal development becomes the prostate gland in the male, which later contributes to the male ejaculation." (Ladas, Whipple, and Perry, *The G Spot*, 1983) It is believed that only about one out of ten women actually ejaculate.

As orgasm approaches, feelings and sensations become more intense and urgent, heart rate and breathing become more rapid, blood pressure and pulse rate rise. Men may have an urge to penetrate and thrust deeply. Woman often contract their vaginal muscles and grip tightly. The colors and vibrancy of both male and female genitals intensify with the increased charge and blood supply.

How a person experiences orgasm depends on the force of the release as well as the height and depth of the charge and how fully it spreads throughout the body. Arousal at different centers of the body can create many different and delightful orgastic experiences:

- Some people reach a high peak of ecstatic excitement that lasts for some time; for others an orgasm is over quickly.
- Some feel a deep and widespread heat moving through their body. Some feel sexual energy streaming in undulating waves. Some feel both.
- Some feel their body move in involuntary rhythmic, orgastic reflex movements—the back-and-forth rocking of their pelvis with the reciprocal thrust of the upper body and head.
- Some feel strong genital muscular contractions.
- Some release sounds—groan, moan, cry out, grimace, laugh, or cry.
- Some feel a melting, a complete release of tension and muscular holding patterns throughout their body, a deep letting-go.
- With release, many people can feel soft or strong vibrations, or trembling, as body holding patterns release.
- Some feel an altered state of consciousness, when perceptions of time, space, thoughts, and images become confused. They may feel whole and complete as a person and/or an openness that is mystical, a joining with a higher consciousness or with their partner as never before. And some people, unfortunately, become frightened or fragmented by the awesome experience.

CHAPTER FOUR

Energetic Charge-Release Cycle

THERE ARE INFINITE VARIATIONS for sexual lovemaking. The Energetic Charge-Release Cycle diagrams in this chapter will show you how different people build, spread, and contain a charge of energy in their body and then release this energy into orgasm. We will use these diagrams to show you how you can alter or enhance your sexual lovemaking through showing you five common patterns. To do this we have divided sexual lovemaking into eight phases: intimacy, desire, approach, charge, containment, orgastic release, satisfaction, and then, again, intimacy. As described in the introduction, each phase or ingredient has its own potential for excitement, joy, and pleasure; its own physical-energetic and psychological-emotional requirements; and its possibilities for disruption.

The way you breathe and move to build a high charge and release into orgasm is your orgastic pattern, which determines how effectively you can accomplish the energetic tasks of each phase of this cycle. Psychological and physical influences can create energetic holding patterns and inhibit this natural process. The breathing and movement orgastic pattern you will be learning in the later chapters sets up the preconditions for your orgastic reflex.

An orgastic release is similar to a reflex in that when the physiological components are set up, the response is inevitable. When you set up the right conditions you can trigger an automatic orgastic release or reflex. The exercises in *The Intimate Couple* are designed to remove the old inhibitory holdings and help you repattern your natural orgastic response for erotic sexuality. More than learning a new response you are unlearning an old defensive ineffective response.

The energetic charge-release diagrams and the sexual relationship assessment guide will help you understand the mind-body process of your lovemaking in each phase. To influence an orgasm, you must understand and work through all phases. Remember, orgasm is just one of the sexual lovemaking phases, and the other seven promise just as much potential for pleasure.

ENERGETIC CHARGE-RELEASE CYCLE VARIATIONS

YOU CAN SEE in the illustration on the next page that with this typical orgastic pattern a charge begins to build, and when it is contained and heightened it reaches a peak. With the body container full, the brimming charge will spill over, triggering the orgastic reflex, and the energy bursts into an orgastic release. You will soon see that there are many possible orgastic patterns that people utilize to build and release energy during this cycle.

The horizontal axis illustrates how people form distinct charge-release orgastic

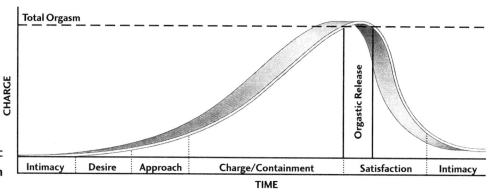

typical energetic charge-release pattern

CHARGE (vertical axis)

Total Orgasm

Orgastic Release

| Intimacy | Desire | Approach | Charge/Containment | Satisfaction | Intimacy |

TIME

patterns by showing how much time they spend in each phase. The vertical axis on the diagram represents the amount of charge built, which is the determining factor influencing your lovemaking.

The release of a high charge of sexual energy is called an orgastic release or orgasm. Some people do not build a very high sexual charge or do not fully let go and allow the sexual energy to release. Either will result in a low-intensity orgasm. Together these elements are also responsible for most of the nonpathological, physical sexual difficulties people have.

Different Patterns

In the past, it was thought that women tended to become aroused more slowly than men, but we now know that both men and women who are free to express their natural enthusiasm and sexual excitement build their own charge when and as fast as they wish. There are fewer differences between men and women than there are variations amongst members of each gender. There are many gender misconceptions concerning sexuality, including which gender has more affairs, who wants sex all the time, and who wants more intimacy. We've seen these issues split fairly evenly between men and women.

The differences in pattern depend more directly on the following:

- how energetically alive you are in general, and how alive you are when beginning your energetic orgastic cycle in particular;
- how sexually aroused you are before you even approach intimacy or sexuality and whether you choose to be there for yourself;
- how present you become, whether or not you really "show up" for the experience;

body-mind awakening

- how comfortable you are in making emotional and physical contact with your partner in intimacy and sexuality;
- how physically and emotionally defended you are and whether or not you have an ability, natural or learned, to pass quickly through your defenses or armoring. This includes how caught up you are in old fears and body-mind patterns;
- how able you are to build and spread a charge of energy;
- how long you can tolerate and contain excitement;
- how well you are able to relax and give in to involuntary rhythms;
- how conducive the environmental surroundings are to lovemaking;
- how much time is spent in each phase of the orgastic charge-release cycle. Since each pattern looks different when you vary the time period, the cycle may involve three minutes for a quickie or all day, night, and the next day for intense lovemaking.

Energy that is inadvertently dissipated as a person is trying to build to a full charge is called a discharge. Consistent or sudden small discharges of energy are a major factor in interrupting a person's ability to reach a full or total orgasm. But remember, to focus exclusively on orgasm is to miss the joy of heightened sexuality in all the other phases. Many people enjoy full sexual and sensual pleasure and are relatively indifferent to their orgasm. The energetic perspective we present here is a shift from how the sexual response patterns of men and women are usually viewed. This energetic approach will make it easier for you to understand and be in charge of your own orgastic pattern.

As you examine each variation, note which is most familiar to you. This alone may show you where your difficulties, strengths, and potential lie. It will also help you to understand the differences between your and your partner's orgastic patterns. Energetically, these different patterns can easily be adjusted so that each person's pattern can "dance" with the other's. Later, as you learn more about your breathing, movement, and charge, you can experiment with not only the time you spend in each phase, but with attuning your own styles to complement each other, creating even more excitement through diversity.

With the following diagrams, you will see how and why some people get what they are looking for and others don't. Remember, an orgasm cannot be seen as separate from building and containing a charge.

TYPICAL CHARGE-RELEASE PATTERN FOR BOTH MEN AND WOMEN

AS YOU CAN SEE in the illustration on page 64, Lenny's orgastic pattern is the most typical. His cycle starts with intimacy, he begins to feel desire, then approaches Mary Jane for sex. As his excitement rises at a consistent pace to a full charge, it is contained until he is ready for an orgastic release. He allows himself to feel a sense of well-being in his body. With release, his state of satisfaction opens him to a feeling of greater intimacy with Mary Jane. The satisfaction and well-being he experienced during sexual intimacy will surely lead him to seek intimacy again, to feel desire, and then to approach, etc., all in a cyclical fashion.

For Lenny and Mary Jane there is a lot of sex play and variation along the way. Notice on the diagram that the energy level, or charge, remains higher after orgasm than it was before the sexual charge began to build. Contrary to popular belief, sex does not deplete one's energy level. The more you have, the more alive, loving, and sexual you may feel.

Each phase can be shortened or lengthened by the amount of time allotted and enhanced just by increasing the amount of charge. Sometimes in the morning the approach is very short as Mary Jane knows that Lenny likes it when she awakens him with gentle oral sex. Other times they extend the approach and heighten their charge all day long with fantasies and phone messages, not actually making love until evening. Sex with the same partner never has to be boring if you learn to focus consciously on different phases and vary the time, charge, and playfulness. The possibilities are unlimited.

People start at different points in the cycle. While some need to feel intimate to feel sexual, others need to be sexual and have a release before they can really feel intimate. If these two types of people become sexually involved, they can remain locked into a sexual "Zen hell" standoff, arguing which way is right. One says, "If only we were more intimate, then I'd feel more sexual." And the other says, "If only we had more sex, I would feel more intimate and loving."

What they are really saying is, "I want to do it my way." Then they use their bodies to prove their stance: "See, I can't get an erection unless you will be sensual and loving with me first." And the other answers, "If I could just have an orgasm, then I would feel closer and more loving." This character style battle is often played out in many areas of the relationship, but when it is brought to the bedroom, it is the kiss of death to lovemaking.

DISCHARGE OF ENERGY BEFORE REACHING ORGASTIC POTENTIAL

THE DIAGRAM BELOW shows three out of many ways that a man or woman can build a rather high, rapid charge or a slow, low-level charge. But a *lack of containment* may cause a man to have an ejaculation and a minimal orgasm *before* his charge is extensive enough to trigger a total orgasm, and a woman to have a small orgasm and say, "That felt good, but did I have an orgasm or not?"

**Discharge of Energy
Before Reaching
Orgastic Potential**

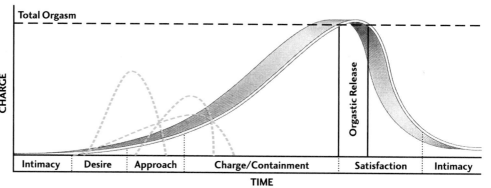

Paul becomes excited very quickly then splits off. This causes somewhat of an ejaculation and a discharge of energy, but not an orgasm. His frustration is as uncomfortable as if he had no satisfaction at all. Although he has had some pleasure, ejaculation alone does not give a full-body release, nor does it replace the sensations specific to orgasm. This is sometimes called rapid or premature ejaculation.

There are different definitions of premature ejaculation. It is often defined in terms of whether a man lasts long enough to please his partner, what percentage of time she has an orgasm, how long he can keep his erection, or how many thrusts he can maintain before ejaculation. We believe that these are ineffective, often damaging definitions. From an energetic point of view, we say that an orgasm is premature *when a man can't contain his excitement long enough to build a charge sufficient for him to achieve a satisfying orgasm.*

Once redefined by this energetic view, it is relatively easy to show a man how to change his orgastic pattern by changing his breathing and movement. This redefinition of premature ejaculation frees him from defining his own sexual process in terms of his partner. It actually lets both partners off the psychological hook—he can be in charge of his own energetic process, pleasure, ejaculation, and orgasm. This psychological hook is usually found in the agency and character style arenas.

> Victoria passes quickly through the intimacy, desire, and approach periods feeling excited. As her excitement builds, so do her longings. She wants nothing more than to merge with Scott. Merging causes her to split off and lose her boundaries. No longer present, as her charge disappears, she tries to regain it by wiggling, squirming, and pretending. Her splitting off and small discharges do not allow her to contain enough charge for a full orgasm. She is disappointed once again, done with sex before she feels satisfaction. A "what's the use?" attitude sets in, severely diminishing any future desire for intimacy and sexuality.

The difficulty for a man to gain or maintain an erection, may not be combined with early ejaculation, but it is also most often due to splitting off, which causes the same lack of containment. Women are not usually thought to experience premature ejaculation, but when we redefine this process energetically in terms of containment, you can see that it is the same process.

Like a boat with a slow leak, Paul and Victoria are unlikely to reach their final destination. They unwittingly discharge their energy as fast as they build it and never get to orgasm. Both of them split off in their own ways as their excitement begins to grow.

People, when extremely nervous or excited, can't contain their energy. They are often overwhelmed by desire and performance anxiety and lose their body experience of erotic sexuality. This pattern is easily corrected by simply slowing down the charging process and getting present. This lets you contain the charge and spread it throughout your body, making it easier to build a sufficient charge. The psycho-sexual aspects to this orgastic pattern are agency, character style, and primary scenario secret themes.

INNSUFFICIENT CHARGE FOR ORGASM

THIS TIME THE PERSON, whether man or woman, never builds a charge beyond a low level (see illustration on page 69). When they don't reach orgasm they just get tired and give up. In this type of cycle, people can pass

The Lost Erection

Impotency worries both men and women more than need be. Every man will have difficulty maintaining his erection at some time in his life. This is normal and is most often just a symptom that he is not present or not paying attention to something emotionally important to him.

Impotency is usually divided into two categories, primary and secondary. Primary means that the man never has an erection, either when he feels aroused and desires contact with a partner, or when he is alone. Nor does he have an erection during the night or upon awakening. Since this is most often due to a physical dysfunction caused by medications or other physical problems, it should be brought to the attention of a competent physician.

Secondary (or intermittent) impotency means a man can have an erection, often in the morning or during sleep, but not always when he wants to, and/or he can't maintain it for as long as he would like. This can also be a side effect of medications but is more often due to psychological issues like the following:

- An underlying fear of impotency. If a man has had difficulty at one time, fears that he will the next time are likely to make them come true.
- Splitting off, the primary cause of intermittent impo-

tence. It is not unusual for him to lose an erection if he is uncomfortable with the intensity of sexual excitement and intimacy and is split off from anxiety-producing emotions and sensations. Splitting off also can be related to overeating, the use of alcohol, marijuana and other drugs, performance anxiety, or other psychological issues of the primary scenario, character style, and agency.

- Lack of adequate birth control combined with a fear of pregnancy. And if he has a history of abortion, his hesitancy may escalate dramatically.
- Inauthenticity in the relationship. For example, if you are upset with your partner, consciously or unconsciously, your body will not perform.

Intermittent impotence is not a sexual crisis. With a little understanding, it can be resolved quite easily. To find your own answers try the following exercise in your journal. Silly as this may seem, imagine that your penis has a voice and can speak to you. Now ask, "Why won't you stay hard? What are you trying to tell me?" Imagine what your penis might say and write the answer in your journal. Then respond, as in a conversation, to what your penis "says."

---

through the first three stages—intimacy, desire, and approach—fairly well, but when they come to charge-containment, they only build a partial charge.

When Becky approaches Mark for sex, he decides to go along, but he doesn't generate his own excitement in his body. He breathes very shallowly, moves his pelvis stiffly, and his mind is stuck thinking about his new computer. He doesn't tolerate intimacy very well, so, energetically and emotionally, he is very cautious. Much of the time he is left feeling, "This sex stuff is not really a big deal. I get more excitement and satisfaction out of closing a deal at the office."

Cindy has a similar problem, but she sees it as "the way it is." She simply doesn't know how to build a charge. She focuses on the loving and the closeness and feels quite satisfied.

Both men and women tend to disappoint themselves in a similar way. When

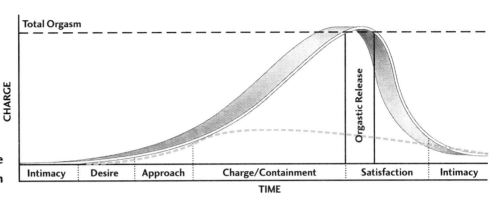

| Intimacy | Desire | Approach | Charge/Containment | Satisfaction | Intimacy |

CHARGE

TIME

Total Orgasm

Orgastic Release

Insufficient Charge for Orgasm

an orgastic charge is small, even when they do have an orgasm the corresponding release is small. The woman may be left with tension, frustration, and possibly engorgement in her pelvic region. This often results in a feeling of irritability, which can undermine future desire. Some people achieve minimum satisfaction despite this pattern, but their pleasure usually comes from the sensuality and closeness, not from sex and sexual orgasm. If a man continually holds his ejaculation back by keeping his charge low it can cause problems with his prostate gland, in addition to not being very satisfying for either partner. Also, holding back an ejaculation is not a dependable form of birth control as proven by the number of babies conceived using this method. The exercises for building, containing, and releasing a charge can radically change this pattern. Your pattern can also be affected by working with the psycho-sexual components of character style, agency, secret themes, speed limits—and your fear of losing control.

CHARGE WITHOUT (OR WITH DELAYED) EJACULATION AND ORGASM—FOR MEN AND WOMEN

IN THIS PATTERN (see illustration on page 70), whether man or woman, a charge is built, but there is neither an ejaculation nor an orgasm.

Marla enjoys sex and is able to build an orgastic level of charge, but she just can't or doesn't know how to let go and release the energy into an orgasm. It is important to her that she look attractive to Don, so she works out regularly. During their lovemaking, she tightly holds in her stomach muscles, fearing to show the slightest bulge. She wants to look good during orgasm.

But more to the point, Marla tries to be in control of everything. She is afraid to allow her emotions and sensations to involuntarily control her movements in sex. As a child, her parents' "out of control" emotions frightened her, and she swore never to be like them. Thinking instead of feeling keeps her cool and composed, but she can't seem to think her way through an orgasm.

Steve has plenty of sexual desire and enjoys making love with Jenny. He feels excited and builds a rather high charge. But he just can't release into orgasm when he is with her, particularly not with his penis inside of her. When he first started having difficulty releasing—sometimes called retarded ejaculation—he and Jenny both enjoyed how long he could last without having an orgasm. It gave them added time for sexual love-play and for Jenny to have numerous orgasms. But when the novelty wore off and they both became focused on bringing him to orgasm, frustration and tension crept in. In therapy he realized that he could have an orgasm when he masturbated; it was when he was having sexual intercourse with Jenny that he couldn't ejaculate. He also realized that his difficulty started soon after he and Jenny had an abortion and that he had been worried about creating another pregnancy before they were prepared to start a family. After checking out their birth control, talking to his therapist and Jenny about his feelings, and learning to aid his release through breath, movement, presence, and stress positions, he was able to have an orgasm when he wanted to, even with sexual intercourse.

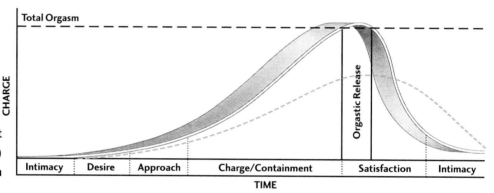

Charge Without (or With Delayed) Ejaculation and Orgasm

If the problem stems from not knowing how to physically trigger an orgastic release, the solution is quite simple. You will learn how to use stress positions in the masturbation and sexual lovemaking chapters. If the problem has a psychological basis, it is more difficult. A fear of letting go can come from many sources, such as punishment for enuresis (bedwetting). Having had an abortion—for both men and women—is commonly a source for this difficulty as is any fear of pregnancy. Retarded ejaculation is also a symptom in the acting out of secret themes and character style.

THE QUICKIE

THE WHOLE ORGASTIC CYCLE, for either men or women, is consummated, but in a short period of time (see page 71, top illustration).

Jamie turns and catches a glimpse of Bill washing himself in the shower and, even though they must leave for work soon, she climbs into the shower, delightfully surprising Bill. This shift out of their daily routine, her willingness to act on her erotic excitement, titillates both of them to a quick, full charge and orgasm.

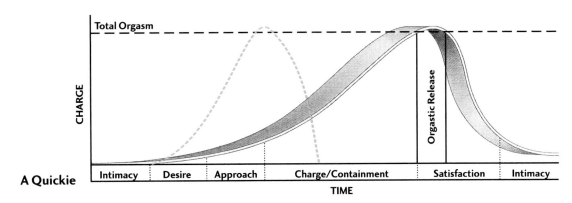

A Quickie

Quickies are great fun as a variation and when time is limited, but if this is all the sex you get, it's like always eating at a fast-food restaurant. These quickies place a limit on satisfaction and can be an avoidance of intimacy. Quickies are a physical necessity only if you split off, don't know how to last longer or spread out your charge. The psycho-sexual component of this problem is almost always character style (chapter 12).

MULTIPLE ORGASMS—
FOR WOMEN AND MEN

MANY WOMEN CAN BUILD to a high charge and release and then, because their bodies remain charged, with a little breathing and movement are open and ready for another wave of orgasm (illustrated below). Some women build a charge and, because it feels so good, try to maintain it just under the orgastic release level. But this reduces her charge. If a woman allows herself to have the orgasm, she can, with a little bit of charge-building, breathing, and movement, quickly be back up to the orgastic level. With each consecutive orgasm, her body softens and her body-container can hold more and more charge. Each consecutive orgasm is more and more satisfying.

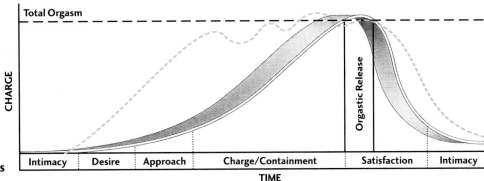

Multiple Orgasms

MEN CAN HAVE AN ORGASM or multiple orgasms without ejaculation. Many men have never experienced this extraordinarily exciting and satisfying variation. It is similar to the orgasm of many women, a release of a wave of energy but without an ejaculation.

Once learned, this makes possible multiple orgasms without multiple ejaculations. After each ejaculation, a man's charge drops significantly, and there is a waiting period before he is comfortable with more sex play and ready for another orgasm. By having multiple orgasms without ejaculations, his body will remain partially charged, and he can immediately build right back up to full charge and pleasure. This can reduce his charge enough to delay his ejaculation, enabling him to "last longer." It is also extremely pleasurable. By focusing on higher charges, both genders can more easily learn to have multiple orgasms.

The secret of multiple orgasms for men is to separate orgasm from ejaculation by learning how to delay ejaculation and heighten a charge in ways other than stimulating his penis. (See Masturbation, chapter 8.)

Having orgasms without ejaculating doesn't in any way interfere with a man's building a charge again and having another orgasm with ejaculation when he wishes. Most men are unaware of their ability to have multiple orgasms. The higher your charge, the easier it is. Be aware, however, that orgasm without ejaculation is not an effective form of birth control, because a small amount of ejaculate may be in the pre-ejaculatory fluid.

It is easier to have this type of multiple orgasm after a man has already had one or two regular ejaculation-orgasms. This is because, from the previous orgastic releases, his body will be more open and able to hold a larger charge, and he doesn't have the pressure of imminent ejaculation to deal with. It is more difficult to have an orgasm without an ejaculation if he hasn't had an ejaculation for a long while.

Delay-Time Between Ejaculation and Next Arousal   body-mind awakening

Most men report that fifteen minutes to a half hour is an average delay time. So if your belief is that you need more time than that, check it out. What you believe is what you get. When you learn to build a charge in a way other than pulling on the trigger, the delay time is greatly reduced, and you'll be surprised at how much fun you can have. In truth, the second or third ejaculation is often accompanied by a more intense orgastic release.

When couples are asked, "How many times did you have sex last night?" some answer by reporting how many ejaculations the man had. Their sexuality is measured by the man. These couples think sex is over when the man ejaculates—whether the woman has had her orgasm or not. An ejaculation is not a sleeping tablet, although many act as if it is. When both partners believe this is true, women go unnecessarily unfulfilled, often leaving the bed in a frustrated rage, to cry or masturbate in the bathroom.

The man can, of course, still participate in the woman's orgastic release during his satisfaction and intimacy phases. He can do this by stroking her body and through oral or manual stimulation of her clitoris. This type of participation will also serve to heighten pleasure for him during the satisfaction and intimacy phases.

WE ONLY BREAK SEX into phases in order to talk about them. For instance, intimacy and desire don't stop when you begin approach. In fact, if you don't keep the phases going simultaneously you won't find your approach as effective. You are always choosing whether or not to fully participate and fire up your own excitement for sexual joining. If you stay conscious, moment by moment you are deciding whether to use your own volition. This active participation must continue throughout the phases as much as in the first approach step. Charge and containment must continue all the time, even in the intimacy phase. Each phase affects desire. If any phase doesn't work or brings hurt feelings or disappointment, it will affect desire the next time around.

While traveling in an airplane, the most dangerous or difficult time is during takeoff or landing: both are times of transition. Approach and satisfaction are also times of transition. Once intimacy is established and there is enough closeness, desire gets going rather easily. But approach, actually doing or saying something to make a commitment to engage in sex, can still remain a problem. Satisfaction is also a time of transition. After orgastic release, the body is more open and the stage is set for tremendous feelings of well-being, loving, aliveness, the softening of the body—and for unmet longings from childhood to emerge. At these times of increased vulnerability, lead with love, compassion, and optimism, and be kind to your partner, or the loving may quickly, without intention, turn to disappointment and dissatisfaction. When this is not understood, the body experience of hope can be last. The character style chapter will help you through these transitions.

Charge-containment variations during sex are very common and needn't be a source of crisis, particularly since simultaneous orgasms are not a goal. One person can go at a faster pace and have two or three orgasms while the other goes at a slower pace. This is not a problem if both lovers agree to stick around until both reach satisfaction. With the breathing and movement chapter (chapter 6) you will learn how to play with building a faster charge and slowing down. This does not have to happen simultaneously for each partner. And it is not a sign of whether a person loves you or cares about you if they don't have an orgasm when you do. Enjoy your partner's orgasm and satisfaction. If you have already had an orgasm and feel satisfied, stick around for your partner's enjoyment. Differences can be adjusted when you know how to heighten or maintain and support your charge. The one whose charge is lower can focus on building his or her charge, while the one with the higher charge can enjoy the phase and, as you will see, help his or her partner catch up.

All day long Tim was thinking about making love to Georgia. When he got home from work he approached her amorously, but Georgia was still in a spin over a new project she was trying to put together at work. Georgia was caught a little off-guard, and it took a few minutes for her to become interested in sex and join Tim in his excitement. She felt the spark but told him she had to make a few notes that would only take five minutes, then she would join him.

Tim began to set the environment as a way to keep his excitement going. He put on the music she liked and turned down the bed. When she returned to meet him in the bedroom, there was a little awkwardness: he was charged up and ready to go, but she wasn't quite ready to engage in sex. But Georgia took responsibility for her own sexual desire and began to build a charge so that she could catch up. Tim took responsibility to slow down so as not to overwhelm and inundate her. He focused on his pleasurable sensations while she built her charge.

Use the energetic orgastic charge-release cycle diagrams below, one provided for each partner, to help you draw your own typical orgastic patterns.

It is essential to think of your body and your partner's body as a constantly changing energetic system. The art of making love is very subtle, but understanding it through the energetic model is relatively simple. Most often, what looks like a difficult problem can be identified and solved with relative ease. By working from an energetic point of view and using our psychological

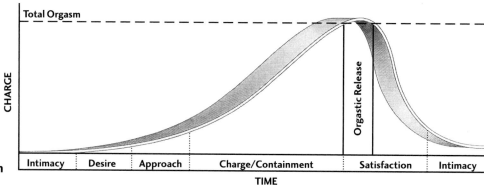

Your orgastic pattern

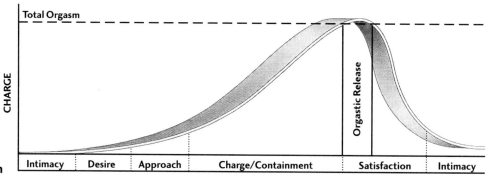

Your orgastic pattern

arena format, the cause and the solution soon become evident. You will find answers throughout the book for enhancing your orgastic pattern. You have unlimited options to deepen the romance and intimacy and make each phase of the orgastic cycle more exciting and alive.

SEXUAL RELATIONSHIP ASSESSMENT GUIDE

AN INTIMATE PARTNER always knows when there is a lie even if they do not know the content. And they know if you are really present or not. If you are close enough to your partner to engage in heightened sexuality—an affair of the heart, body, and soul—you need to be authentic. Because you are seen, an intimate relationship allows you to face yourself and know who you are at a deeper level.

There are some people who take responsibility for any problem that arises, while others tend to place blame, never taking responsibility. The survey that begins on page 76 is not meant to support either stance. Either stance can undermine the relationship. If you beat yourself or your partner up with the insights you gain, you will lose both the advantage of the insight and your ability to bring about change.

This survey will provide a better understanding of the psychological-relationship issues that may be troubling your sexual relationship. This is not a test. The questions are designed as a personal checklist. Any question that you can't answer yes indicates a possible problem area in that particular phase. Write in your journal about anything that required a no answer. Before you discuss it with your partner, resolve your part of the problem. Think about what would have to happen for you to be able to change each no to a yes. Watch the judgments and assumptions you make.

INTIMACY:

_____ Do you feel close to your partner?

_____ Do you like your partner?

_____ Do you feel comfortable and safe with your partner?

_____ Do you trust your partner?

_____ Do you feel that you really know your partner?

_____ Are you glad to see your partner when he or she walks into a room?

_____ Do you offer love and physical affection to your partner?

_____ Do you receive love and physical affection from your partner?

_____ Do you reveal your internal emotional life to your partner and let yourself be known beneath the surface?

_____ Do you refrain from making your interior emotional life your partner's responsibility or fault?

_____ Are you honest, real, and authentic with your partner?

_____ Can you be a follower in the relationship as well as a leader?

_____ Can you follow through on your partner's requests and do it the way she or he wants it to be done?

_____ Do you join in mutuality rather than just living parallel lives?

_____ Do you sustain a positive intention toward your partner, especially when there is a problem?

_____ Do you believe your partner has a positive intention toward you?

_____ Can you tolerate not always having to be right?

_____ Do you refrain from trying to get even when you are hurt?

_____ Do you feel seen, heard, and understood in this relationship?

_____ Can you get what you want from your partner on a fairly regular basis?

_____ Do you have intimate "skin time" (see chapter 1) on a regular basis?

DESIRE:

_____ Do you ever feel sexually turned on?

_____ Do you generate sexual excitement in your body for yourself?

_____ Do you feel sexually attracted to your partner?

_____ Do you feel the same entitlement as your partner in this relationship?

_____ Do you ever feel sexually attracted to anyone else?

_____ Do you ever have sex with your partner just for your own satisfaction?

_____ Can you use your volition in this relationship?

_____ Do you refrain from seeing your partner as needing to be helped, changed, or fixed when you approach for sex?

_____ Do you ever masturbate?

_____ Do you feel comfortable with masturbating?

_____ Do you keep yourself from being too busy (overworked, overextended, or exhausted) to feel desire?

_____ Can you let go of old grudges or betrayals so that you can be turned on?

_____ In your eyes, can your partner do anything right when it comes to sex?

_____ Do you refrain from taking drugs or medications that can interfere with your presence and desire?

_____ Are you sexually exclusive with your partner?

_____ Do you refrain from harboring secrets that keep you in fear of being discovered?

APPROACH:

_____ Dare you ask for what you want?

_____ Can your partner ask for what he or she wants and get it the majority of the time?

_____ Do you make sure you have a feeling of erotic excitement in your body as you approach sex?

_____ Do you initiate the approach for sex at least half the time?

_____ Do you have more than one style of approach?

_____ Does your style really work?

_____ Can you translate your desire into approach rather than playing, "If you really loved me you'd know what I want," or making your partner guess your wishes?

_____ Can you use words to ask for what you want sexually? (Physical gestures can be invasive or misconstrued.)

_____ Do you avoid euphemisms? (They can be misinterpreted, annoying, or a way of maintaining emotional distance. "Will you sleep or cuddle with me?" may get you only that).

_____ Do you avoid hostile humor in your approach?

_____ Do you set up an atmosphere inside yourself that makes you approachable?

_____ Are you available for loving even when you are not sexually aroused?

_____ Are you approached frequently enough that you feel desired and wanted?

_____ Can you turn your own erotic feelings on?

CHARGE:

_____ Do you have a way of heightening your charge other than stimulating genitals?

_____ Do you get turned on by your senses (seeing, kissing, touching, tasting, smelling, hearing, feeling, talking, dancing, or being close to your partner, etc.)?

_____ Do you feel comfortable breathing fully during sex?

_____ Do you have a way to come back to presence when you are mentally, emotionally, or energetically absent during sex?

_____ Is your body reasonably toned and flexible?

_____ Do you respond with enthusiasm?

_____ Do you make sounds rather than remaining silent during sex?

_____ Do you make love with adequate lights on to see and be seen?

_____ Can you get turned on without having a fight or crisis and then making up?

_____ Can you be turned on with a partner who is present and available rather than abandoning or withholding?

_____ Do you keep your sense of humor when you find yourself more interested or turned on than your partner?

_____ Do you make sure that you are not too inundated by yourself, your partner, family, kids, or work to feel turned on?

_____ Can you build a high charge without doing something physically or emotionally painful or dangerous?

_____ Do you avoid creating emotional distance (treating your partner as an object so you can be more turned on)?

_____ Do you know the difference between your emotional longings and sexuality?

_____ Do you know the difference between aliveness and crisis?

_____ Have you ever decided to be fully sexual?

_____ Have you decided to live, to be fully alive?

CONTAINMENT:

_____ When you feel a charge of excitement, can you savor it rather than immediately relieving your tension?

_____ Can you tolerate the emotions of intense intimacy?

_____ Do you delight in the charge itself?

_____ Do you avoid excessive wiggling, talking, scratching, laughing, yawning, screaming, biting, etc., which would lower your charge?

_____ Do you stay present and in contact with your partner?

_____ During sexual lovemaking do you avoid holding your breath (which lowers your charge)?

_____ Do you avoid lowering your charge by continually thinking or fantasizing about other things?

_____ Can you delay your orgasm until you are ready?

_____ Can you tolerate it when your partner is not as turned on as you are?

_____ Can you contain the fleeting thoughts that come to you during lovemaking that if spoken are certain to upset your partner?

RELEASE:

_____ Can you have an orgasm when you are with your partner?

_____ Can you bring yourself to orgasm when you masturbate?

_____ Men, can you have a full orgasm with your penis inside your partner?

_____ Women, can you have an orgasm with your partner's penis inside you (even though you may need additional manual stimulation)?

_____ Can you have an orgasm with manual or oral stimulation from your partner?

_____ Do you bring yourself to orgasm when you want to?

_____ Do you have more than one position in which you can have an orgasm?

_____ Can you have an orgasm without having to squeeze, push, struggle, get angry, bite, scratch, hurt, or be hurt?

_____ Do you avoid splitting off, tightening up, or holding your breath just at the moment your orgasm is imminent?

_____ Do you stay present as you approach orgasm?

_____ Do you stay with your orgasm instead of letting anxiety stop you?

_____ Does your heart open when you have a release?

_____ Do you avoid faking orgasm or enjoyment?

_____ Have you avoided falling in lust with your vibrator so that no person can live up to its triggering effect?

SATISFACTION (after release):

_____ Can you stay present after an orgasm so that you can feel the emotional fulfillment and closeness?

_____ Do you stay present and feel your own physical sensations?

_____ Do you stay in contact rather than falling asleep or going off to the bathroom, smoking a cigarette, eating, picking up a book or the telephone, turning on the TV, or worrying about the kids or tasks at the office?

_____ After orgasm do you avoid picking a fight to close your heart? ("Honey, I need to tell you what I was upset about last Tuesday," or, "Haven't you gained a little weight, darling?")

_____ After orgasm do you lean toward the good feelings (rather than the interruptive, bad ones—guilt, anger, sadness)? Are you happy, more relaxed, and loving, with a sense of well-being?

_____ Do you take care of any feelings of being inundated rather than pushing your partner away with words, thoughts, or deeds?

_____ Do you take care of any feelings you have of being abandoned rather than clinging or blaming?

_____ Do you feel more alive rather than drained?

_____ Do you have a feeling of satisfaction or completion rather than more longings?

_____ Do you avoid rating yourself or your partner on performance?

_____ Do you ever feel fulfilled? Is it ever enough?

INTIMACY (after release):

_____ Do you feel closer to your partner and more loving?

_____ Do you retain the loving feeling for long?

_____ Do you find yourself less, rather than more, irritable with your partner after sex?

_____ Do you look forward to the next time you will have sex rather than feeling relieved that sex is over for now?

When you complete the survey, look back and identify the issues and phases that show room for improvement.

Solutions will be found through studying and applying the information you gain from the four arenas (psychological), and by practicing the exercises (physiological) for maintaining your energetic presence, charge, and containment. This two-tiered approach will help you to increase sensuality, alter your orgastic patterns, and open, emphasize, and charge different parts of your body.

SECTION III

PRACTICING ALONE
for the
INTIMATE COUPLE

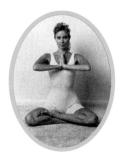

CHAPTER FIVE

Preparing to Practice Alone

BODY-MIND
COMMITMENTS

WE OFTEN LIMIT our sexual capacity because of a sexual self-image developed at an earlier time in life. At a time of youthful feelings of inadequacy and little sexual experience or knowledge, we give ourselves a "grade." As sexual adults we unconsciously respond more to the old grade than current feelings, growth, or capacity. Your success with these exercises depends on whether you allow yourself to have a new experience—a heightened awareness of your body, emotions, and sensations and a commitment to establishing a new grade.

Because of outmoded, no longer valid beliefs stored in our bodies, we limit what we can do and how we can be. Body-mind commitments such as "I can't learn to dance," or "I'll never understand mathematics," establish rules that can limit your life.

With the movement exercises in *The Intimate Couple* you can release these old body-mind commitments and have a new experience of your sexual self in lovemaking and orgasm—as long as you are willing to set aside your preformed assumptions.

LETTING GO

IF YOU DO THE SAME THINGS you have always done, you'll receive the same results you've always gotten. When you do something new, just because it's a change, you may feel anxious or afraid of losing control.

Lovemaking, particularly orgasm, presupposes *some* loss of control, both psychological and physiological.

Yet there is a certain comfort in the old way even when it doesn't work. Often people are surprised by the strength and the sudden appearance of feelings they didn't know they were harboring. Taken off guard, their response is to tighten their body, resist feelings, pull back to more familiar ground. This attempt to create the illusion of control makes it difficult to heighten aliveness, intimacy, or sexuality.

To communicate well with others, you must first be able to recognize and accurately interpret your own interior feelings. To disregard your feelings is to disregard your inner guiding force, the guide to self-awareness and self-protection, and to a life unmistakably your own.

Interior signals have a function. Some of them are meant to protect and guide us toward aliveness, well-being, and growth, but others are self-destructive and are meant to enforce old "speed limits." You must learn which to follow.

Try this experiment: Take five full breaths through your mouth. Tell yourself, "I am in control." Then close your eyes and notice how this feels, particularly in your body. Let yourself get the feeling of being in control.

Now, take five breaths, and then tell yourself, "I am in charge." See how this feels. Then, once more, tell yourself, "I am in control." What do you notice? What is the difference between these two statements? What is the difference in your body? When you think you are in control, it is an illusion. It also closes your body and thereby restricts your ability to hear your body voice. Being in charge of your life is possible.

With the exercises in this chapter you will have a sense of self as an experience in your body. When your sense of self is felt and known as a feeling in your body, a place that is a witness to your life, and is felt over time, then you will always know that you can find your way home. You will know there is nothing that can be lost, taken away, or forgotten. Only then can you feel the superficiality and futility of trying to be in control.

The exercises that follow will work as your guide to achieving a natural state of physical and emotional consciousness and well-being. This level of aliveness will help you establish new patterns. You will be able to move beyond your previous limitations so that you, too, can experience a total orgasm.

HOW AND
WHERE TO WORK

IT'S BEST TO DO YOUR INDIVIDUAL WORK in a place where you will not be observed. You will be practicing alone for a week or more before you begin practicing with your partner. Plan it so you and your partner begin your individual work at the same time so you will be ready when it is time to practice together.

This is a special time for you to experiment unself-consciously while exploring and learning about yourself, your body, and your sexuality. It's a time to enjoy pleasing yourself and to learn to feel comfortable with building a higher charge without the expectations of another person to influence you. Such an attitude may be a luxury for you; you may not be in the habit of being so independent and directly good to yourself. It's a fine habit to cultivate, though it may take time to feel really comfortable. But start now. Being able to pleasure yourself is the first step, and an absolute must, for better sex. Be greedy!

Doing the exercises in this book may make you feel turned on. It is quite natural for you to want to use your excitement as a form of foreplay. If you can, though, keep the exercises and your sexual lovemaking separate. Going from the beginning exercises directly to sex doesn't allow enough time for you to develop a new pattern. You will tend to revert to your old ways.

PLACE

PICK A ROOM or place that you like. It should be somewhere that you will not be disturbed. The temperature should be "body warm" so you can practice without goose bumps and can move without sweating.

The floor is the best place to work since it allows more room for movement and more stability for the grounding exercises. It also separates the place you exercise from where you conduct your sex life—for most people, usually in bed. If the floor isn't carpeted, a mat or folded blanket or two will make a comfortable but firm support beneath you.

Once you are comfortably settled in this room, lie down on your back. What do you hear? Music, traffic, conversations? If you focus on these you will miss your internal rhythms. Learn to focus on what is going on *inside your body* rather than outside interruptions.

Now, without allowing distractions, tune in to your own inner music. Remember, the volition, energy, sensitivity, and sense of self you need is within you, not your partner. To increase your sexual aliveness, you must listen to your body voice.

TIME

WHAT'S A GOOD TIME OF DAY to begin exercising? Any time that suits you and takes into account the following: If you must rush to an appointment in an hour, do not start exercising, because you are not likely to be very present. Also, a tired body naturally closes up and working at such times will be frustrating. If you are consistently tired, you are treating yourself poorly and need to find a way to rest before you begin. If you want these exercises to work, create a comfortable niche of time and space around yourself. If you can't find time to do the exercises, you probably are not finding time for sex either.

It's best to work consistently for several weeks. Allow time to work at

How to Deal with Internal Interruptions

You have probably had the experience of trying to do a task only to feel hungry, thirsty, or sexual, or perhaps to start thinking about other things that have to be done. The following is a guide to help you deal with interruptive thoughts, emotions, and sensations while you are doing the exercises. Practice this guide for monitoring and understanding your inner voice while you are alone, and you will be prepared when you are with your partner. Be sure to note your observations in your journal.

1. **Notice when a thought, emotion, or sensation is interrupting you from being present while doing the exercise.**
   - See if you can easily set the distraction aside and bring your attention back to the exercise. If the distraction is persistent, continue on to the steps below.

2. **Identify where the interruption registers in your body.**
   - What are you feeling and where do you feel it in your body? Every thought, emotion, or sensation is felt in your body somewhere.

3. **Identify the function of the interruption.**
   - Recall what you were feeling and doing *just before* the distraction occurred. (For example, "I was feeling good, uncomfortable, scared, frustrated, sexual, excited." "I was just getting into a nice rhythm." "I was feeling more open or vulnerable.")
   - Identify the function the interruption served. (For example, "It gave me time to calm down and reconnect to myself." "It kept old holding patterns of hurt, anger, or righteousness in place.")
   - Once you have identified the emotional-body component and the function of the distraction, follow the next step.

4. **From the primary scenario chapter (chapter 2) identify the Good Mother Messages (page 27) you are seeking.**
   - Which of these messages could support and calm you so that you could feel comfortable continuing with the exercise? Give these messages to yourself.

5. **Bracketing off.** If, after doing the first four steps, the interruption persists, write it down in your journal, promising yourself that you will work on it later. Then continue with your exercise routine.

Follow this procedure to deal with all interruptions—physical, emotional, and mental—that persist. It is much easier to identify and overcome internal interruptions while you are practicing alone. We usually have only a few favorite psychological or physical themes that we use again and again to distract ourselves. (See Secret Themes, chapter 11.) Unconsciously we know these are surefire ways to upset ourselves. Their primary purpose is to maintain old holding patterns. Figure out what your interruptive patterns are and develop a little sense of humor about them while you are working alone, for they will surely follow you when you begin to exercise with your partner. If you don't solve this problem now, when you are with your partner, the interruptions are likely to look like a relationship problem. Then they can turn into one.

least once a day for two weeks, three weeks, or however long you need until you feel you "have it"—when conscious effort is less necessary and the results feel more natural. Once you get started, you'll understand what "having it" means. Bear in mind that every person is unique; each goes at his or her own right pace. Some people will need go through only one series of breathing exercises and they will "have it." Others will be slower getting their movement and breathing in sync. In fact, going slower is often faster in the long run. The more relaxed you are and the more frequently you practice, the sooner you should be ready to work with your partner.

CLOTHING

MAKE SURE THAT YOUR CLOTHING is not binding. If you are wearing a bra, belt, or tight waistband, remove or loosen it. Tight clothing can create a block that will hinder energy flow in your body. Clothing you might use for an exercise workout will do. Make sure that your clothing or jewelry is not distracting and that you are neither too cold nor too warm to be comfortable.

CHEMICALS

CHEMICALS SUCH AS ALCOHOL, tobacco, or drugs can mask your body-voice and internal rhythms. *Do not use any drugs, particularly marijuana, stimulants, or depressants before exercising.* They will just take you away from yourself and interfere with your natural charging process. Your efforts will be wasted if you cloud your ability to know your somatic self. If you have difficulty in building a charge, check any chemicals, drugs, or medications that you are taking. Even over the counter antihistamines can reduce your ability to build a charge.

SPECIAL HEALTH PROBLEMS

IF YOU ARE CURRENTLY UNDERGOING TREATMENT for a psychological problem or serious illness, and excitement is prohibited, show this book to your doctor before you begin. These exercises will release feelings and emotions and increase your breathing and excitement. If your doctor or therapist feels that this could work against your professional treatment, follow his or her advice.

If you have any of the following, check with your doctor before proceeding with the exercises:
- If you have ever had asthma or other breathing difficulties, the breathing exercises may cause temporary breathing difficulty. If you have an inhalator pump, keep it nearby.
- If you are prone to fainting spells it is not advisable to do the high-charge breathing while you are alone. If you have ever had epileptic seizures, higher charges could cause a seizure to occur. The movement parts of the exercises are okay, but do not do the extended breathing.
- If you have heart disease, particularly arrhythmia, or low blood pressure, check with your doctor. These exercises tend to lower your blood pressure.
- If you have had back problems, go slow with the movements and don't do anything that will cause a strain. When you do the cross-crawl exercise, for instance, be sure to bend your knees.

SELF-OBSERVATION

A LARGE MIRROR is extremely useful to observe yourself while doing the exercises. It can help you stay present. A video camera with an immediate feedback monitor is even better. But do not become so absorbed in watching yourself that you miss your internal experience. As you do the exercises, be aware of your senses: sight, smell, taste, touch, hearing. The olfactory senses are very easily influenced. If you use a little incense or perfume when you exercise alone, use the same scent when you work with your partner. The smell will bring back all the body memory of the exercises.

DOING IT YOUR WAY

AS YOU WORK WITH THE EXERCISES, you may get an impulse to do a certain thing differently from how we suggest or to try something new. Do it, but keep in mind that your urge to change an instruction or exercise is likely an attempt to avoid a new experience—the very experience the exercise is set up to provide. All too often what feels "right" or attracts you most are the old, ineffective patterns.

To maintain your body's sense of self, learn to stay aware of your full body, your sensations and emotions, not just the thoughts in your mind. As you become more familiar with your deeper feelings, the intensity of your emotions will diminish.

If you work on these exercises and feel nothing, it may just be part of your character style. It is classical for some people to respond to suggestions or directions with a defiant, "No one can tell me what to do." If this is true with you, this reaction can sabotage your efforts even though you are doing something positive for yourself. Having a strong belief about what the exercises will or won't do, can prevent you from having any other experience.

Charge, Breathing, and Movement

WITHOUT BREATHING, all other systems of the body fail. It is the first self-supporting activity that you do for yourself when you enter the world. Most people, however, take this vital activity for granted and do not realize the central role that breathing plays in their sex life.

When you increase your breathing, you are increasing the level of excitement in your body. The experience of this excitement is what we call "charge"—the feeling of energy or aliveness in your body that occurs when you are "turned on" by feeling a strong interest, attraction, anticipation, attunement, love, sexuality, lust, infatuation, joy, etc.

How you breathe and the volume of oxygen you take in determines whether you increase, maintain, or decrease your charge of energy. *When your excitement is growing, your breathing will increase naturally unless you restrict it.* Yet, during sexual excitement many people hold their breath. They shut down just at the time they naturally need more air and a higher charge. To be wholly sexually alive is to breathe fully, move freely, and feel deeply.

When your excitement and breathing take you past your speed limits, you might very well feel anxious, a little "out of control," and have difficulty in breathing. This is the body's attempt to control excitement. If you constrict your chest and diaphragmatic muscles, you immobilize your lungs and they can't allow enough air in. The word "anxiety" describes the condition of the involuntarily constricted chest. (The Latin origins, which are associated with "anguish," are derived from the words *angustus,* narrow, and *angere,* to constrict.)

Because breathing amplifies sensations and emotions in your body and brings them to your attention, many people try to control excitement by holding or limiting their breath. Feelings can be unsettling; yet, they are just internal messages that let *you* know what is safe or dangerous, what is satisfying or "just not you," what is historically familiar or conspicuously new.

We eliminate uncomfortable feelings either by constricting our chest and diaphragm so that we breathe shallowly or by holding our breath. Many children who are abused learn to turn their energy down in this way so, like shadows on the wall, they are barely noticed. They hold their breath and restrict their movements, lowering their energy to create "invisibility" in order not to attract attention. Others tend to puff out their chests, trying to look and feel more powerful.

When we feel safe our muscles are relaxed and our breathing is steady and even. When we are happy, our entire being can fill with the feeling of elation (from the Latin word *elatus,* to carry out or away, to lift up). Our movements become more animated and our breathing deeper and fuller. Think of something that makes you happy (try it now) and a smile will come to your face and you will inhale a deep satisfying breath; and if your happiness carries you to laughter, you might notice (try this now, too) how laughter and breathing are nearly the same thing. In fact, with each chuckle or guffaw we are practically panting!

Unfortunately, restricting your breath to feel "cool, calm, and collected" will lower your charge and limit pleasurable feelings as well. You don't have to make pleasure a crisis. Enjoy yourself. Having a full charge of life energy is normal and healthy. Uncomfortable, injurious, and fear-filled experiences in our lifetime influence and establish our reactive physical responses and patterns, including restricted breathing and movement—energetic holding patterns—and limit our energy.

Sense of Well-Being

A sense of well-being is *an experience of self felt in the body*. It is not the same as a feeling of "happiness," which, like other emotions, can be fleeting. Sensory-emotional states are signals or messages about *how you are feeling at the moment*, in relationship to either your inner or outer world. A sense of well-being, on the other hand, although often hidden beneath the surface, is consistently available in your body. It emanates from a core essence of self. It is a feeling that "someone is home" within you that you can count on. It is a good feeling in your body that lets you know that you will be okay no matter what else is going on. It is a steadfast feeling that you won't stray too far from your being—a feeling of continuity.

The *Practicing Alone Exercises* will help you develop a somatic experience of self—what we call the "I am" experience. This interior sense of self and well-being will help you find your authenticity, sustain your inner balance, and witness the unfolding of your life.

body-mind awakening

Therefore, you can maintain a sense of well-being whether you are feeling sad, happy, angry, or passionate. You will find that this state is just beneath the surface of your body. The breathing and movement work will intensify this inner state so that you can feel it more easily. But it is up to you to make it last and find it when it seems to disappear. We provide the tools—only you can provide the desire, focus, and practice.

For many people, their sense of well-being remains elusive and fragmentary, which is unfortunate, because much higher charges can be built when each person can sustain their own sense of well-being. When you don't take charge of your well-being, you are apt to reach out to your partner sexually to fulfill your core needs. Dependency, at best, provides short-term highs but long-term deadness to sexuality. All of our breathing exercises focus on building an internal sense of well-being and the "I am" witness experience as a constant in your life.

MOVEMENT

MOVEMENT IS A NATURAL PART of being alive. If you don't move, it is difficult to feel your body at all. If you immobilize a limb, it becomes less sensitive to feeling. It may even become numb. You must keep moving to stay aware of feeling alive.

How you move—whether you are flexible or rigid—determines whether your body is open or closed to a charge of energy and whether this energy spreads through your body, remains locked in a small area, or is lost altogether. In the practice exercises you will be learning to move your body in a way that is open and free and that stimulates the natural orgastic reflex. Old speed limits—especially those for eroticism and sexuality—cause us to tighten our bodies and even to reverse natural body rhythms. Through movement exercises you will be relearning to coordinate all the segments of your body so that you do not inhibit the flow of energy as it passes through. You will also be learning to coordinate your breathing with your movements to enhance your ability to build a charge and free your erotic energy.

Excessive movement can dissipate or interrupt the building of energy. A race horse, for example, that is dancing and prancing may look like a champion, but he is likely to use too much energy before leaving the starting gate and not have enough to finish. Likewise, a runner knows that extra body twisting, swinging, or sideways motions will waste the energy he or she needs for forward motion.

In making love there can also be smooth and flowing movements reaching a crescendo of excitement, then gradually decreasing to stillness and complete satisfaction. But you can disturb this process if you dissipate the energy as you build it. Then little is left contained in your body for enjoyment and orgasm.

FEELINGS

FEELINGS—EMOTIONS AND SENSATIONS in your body—can be changed by the way you breathe and move. In turn, emotions will immediately alter your breathing and movement patterns. And both breath and movement affect your level of energetic charge. This principle obviously applies to your lovemaking.

As our bodies begin to feel open, many of the first emotions and sensations to surface are apt to be clouded with childlike feelings and memories,

Body Memories Arise

body-mind awakening

As you practice these exercises, continue to pay attention to sensations and emotions you feel in your body. It is important to be aware that when you do any kind of body-opening exercises, or if your body is worked on, as in massage, old memories are likely to loosen and come to the surface.

You may not recognize at first that these are messages from the past and you might assume that they describe your current self, life, or intimate relationship. The releasing power of these exercises can relieve the pressure of stored-up emotions, negative or positive.

At first the interruptions are more physical. You may start to yawn, scratch, wiggle, laugh, become dizzy, nau-

seous, etc. Then come the psychological interruptions. You may wonder, "Why am I doing this?" or even, "Should I be doing this?" You may find yourself getting lost in old fears or problems, plans or fantasies. You can't use the excuse that you'll scare your partner with your heightened excitement because there is only you.

Remember, when you let go of some of the tightening in your body, whatever was stored in the holding pattern is likely to come to the surface as thoughts, images, dreams, sensations, or emotions. This can make you a little anxious or it can fascinate you. This is not a crisis. It's best to feel what emerges for a few minutes, acknowledge it, and then let it pass with an outgoing breath.

"ghosts" from the past. It is not dangerous for these body-memories to arise momentarily, reminding us of *what was* unless you mistake the message for *what is*. As you exercise alone, it will become clear what type of interruptions are apt to originate within you and are not caused by your partner.

BUILDING A CHARGE: BREATHING AND MOVEMENT EXERCISES

FIRST READ THE INSTRUCTIONS for an exercise, then imagine yourself doing the exercise. Collect all of your beliefs about what is supposed to happen, about what you can or can't do, and set them aside. Then begin. Use your journal to record your thoughts, feelings, and bodily sensations after you complete an exercise. Each exercise set should be done in the sequence presented. As breathing and heightening your charge can cause your mouth to feel dry, you might want to keep some drinking water nearby.

How You Breathe

Remember, each person has his or her own characteristic way of breathing. How a person breathes is a metaphor for how he or she lives life.

For building a deep charge, it is important not to restrict the breathing passages. This means breathing with your mouth, jaw, and throat open and relaxed during both inhalation and exhalation.

- Some have trouble taking in; others have trouble letting go. Breathing is not just inhaling, it is the full cycle of inhaling and exhaling.
- Some breathe cautiously, tenuously, or actually hold their breath.
- Some work hard at everything—pushing both inhalation and exhalation.
- Some are stingy with themselves and don't take in enough air for higher states of aliveness and well-being.
- Some don't allow their chests to relax enough to expel the air completely. An exhalation is very much like "letting go." It is a passive process,

Dizziness Versus Overcharge

As you practice extending your breathing, you might feel a little dizzy. This is a form of splitting off in an attempt to avoid the experience of increased aliveness in your body. Increased practice will raise your tolerance level. Any time you feel a rush of energy, you can let it spread through your body rather than allow it to carry you off into dizziness.

If you feel split off—dazed or distracted by increased energy of aliveness—simply use your eyes: focus on colors and objects by doing the presence exercise on page 56. You can stay present and have a higher charge at the same time.

As you begin to develop the capacity to tolerate higher levels of excitation and oxygenation through charge breathing, the light-headed feeling will diminish or disappear, leaving only a charge of energy and a sense of well-being. The excitation that you experience during

body-mind awakening

charge breathing is very similar to the feelings of excitement that go along with orgasms and with being fully alive. Thus, by concentrating on charge breathing, you will be allowing yourself to tolerate more excitement, without shutting yourself off.

If you breathe so much that your hands or the muscles of your mouth, eyes, vagina, and anus begin to contract, you are overcharged and you've gone too far. It's not dangerous, it's just not necessary.

Overcharge occurs when too much carbon dioxide is discharged from the blood due to a rapidly increased breathing rate. If this happens, just stop the exercise and hold your breath for a moment or two. Your charge will drop and the discomfort will subside. This much breathing is beyond what you need. Slow your breathing pace.

Charge Breathing Exercise

The purpose of this first exercise is to introduce you to charge breathing. The focus of charge breathing is in your upper chest, with an emphasis on the inhalation. The exhalation is relaxed, much as a sigh of relief. With this type of breathing you inhale a maximum amount of air with a minimum amount of effort, using both your chest and your diaphragm. Your chest expands first, then your diaphragm pulls down. Try not to use your belly.

There are no right or wrong ways to breathe, only different results. Belly breathing is more calming and soothing; high-chest breathing builds excitement and aliveness. Therefore, if you want to calm down, breathe in your belly. *If you wish to build a high charge of excitement, breathe in your upper chest.* With each full-inhalation breath, you will be training yourself to build excitement. By learning to relax and let go of tension with each exhalation, you will be spreading your charge and preparing to let go more deeply into orgasm.

Begin: Sit up straight on the floor or on a chair.

Step 1. With your index fingers high on your chest, find your clavicle or collar bone. Move your fingers around until you find little indentations just below the middle of this bone on each side. Place two fingers on each indentation under the clavicle bone; press and hold. These pressure points are usually a little tender to the touch.

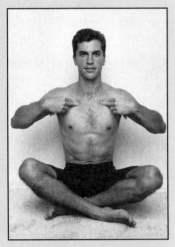

Step 1:

Step 2: Keep your eyes open. Breathing with your mouth open, use your upper chest to take in a full breath. Hold it for a moment at the top of the inhalation, then let the air go. Don't force it. Remember, the emphasis is on the inhalation. Take five of these full breaths. As you inhale, see if your breath can make the fingers you have placed on your upper chest move. After even five breaths, some people feel a slight rush of energy. Don't worry, a little oxygen won't hurt you.

Step 3: Now, take two sets of five breaths. Pause between each set of breaths just long enough to notice when the rush comes in. Notice where this energy sensation travels to in your body—eyes, head, chest, belly, stomach, pelvis, hands, feet, etc. You may notice the energy as a tingling, as heat, or as other body sensations. Notice if there is a place in your body that feels tight and doesn't feel open to the inrush of air and energy. Try to relax that part of your body in order to welcome the extra rush of energy and its flow. Don't feel concerned if you don't feel the charge of energy yet.

Step 4: Now, take four sets of five breaths. On a scale of one to ten, how much more alive do you now feel in contrast to before you began the breathing exercise? Is there any part of your body that doesn't feel tingling or more alive?

allowed by relaxing the muscles in the chest, diaphragm, and abdomen. If the chest and diaphragm muscles are not relaxed fully but are held tensely, air retained in the lungs restricts the subsequent inhalation.

- If air is blown out rather than let out, muscles become tensed rather than released. This causes a restriction rather than the softening and opening needed for building a charge. For trained wind instrument musicians or singers it is often more difficult to learn to relax the chest for exhalation.
- Some people breathe in uneven spurts. This type of breathing is often a result of anxiety.
- Some restrict the volume of air by filtering it through their lips or teeth.

New Sensations

When you breathe deeply, you'll probably notice new body sensations. You may develop tingling sensations in different parts of your body, usually starting in your hands, feet, and face, particularly around your mouth, and very often extending over your whole body. The tingling is a sign that your body is becoming more alive. As the charge deepens, you may feel heat and muscular vibrations as holding patterns begin to release. You may be more aware of your heart beating, the peristalsis of digestion, energy moving through your body, sensations of hunger, of wanting to urinate, and of emotional longings.

Don't be alarmed; this is supposed to be happening. If you are paying attention you will notice this same tingling during heightened sexuality and orgasm unless you shut it off by restricting your breathing. This feeling of tingling (aliveness) is present in your body all the time when you let go and pay attention to it. It merely means that you are alive! In these exercises you are beginning to learn to tolerate excitement and are feeling an exaggeration of your natural awareness of being alive.

The sensations you may be experiencing, if they are this close to the surface, are not new. You probably have just been holding them under control by limiting your breathing. Let them happen. Pay attention to them as though they were just an interesting phenomenon. Let yourself experience them, but avoid thinking about or analyzing them.

As you work on these exercises, you may experience body sensations and emotions that seem to spring from nowhere. You may encounter feelings that surprise you such as joy, excitement, loneliness, fear, anger, grief, and more. Because you are trying to open your body and allow yourself to feel, these emotions can be viewed as signs of success, clear markers that you are becoming more in tune with yourself.

Once you are experimenting with the individual exercises, you may begin to feel changes both in your body patterns and in the way you move. The changes may be slight at first, but they'll be enough to help you feel what this energetic approach is all about.

Moving Heightened Energy Exercise

The purpose of this second exercise is to build a sensation of energy in your body so that you can feel, then mobilize and move it from one part of your body to another. If at first you can't feel the energy at all, or if you feel only a slight amount of energy, do not feel discouraged. Even a small sensation of energy will provide you with a body experience to build upon. With experience, you will learn to heighten your charge further. As you do the exercise, the movement of energy will take place at the bottom of the exhale, in the quiet place before the next inhalation.

Begin: Sit upright, either in a chair or on the floor. If you are on the floor, place a pillow, blanket, or rolled towel under your tailbone so it slightly lifts your torso. This will relieve strain on your back and help you remain upright. If you are on a chair, make sure your feet are flat on the floor.

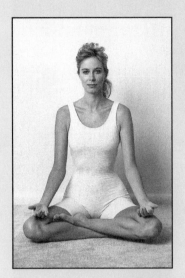

Begin.

Set 1: Step 3.

Set 1: Right-hand, Left-hand, Heart Triangle

Step 1: Take five big, sighing, letting-go breaths, high in your chest with your mouth open. Take these breaths through your mouth, using your breath to lift your upper chest. Rest for a few moments, then take two more sets of five breaths, resting between each set. You may feel a little rush of energy between each set. If so, let the energy settle in, then continue.

Step 2: Now, rub your hands together in a quick back and forth direction to create friction. Continue this for about one minute. Then hold your hands apart and see if you can feel the tingling or energetic density between them. Vary the distance between them from about four inches to a foot, moving your hands in and out to intensify the feeling. You can also move one hand up and down, passing the other. Can you feel the ball of energy you have created between your hands? It is similar to the sensation of sensing another person standing near you though you are not touching.

Step 3: Once you can feel this ball of energy, rotate your hands so that your palms are facing, one above the other—right hand on bottom and left on top—as though the ball you are holding is resting in your right hand and held in place with your left. With both hands, place the ball on your right knee. Remove your left hand, leaving the ball in your right. Can you feel the tingling of the energetic ball in your right hand? Now, again take three sets of five breaths.

Step 4: Next, bring your left hand back, pick the ball up with both hands—this time holding it in the palm of the left hand—and place the ball on your left knee. Return your right, upright palm back to your right knee, assuming the beginning pose. Now both of your palms are upraised, resting on their respective knees. Do you notice that you can now feel a ball of energy in both hands?

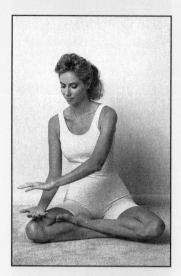

Set 1: Step 4a.

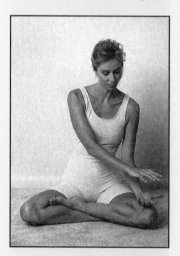

Set 1: Step 4b.

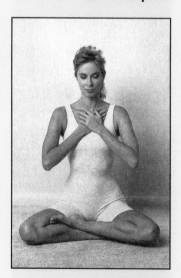

Set 1: Step 5.

Step 5: When you can feel the energy strongly in both hands, again take three sets of five breaths. Raise the energy balls in both hands, bringing them together to form one ball. Bring this new ball to the center of your chest, just below the collar bone. As you hold your hands on your upper chest, notice if you can feel the ball of energy penetrating into your chest about an inch and a half. Notice if there is something that you need to do or are doing to allow the energy in—to feel the charge in your chest.

Step 6: Return your hands, palms up, to your knees as in the beginning position. Notice that an energetic triangle has been formed that extends from your hands to your chest or heart. Now with a little imagination and practice, you can circulate the ball of energy around this triangle. To do this, take a large inhalation through your mouth, expanding and lifting your upper chest. Hold it for a moment, then exhale all your breath. Hold your breath out for a moment when you reach the bottom of your exhalation. Then imagine that you feel the energy in your right hand. Allow it to move to your left hand; allow it to continue to return to your heart (upper chest). Repeat this routine several times until you feel a smooth rhythm of energy moving from hand to hand to heart at the bottom of each exhalation. Repeat silently to yourself, right hand . . .left hand. . . heart. Repeat this practice at least ten times.

Note: What do you feel in your body? Are there any changes in sensation? Do you feel any tingling, temperature change, or emotion? Remember, feeling your energy does not necessarily mean you are already feeling it intensely. If you can sense it at all, you can move the energy; it will grow over time.

Set 2: Right-hand, Left-hand, Genitals Triangle

Step 1: This is the same exercise, but instead of bringing your hands to your heart, bring your hands with the ball of energy to your genitals. Again, as you did in set 1, take three sets of five breaths, rub your hands together, feel the ball of energy, then place it first on your right knee, then on your left knee. When you can feel the two balls of energy in your hands, bring your hands together forming one ball. Bring this ball of energy to your genitals, touching them.

Notice if you feel the energy in your genitals. Notice what you have to do to experience this energy.

Step 2: Once you can feel the energy in your genitals, take a full inhalation through your mouth, expanding and lifting your upper chest. Hold it for a moment, then exhale, again through your mouth. Hold your breath out at the bottom of your exhale. Imagine that you feel the energy in your hands move into your genitals and through your pelvis. Inhale and place your hands back on your knees. At the bottom of your next exhalation, allow the energy to flow back around the triangle again. Repeat this routine several times until you feel a smooth rhythm of energy moving from hand to hand to genitals. Repeat silently to yourself, right hand…left hand…genitals. Repeat this exercise at least ten times.

Note: What do you feel in your body? How is this the same or different from when you enlivened your heart? Which is easier for you, enlivening your heart or your genitals? Do you have any thoughts, emotions, or fears that have arisen in association with enlivening your genitals and pelvis?

Set 3: Right-hand, Left-hand, Heart, Genitals Pattern

Step 1: This time, after doing your three sets of five breaths, rubbing your hands, and placing them on your knees palms up, take a breath and, while holding the exhalation out, imagine the energy ball moving from right hand to left hand to heart, then allow the energy ball to drop down from your *heart to your genitals and through your pelvis.* Repeat silently to yourself, right hand…left hand…heart…genitals. Practice this at least ten times.

Note: What do you feel in your body and where you are feeling it? Is it easy or difficult to move your energy from your heart to your genitals?

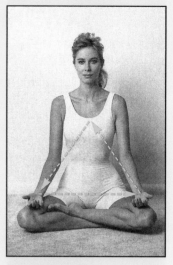
Set 1: Step 6.

Set 4: Right-Hand, Left-Hand, Genitals, Heart Pattern

Step 1: Again, after doing your three sets of five breaths rub your hands, place them palms up on your knees, and take a breath. Now, while holding your exhalation out, imagine the energy moving from hand to hand to *pelvis, then allow it to move up into your heart.* Repeat silently to yourself, right hand . . . left hand . . . pelvis . . . heart. Practice this at least ten times, then end with salutation.

Note: What do you feel in your body and where do you feel it? What is this experience like for you? Can you move more easily (set 3) from heart (loving) to genitals and pelvis (sexuality), or is the reverse (set 4) easier—from sexuality to loving?

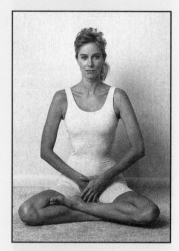
Set 2: Step 1.

Some find that they can move from heart to genitals more easily than from genitals to heart. For others it is the other way around. We find the ease about evenly divided in number and between genders. Neither is "correct" or "better"; yet many couples argue about whether sexuality should lead to intimacy or intimacy to sexuality. With this struggle over where to begin, getting started becomes impossible. After experimenting with this exercise, you will see that after a while, by moving energy, you can shift from heart to genitals or the other way around with ease.

We recommend that you use this energetic charge breathing exercise each time you begin the exercises that follow. When you begin the sessions with your partner, we will show you how to exchange this energy between you. This energetic practice is useful for becoming present and creating an energized inner calm. When you look around, you may find that everything looks clearer and more colorful. You may also find other senses to be more acute. Many people can feel a heightened sense of their well-being after only a short time doing this exercise but, to sustain it, continue to practice.

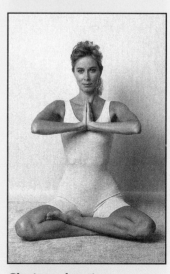
Closing salutation

Pelvic Movement

The purpose of this series of exercises is to bring to your pelvis the awareness and aliveness that you became familiar with during the energetic charge breathing exercises. Now you will begin to integrate breathing and rhythmical pelvic movement. These exercises emphasize coordination of your pelvic movements and your breathing. This is an integral aspect of building a high charge. These exercises are to be done in front of a full-length mirror.

Set 1: Pelvic Circular Rotation
Begin: Stand in front of the mirror with your hands on your hips.

Step 1: Move your pelvis in a smooth circle . . . forward, side, back, side . . . again and again, for about a minute. (This is also a warm-up exercise used in Tai Chi.)

Step 2: Check your breath. Most people hold their breath when they start to move their bodies, particularly their pelvis. Now see if you can move your pelvis and breathe fully, through your mouth, at the same time.

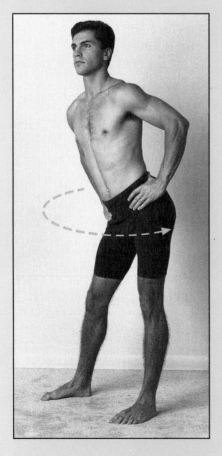 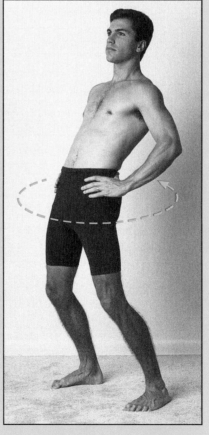

Set 1: Step 1A.   **Set 1: Step 1B.**

Set 2: Pelvic Rock Rotation

Begin: Stand in front of the mirror so that you can watch yourself from the side.

Step 1: Bend your knees slightly and plant your feet firmly on the ground. See if you can *isolate* your pelvis by rocking it forward and backward *without* moving your upper body. Breathe out as you rock your pubic bone forward and up toward the ceiling, then breathe in as you rock your tailbone back and up toward the ceiling. Do this eight to ten times.

Step 2: Check your breath. Have you been breathing or holding your breath? Can you move your pelvis without moving your body from the waist up or from your knees down?

Note: In order to build or maintain a charge, you must inhale when your pelvis swings backward and exhale when your pelvis swings forward. If, instead, you inhale during forward movement, your abdominal muscles contract and prevent the "letting go" necessary for orgastic release. Further, if you hold your pelvis rigidly, you can't breathe fully because the pelvis participates in every breath cycle.

Set 3: Pelvic-Genital Rock Rotation

Begin: Stand facing the mirror.

Step 1: Every time you rock your pelvis forward, breathe out and imagine you are releasing the air out through your genitals. Notice how you feel when you move and breathe in this pattern.

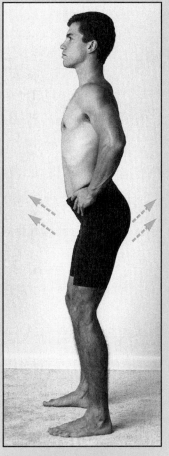

Set 2: Step 1.

Step 2: Notice if your neck is stiff. Often when your pelvis moves freely, your neck will compensate by becoming rigid. Pelvis, neck, and breath must coordinate smoothly to heighten the charge and enable full orgastic release. If you have trouble breathing in, try emphasizing the inhalation every time you rock your pelvis back. If you have trouble letting go, emphasize the exhalation when you rock your pelvis forward.

Note: To assess your breathing pattern, notice if you stop yourself from full inhalation, exhalation, or rotation; that is, which muscles, if any, do you contract to inhibit full breath and movement? The work of awareness and change is slow and requires practice. Pay attention to how you're moving and how you're breathing. This awareness will pay off very quickly in your lovemaking.

Awakening Your Body

EACH PERSON HAS A UNIQUE SET of energetic holding patterns—parts of the body that are tight and rigid or flacid, numb, or sometimes overly tender to the touch. As discussed earlier, *these holding patterns are body tissues that block the build-up and spread of energy throughout the body,* from top to bottom and back again.

These holding patterns cut off access or—like armor—protect your body and mind against feeling, moving, and experiencing the energy in your body to the fullest. To work with awakening your body, it is best to imagine it as divided into segments; each segment going all the way through and around the body—from side to side, front to back. And each of the segments represents an area in which energy can become blocked or held. But once each segment of the body is freed from its holding pattern, your body will be more open and awake and more easily aroused. Opening your body is the secret to more aliveness and better sex; and the more open your body is, the better you can experience a higher charge, more intense and deeper feelings, greater orgastic release, and more profound satisfaction.

Heightened Sensitivity

Holding on to old patterns or feelings is often reflected in your hands: the way you hold them indicates what you're holding on to. For example, a closed fist may represent anger or that you are holding something in. Let your hands rest open, palms up, in a receptive position.

body-mind awakening

Many people grasp at the bed and hold onto it as they approach orgasm. A tight or clenched jaw, rigid back, shoulders up around your ears, flexed or grasping toes, tight anus, etc., are all indications of holding on. As you practice, try to let go. Practice this with each exhale.

Body segments were first described by Wilhelm Reich, who believed that they contained muscular constrictions, which limited or reduced breathing, movement, feeling, and expression, and that they were the historical remnants of our psychological and physical experiences. He organized the body into seven lateral segments: *ocular*—eyes, brows, and forehead; *oral*—mouth and chin; *cervical*—neck, throat, shoulders, and upper chest; *thoracic*—upper chest, arms, hands, heart, lungs, and upper back; *diaphragmatic*—lower chest, mid-back, diaphragm, and solar plexus; *abdominal*—lumbar area, stomach, and colon; and *pelvic*—buttocks, anus, genitals, ovaries, uterus, legs, and feet.

All the segments are connected, with varying degrees of interdependence. Many common holding patterns are not adjacent but act in a reciprocal fashion:

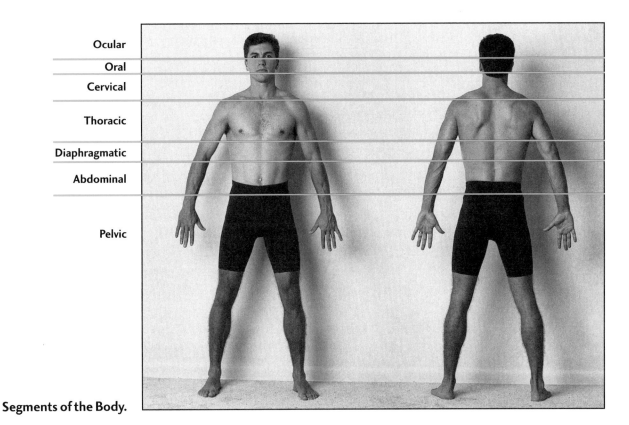

Ocular
Oral
Cervical
Thoracic
Diaphragmatic
Abdominal
Pelvic

Segments of the Body.

eyes-feet—the more present (eyes) you are, the more grounded (feet) you will be and vice versa.

neck-pelvis—holding in one may cause a block in the other, and releasing one can release or tighten the other.

head-heart—sometimes people can think very well but can't feel their emotions, or the other way around.

head-heart-pelvis—when these are not balanced they will affect your sexuality and intimate relationship.

anterior-posterior (front-back split)—holding in the pelvic segment—your anus, for instance—will affect your genital holding patterns and vice versa.

right-left or top-bottom—these splits can make you feel off-balance, stronger, weaker, or more sensitive on one side than the other. Ticklish areas, usually a sign of a holding pattern, may be in just one area of the body.

As you felt in the energetic breath pattern, it is not difficult to move energy from one part of your body to another. When there is a lack of energy in any part of the body it can be seen as coming from two different types of body defenses: one is hyper-, or increased holding of tension in the area; another is hypo-, or lack of muscular tension or tone in the segment. Therefore, even though you work with one segment to release it, you must keep in mind a whole-body concept—that is, as the holding in each segment is eased, you have to work with the associated or adjoining segments to maintain the openness and prevent the holding from re-forming.

Working on one part of a reciprocal pattern affects the other. In fact, a block that is holding emotional trauma or is otherwise resistant to release may be more effectively relieved by working with the reciprocal block. For instance, a neck or throat block can indicate a pelvic block, which may be more effectively released by working with the less vulnerable neck and throat. If, however, a tenacious block is held to maintain an emotional or psychological "speed limit," which is often the case, releasing one end of the block, such as the neck, can actually cause the other end, the pelvis, to close down. In this case, both ends of the block must be released at the same time. (Rosenberg, Rand, Asay, *Body, Self and Soul*, 1985) In addition, as the block's function is to maintain the status-quo limitation, the psychological component must also be worked on for full release.

SEGMENTAL RELEASE EXERCISES

IF YOU HAVE NOT DONE the breathing, movement, and charge exercises (chapter 6), do them now. They will help you become more aware of your body and more physically and emotionally available, and will assist you by building at least a minimal amount of charge to begin these exercises.

Make sure your *journal and a pen* are within reach so that you can write down thoughts and emotions. Later you can process any of these insights that need completion. If you are interrupted and cannot focus, use the procedure in "How to Deal with Internal Interruptions" (chapter 5).

Pleasure

In our culture it is considered "adult" to postpone pleasure and "save" some for tomorrow. In loving relationships, couples who love each other and engage in sexual lovemaking regularly feel closer; their bodies are more relaxed, alive, and healthy than those who have sex less frequently. To deny your sexuality for extended periods in a monogamous relationship is to deny the physical nurturing, healing, and companionship that bonds lovers to one an other.

If you want to know why you don't allow yourself to feel pleasure you can always find the answer by reviewing the history of your childhood. But answers to all the

body-mind awakening

"whys" in the world won't make you more comfortable with pleasure. You have to *do* something different. To increase sexual excitement *you* must allow yourself to feel pleasure.

The object of exercising alone, without your partner, is not only to heighten your awareness of yourself, but also to better acquaint you with any strong resistance you have toward your own pleasure. By noticing what thoughts, sensations, and emotions interrupt your breathing or movement during exercises, you will see that the same patterns of distraction appear again and again.

Basic Exercise Position

All exercises, unless otherwise noted, are to be done in this position: Lie down on your back on the floor on a mat, blanket, or carpet. Let the full weight of your body relax onto the floor. Feel which parts of your body touch the floor. Can you trust that the floor is solid enough to hold you? Figure out what you have to do in your body to surrender and let the floor support your full weight.

Next, bring your knees up so that your feet are flat on the floor. Keep your legs and feet about shoulder-distance apart. Move your feet so that you can feel your heels and toes touching the floor equally. If your feet are too close or too far away from your body, your position will not allow the energy to flow as easily. It can also cause you to feel ungrounded. Without grounding, you will discharge the energy as quickly as you build it.

When you are working with the energy in your body, it is important to be aware of your feet, to bring your attention and energy to them. This helps you feel stable and contain higher levels of charge. On a psychological level it yields a feeling of confidence, trust, and clarity within. On a physical level, the solid placement of your feet allows you to move your pelvis without contracting your abdominal muscles. And your feet serve as a ground, a point at which your energy will return and recycle through your body rather than dissipating.

Your feet and eyes have a strong energetic connection. This means that when you work on one, the other is affected. This also means that if you disassociate from your feet, it is likely to cause you to split off with your eyes. When your feet are grounded you can stay present more easily and tolerate a higher charge.

Pay attention to any area that seems to be tense—your eyes, jaw, shoulders, chest, diaphragm, belly, pelvis, legs, feet. Tighten any tense area as much as you can, exaggerating the tension. Then let it go completely. Do it again, tensing as you inhale, then letting go as you exhale with a big sigh.

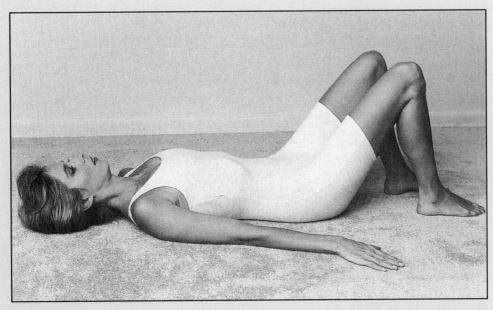

Begin.

In each set of exercises that follows, you will learn to deepen and spread your charge, integrate the segments of your body, and stabilize your sense of well-being. You will probably not complete all of them in your first session. Each time you begin subsequent exercise sessions, start at the beginning. In a short time, you will move through the entire series easily.

Perform the exercises in the sequence presented.

As you did in the last chapter, first read the instructions, then imagine yourself doing the exercise. Collect all of your beliefs about what is supposed to happen and what you can or can't do, and set them aside. Then begin. Do these exercises slowly and consciously, with presence and awareness. Try to imagine that your awareness is a searchlight, so that when we ask you to be aware of something, you can direct your total attention, your searchlight, to the focus area.

Go through the whole sequence, then focus on your body and identify all the areas that are open and alive. Then identify areas you have not mentioned. These are your current holding patterns. Note these in your journal; when you do the exercises again, you will know the area(s) that most need your attention.

Cross Crawl

The cross-crawl exercise is a fine way to keep the neural pathways of the brain open. The cross-crawl balances both sides of the brain and creates a mind-body integration. Your mind and your body will feel more attuned to each another. By working with the ocular and pelvic segments you will feel a great deal more present, alive, and grounded. After doing this exercise, most people feel as if all their body parts are suddenly part of a whole.

You can do the cross-crawl by getting on your hands and knees and crawling around the room, but the following exercise is a quicker and easier way to get better results.

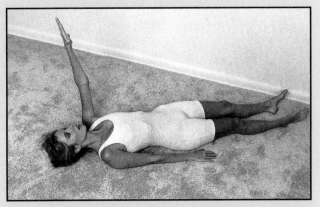

Step 1.

Swinging Alternating Arms

Begin: Lie on your back on the floor with your legs straight out, arms alongside your body. Allow the weight of your body to relax onto the floor.

Step 1: Swing your right arm straight up over your head, almost touching the floor, then back to resting position alongside your body. Next, in the same way, swing your left arm up over your head and back down to your side. Alternating arms, repeat this pattern several times.

Step 2: Inhale each time you raise your arm; exhale as you lower it. Emphasis is always on the inhalation; the exhalation is a soft letting-go sound. Coordinate your breath with your arm movements. Allow the upward swing of your arm to lift and deepen your breath. Try to breathe from the back of your throat with your mouth open wide.

Step 3: Look at your right hand with your eyes as you raise and lower it; then follow your left hand with your eyes as you raise and lower it. Really look at your hand as it swings up and drops down. *Using your eyes without turning your head is very important as this unlocks the holding patterns.* A fixed stare won't do. To help you fol-

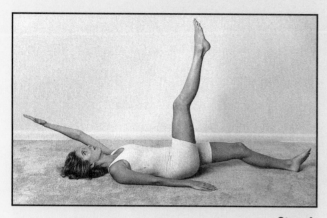

Step 4.

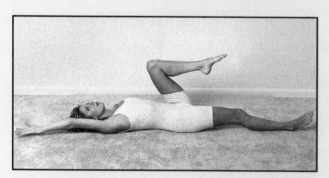

Step 4 alternate.

low your hands with your eyes you can hold tissues or socks in your hands. Alternating arms, repeat this upper-body, arm-breath-eye coordination several times until you feel a free and playful rhythm, as a child might feel on a swing.

Step 4: To add your lower body, as you raise your *right* arm, raise your *left* leg as high as is comfortable, then lower both arm and leg to the floor. Alternate by raising your *left* arm and *right* leg, then lowering both. If a straight-leg raise is too strenuous or uncomfortable, or if you have a back injury, raise your leg bent at the knee. Continue this alternating cross-crawl pattern. Maintain your breathing rhythm, inhaling as you begin each upward swing of your arm. Make sure to focus your eyes on your hands.

Practice this full cross-crawl for about twenty sets. Pick up the rhythm, let go of your mind, and pay attention to the feel of your body swinging. If you are trying too hard to do it right, you won't be able to do it at all. If you find yourself raising the same side arm and leg, forgetting about your eyes or breath, it is probably just a momentary avoidance of self-integration. You are probably just about to let go of your body-mind holding pattern and feel more "together" in your body. Merely go back to the full cross-crawl, breath-eye-hand coordination and allow yourself to feel good.

Note: What you are feeling in your body and where you feel it. If you feel an emotional upset, note it in your journal. Don't dwell on the upset. It's best, if you can, to move right along to the next practice. You can work on emotions later if there is still a problem. Chances are, if you stay with the exercises your feelings will change.

Sit-up Crunches

This next exercise will help you feel more energized and "in your body." Your chest and pelvis are likely to feel more open and connected to each other. As holding patterns release, your energy will spread. Areas that release may tingle or vibrate, indicating a heightened charge.

Crunch A and B together release the neck-pelvis energetic holding pattern and reestablish upper and lower body coordination. To build a charge, the cervical and pelvic segments must not be rigidly held, and the charge must be able to spread from one to the other. These crunches help build and spread the charge and establish grounding—coordinating the cervical segment with the pelvic segment in an orgastic pattern. In crunch B, with the weight of your head back and pushing with your feet, you activate your pelvis. It also works more specifically with holding patterns in the cervical segment. It is necessary for the cervical segment to be open, well, and alive for making emotional, loving contact, for full breathing, and for a full orgasm. Focusing your attention on your feet, once you have the rhythm of the exercises, will help you stay grounded.

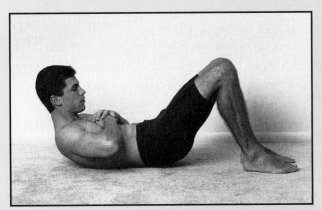

Set 1: Step 2.

Set 1: Sit-up Crunch—Head Forward

Begin: This exercise is similar to doing a partial sit-up or abdominal crunch. Particularly when you are beginning, this exercise should be done in a rather slow, continuous flow of motion, with all of the body movements and breath coordinating. Start in the basic exercise position—on your back, knees raised, your feet flat on the ground.

Step 1: Close one hand in a fist. Place it in the center of your upper chest, several inches below your throat. Place your other hand, palm open, over your fist, keeping the elbows of both arms raised.

Step 2: Take a deep inhalation through your mouth. As you exhale through your mouth, raise your head forward, toward your pelvis, as in a sit-up or belly crunch. At the same time, press down on your chest with your hands, assisting the exhale. This will help both your leverage and assist the forward rocking and rolling motion of your chest. Practice this several times before moving on to the next step.

Step 3: Inhale, and as you exhale press down with your hands on your chest, bringing your head forward and *at the same time* rocking your pelvis toward your head. To do this you will have to press or push with your feet as you exhale. Again, inhale and, as you exhale, press with your hands and feet as your head and pelvis rock toward each other. As you bring your head and pelvis toward each other look at your pelvis.

Step 4: Begin to emphasize and elongate your inhale. Once you can get a feel of this exercise, depending on your ability, do 10–15 of these head forward sit-ups.

Set 2: Sit-up Crunch—Head Back

Begin: Basically, this is the same exercise as above, but this time *keep your head tilted back* toward the floor as you do the crunch.

Step 1: With your hands on your chest, elbows up, inhale through your mouth. As you exhale press again with your hands to rock your upper body toward your pelvis while allowing your head to fall back with your mouth open wide. This will cause your chin to tilt up. As you exhale, as you did in crunch A, use your hands to press your chest, pushing away from your chin, helping to expel the air from your chest. Take your time to get a feel of this upper-body rocking motion. Letting your head fall back causes your upper chest, throat, and neck to stretch and become more open and allows the incoming energy to spread more fully through your body. The weight of your head tilted back also helps your pelvis to rock forward. It is not necessary to lift your head off of the ground. It is most important to remember that you always exhale when your pelvis rotates forward.

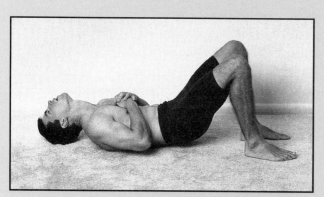

Set 2: Step 1.

Step 2: Once you find a rhythm with your upper-body motion, continue the movement with your head back and your hands pushing on your chest. Then remember to push with your feet upon exhalation, causing your pelvis to rock toward your head. Make sure that, as your head falls back, your pelvis rocks toward your upper body. Remember that to do this, your feet must be firmly planted on the ground so that you can use them to push. If you lift your feet instead of pushing firmly with them, you will unground yourself. Once you establish a rhythm, focus your awareness on your feet and grounding.

Step 3: Elongate your inhalation so that your breath is full and your pelvis can make a full rotation. Once you are comfortable with this exercise, repeat 10–15 head-back sit-ups.

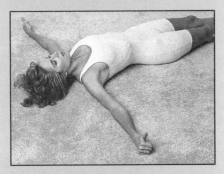

Begin.

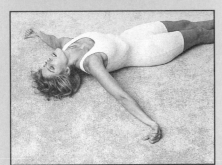

Set 1:
Step 1.

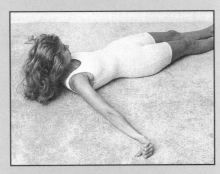

Set 1:
Step 2.

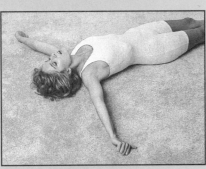

Set 2:
Step 1.

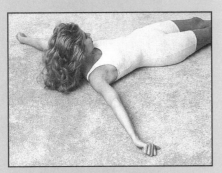

Set 3:
Step 1.

Arm Roll

This exercise opens your cervical segment and frees your upper body, primarily your neck, throat, shoulders, and upper chest. A great deal of everyday pain and tension is usually held here. The whole upper-body area, including arms and hands, is often tense and sore. Study the hand positions in the illustrations, for they indicate the motion of your shoulders.

Set 1: Synchronize Head and Hand Motions
Begin: To begin this upper-body exercise, lie flat on the floor with your legs straight out.

Step 1: Place your arms on the floor, straight out from your body. Make each hand into a loose fist with your thumbs up. Now as you inhale, roll your thumbs, hands, arms, and shoulders as far as you can *toward your head.* Notice that your chest will rotate up. Your back will arch a bit, and your head will roll back with your chin up.

Step 2: As you exhale, roll your thumbs, hands, arms, and shoulders as far as you can *toward your feet.* Notice that your head will now roll forward. If lifting your head is uncomfortable, allow it to remain on the floor and simply rock forward. Do this series about ten times. Remember to breathe with your mouth, deep into your upper chest, emphasizing the inhalation, then let go with the exhalation.

Set 2: Reverse Head and Hand Motions
Step 1: Starting in the same position, with your legs straight and arms stretched out to your sides, make each hand into a fist with your thumbs up. As you inhale, roll your thumbs, hands, arms, and shoulders in the opposite direction as your head. Do this ten times.

Set 3: Repeat Set 1
Step 1: As you repeat Set 1, note how much freer your movements are.

Breathing-Movement Orgastic Pattern

Coordinating your breath and body movements in an orgastic pattern sets up the preconditions for heightened sexuality and your orgastic reflex. The orgastic reflex is your body's most natural involuntary release into a full orgasm. This pattern, although inborn, becomes disrupted through trauma or inhibition. Any way that you inhibit your orgastic pattern and reflex through breath, movement, contractions, or lack of presence, minimizes the expression of your sexual excitement and orgastic release. As you might guess, departures from the flow of this natural body breath and movement are developed unconsciously, but they very actively impose the physical aspects of emotional limitations for sexuality.

The orgastic pattern is a full-body exercise that integrates all the body segments. Your movement will spread the energy as your breath helps it to build. As you will experience, the pelvic rock movement will cause your whole body to move in an orgastic pattern.

Synchronizing pelvic movement with breathing is essential for reestablishing your full sexual potential by releasing holding patterns while spreading and building a charge. It is a little complicated and requires practice to gain the full advantages, so don't be discouraged if you don't get it right away.

During the day, notice the amount of tension you unnecessarily hold in your pelvis while walking, dancing, or performing other activities. Observe the way you hold your pelvis and if this is reflected in your neck through tension. If you can catch this connection often enough, you can save yourself a lot of backaches or tension headaches.

Begin: Lying on the floor in the basic exercise position, place your fingertips just above your pubic bone to see if the abdominal muscles are relaxed. To get a better feel for these muscles, lift your head slightly and you will find that they tighten. It is most important that you keep these muscles soft and loose for this exercise. Tight abdominal muscles block energy and lower or deaden your charge of excitement. (If you have ever tightened your abdominal muscles just before an orgasm, you may have been left wondering where your orgasm went.) The pelvic rotation and breath pattern is the same as with the sit-up crunches.

Step 1: Start first with your lower body. To do the pelvic rock, inhale and, as you exhale, push with your feet into the floor. Use your whole foot so that your pelvis rotates toward your head. Make sure your abdominal muscles have not tightened.

Step 2: With each inhalation, relax the pressure on your feet so that your pelvis is allowed naturally to rock away from your head toward your feet. Your back will arch slightly. Make sure you have not tightened your stomach muscles.

Step 3: To continue a back-and-forth rocking motion with your pelvis, alternately inhale, allowing your pelvis to rock away from your head elongating your torso for a fuller breath; then apply pressure with your feet on the floor, rocking your pelvis toward your head upon exhalation. Make sure to emphasize your inhalation. Practice elongating your inhale. Do five sets of five breaths. Remember, to avoid tightening your abdominal muscles, you must push with your feet to rock your pelvis. In this way you will find that you can rock your pelvis much like a child does on a playground swing. Rotate your pelvis in long, slow, easy, smooth movements. Do not force your movement.

This pelvic rotation is most important in building a charge during intercourse. If you do not let your pelvis

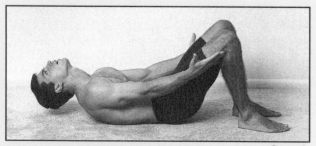

Step 4.

rotate freely, you can only thrust rigidly with your whole torso, tightening your back, which can cause lumbar back pain, and limiting your charge. Once you get the hang of pelvic rotation, you'll prefer it to whatever you've been doing because it is the most natural orgastic pattern.

Step 4: Now, keeping your head on the floor, inhale. As you exhale, reach downward with your arms so that your hands reach toward your knees. This should cause your neck, shoulders, and upper back, or thoracic, area to press into the floor, forming an arch, and your chin to roll up and head back on the exhale as it did with crunch B. Do two sets of five of these pelvic rocks.

Step 5: Now, without the reaching movement, just coordinate your breathing as you rock your pelvis backward and forward about 15 times. Focus on rocking your pelvis with your feet; your head and neck will follow.

Step 6: Imagine as you breathe that the air is flowing through your genitals. Pretend to draw it in through your genitals when your pelvis tilts back (breath in, pelvis away from head), and let it flow out through your genitals when your pelvis tilts forward (breath out, pelvis toward head). Keep your mouth open and keep sighing softly as you exhale.

Step 7: Continue to synchronize your breath with your pelvic rotation. Practice very slowly. *Be sure your breath goes out when your pelvis rocks forward*—toward your head. Pay attention to see if you tense yourself by moving more muscles than necessary to do this simple rocking of your pelvis. Try to release those extra muscles. Once you've got it, you'll begin to see how natural the phenomenon of pelvic movement is. Breathe and do this pelvic rock for at least five sets of five, staying aware of your breath and your abdominal muscles.

Step 8: Notice if you are holding tension in your anus or buttocks. If you are, let go of the tension with each exhale. You may begin to vibrate, shake, or tingle. This merely means that your holding pattern is loosening and more energy is building.

Strange things may start happening now; your neck may become tense or a headache may start, or you may feel pain in some other place in your body. Stop if you feel tension coming into your neck. As your pelvis moves, it is common for your neck to become tense because these areas work together.

Step 9: The way you hold your head and the way that you hold your pelvis are coordinated, so as you begin to loosen your pelvis, the tension may shift up to your neck. If so, start at the beginning. But first massage your neck, then resume breathing smoothly. Paying attention to relaxing your neck, again slowly work up to your pelvic movement. With a little work, your neck should release. Do this same thing—massage plus starting over again—to release tension anywhere else in your body.

AS YOU WORK ALONE and do these exercises, the difficulties you have with your breathing-movement orgastic pattern are sure to show up. When you are with a partner and a difficulty shows up, there is a temptation to blame the other person. You might think: "My chest would be open, and I would feel loving if only she (he) would...," or, "I'd be able to stay present if I didn't feel so vulnerable to him (her)." When you exercise alone you can see that your mind-body difficulty is yours and has nothing to do with your partner.

Don't go any further until you find where your own personal stumbling blocks lie. Here are the most common problems:

Are You Splitting Off?

As you start to breathe and move, you may have difficulty in staying present, especially if emotions or sexual feelings arise. You may find yourself feeling spacey, dizzy, or just thinking about something else. You may be breathing or moving too fast—past your own rhythm or faster than you can comfortably contain and still spread energy. Slow down and find your own rhythm. Because few people are accustomed to tolerating the excitement of sexuality and because these breathing exercises parallel that feeling, it's common to split off.

To avoid splitting off, all you have to do is get present. Don't go away. Don't go into that hypnotic trance. There is no quicker way to lose your charge than by splitting off. To help combat this problem, revisit the presence exercise on page 56 in chapter 3. Keep your eyes open and focus. Look around at the colors and objects. Feel what is going on. Most people split off when an uncomfortable emotion, sensation, or thought surfaces. Go back and find out what happened just before you "left." Learn to track your own presence and your departures.

Do Your Head, Neck, and Chest Lack Movement?

Even though your pelvis rocks, your head, neck, and chest may remain stiff, without motion. Your neck and pelvis may not feel free to move at the same time. This limits sexual excitement. Your neck and pelvis must work together to further your breathing-movement orgastic pattern and reflex.

As you begin to loosen your pelvis, your tension may shift to your neck. If so, massage it a bit or go back and do the arm roll exercise again.

Is Your Chest Tight?

Your chest may become or remain tight, rigid, or puffed out, so that emotions can't be felt. Your breaths may be shallow, without much exchange of air. This can indicate a split between sexuality and loving where you can feel one or the other but not both at the same time. Or it may just indicate the presence of a constant barrier that's keeping you from loving and other soft emotions.

Try to remember a safe and loving time in your life, even if it was just a moment with a pet. See if you can feel the loving in your body. This along with the charge breathing exercise will help to open and soften your chest and diaphragm. In addition to helping you breathe and build a higher charge of energy, the memory can also let you feel love toward yourself as well as others. With your chest closed you are apt to feel isolated, unloved, and alone.

Is Your Pelvis Rigid and Closed?

Your pelvis may not isolate or rotate. It may just move stiffly, like a board instead of a hinge. Most often it is your belief system that keeps you locked in this position. Get out your journal and write. You can review the psychological arenas in chapter 2.

The first thing for both men and women to assess is gender prejudice, especially towards your own gender. When you are prejudiced toward your own gender you don't want to feel its physical embodiment, that is, the feminine or masculine feelings and sexuality that come with moving your pelvis.

Second, if you have a low threshold for excitement or sexuality and they both happen at the same time, you may have gone beyond your family "speed limit." Explore.

Character style is the third thing to look at. It may be just your psychological rigidity, your *idea* of how you think you should perform, or even how you think the exercise should have been set up. You may also have some automatic resistance to being told what to do, which can increase if you view this book as telling you what to do with your body or sexuality. The following exercises will continue to provide help for any pelvic rigidity that persists.

The fourth possibility, agency, is that an open and alive pelvis can provide an experience of a self separate from the needs of others, causing you to feel selfish and sinful.

Are Your Abdominal Muscles Contracted?

If you contract your abdominal muscles, it will cut off or diminish your charge. This may be a remnant of youthful habits established during masturbation. Because masturbation is usually done quickly, people often tense up to be quiet and keep their excitement under control. Then they stress their bodies so they can have an orgasm with the barest amount of charge.

To undo old habits, it may just take a little practice and a reminder to your body that your sexuality no longer needs to be secretive, nor is it dangerous. If you are still contracting your abdominal muscles, go back and repeat step 1 of the breathing-movement orgastic pattern exercise. Try to figure out how you can rock your pelvis using your feet instead of your stomach muscles. Try breathing in your stomach; then alternate to chest breathing; then again to stomach breathing and back again. Massage tight abdominal muscles.

Are You Over-Thinking or Trying Too Hard?

If you try to think your way through an exercise, trying to figure out what is supposed to happen and trying to do everything perfectly, the exercise becomes difficult. This approach won't work when it comes to your body. It's like trying to think your way through an orgasm. You just have to trust that given the right sequence, your body will recognize its natural rhythms.

Going back to the first exercise in the series—the cross-crawl—will help you get back into your body and activate your natural coordination.

To get a feel for your body's natural rocking motion, lie down on the floor close to a wall. Put your feet up on the wall so that your shin bones are parallel to the floor. Push and release with your heels to create a pelvic rocking motion. Feel how easy it is for your pelvis to rock instead of lift. Now slide your feet down the wall so your heels touch the floor. Your knees will be bent. Push with your toes to rock your pelvis. Notice that your upper body participates. Allow your head, neck, and upper shoulders to move freely.

High-Charge Breathing Pattern

exercise six

As you become comfortable with charged breathing, little by little you can increase the level of charge that you can contain by repeating the sets-of-five breaths. This is the same pattern you will use when you want to build or sustain a charge that is dissipating during sexual lovemaking. Remember, to contain these higher amounts of energy, you will have to remain energetically present and your body will have to be fairly open. Take your time; pace yourself. It will not do you any good to try building more charge than you can contain.

Step 1: Lying on your back in the basic exercise position, do about ten sets of five breaths high in your chest with an emphasis on the inhalation. Pause between each set to be sure you stay present and to let the charge spread throughout your body.

Step 2: After each set of five breaths, ask yourself these two questions:
- What am I aware of?
- Where do I feel this awareness in my body?

Pay attention to your sensations, not your thoughts, which are most likely interruptions to your charge. If thoughts continue to interrupt, review chapter 5 about working with interruptions in your journal.

Step 3: Notice any sensations you are feeling in your body, particularly the moving of energy, heat, vibrations, or tingling. Note where you feel these sensations.

Step 4: Inhale and, with your exhale, push with your feet to rock your pelvis as you have done in previous exercises. Exhale as your pelvis rocks forward, toward your head, and inhale as your pelvis rocks back to the open position. Any time your charge drops, repeat this rocking and breathing pattern. Notice that the rocking of your pelvis, using your feet, will probably cause your whole body to rock.

Step 5: If you find that any emotional or physical holding pattern persists, identify it and note it in your journal for further work. A lack of sensations, such as no tingling, can often indicate a holding pattern. An intense tingling or heat sensation can indicate an area of your body that is "thawing out" or coming back to life. Repeat this basic rock after any interruption in your exercises to quickly regain your previous level of charge.

Strap and Ball

The strap and ball exercises are designed to further open and bring aliveness to your pelvic area. There are three stages, first the strap, then the ball, then the pelvic lift or bridge. After completing the previous exercises, your body is now prepared for exercises that specifically spread the energy more deeply into your pelvis and from your pelvis to your legs and feet and back again.

Set 1: Strap

Begin: You will need an old belt, tie, or strap that is strong enough to hold your legs as you stretch against it.

Step 1: Lie in the basic exercise position. Place the strap around both lower thighs, just above your knees. Keeping your knees about 3 inches apart, buckle or tighten the strap so it can't open as you strain your legs against it. Breathe in as you arch your back and your pelvis rotates back.

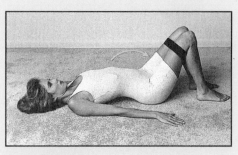

Set 1: Step 1.

Step 2: With this pelvic rock exercise, take a breath in, then, as you exhale, push with your feet, which will cause your pelvis to rock toward your head. Keep your eyes open and your stomach muscles relaxed. You can use your hand to feel if you are keeping these muscles relaxed. At the same time, try to spread your legs outward against the strap. Then, as you inhale, ease the pressure on your legs and feet so that your pelvis can rock in the opposite direction and your back will arch. Repeat this pelvic rock, pressing with your legs against the strap with each exhale. Don't forget to breathe fully, emphasizing the inhale. Do three sets of ten.

Step 3: Revove the strap and proceed to set 2.

Set 2: Ball

Step 1: Use a ball (preferably not inflated to its maximum) or a pillow, about the size of a volleyball. Lie in the basic exercise position and place the ball between your knees. Breathe out as you rotate your pelvis forward.

Step 2: Do the same pelvic rocking motion you did with the strap. Take a breath in; then, as you exhale, push with your feet, rocking your pelvis toward your head. Keeping your eyes open and stomach relaxed, squeeze the ball with your legs as tightly as you can with each exhale. Continue this rocking motion by pushing with your feet as you exhale and releasing as you inhale. Use your legs, not your abdominal muscles, for squeezing. Don't forget: this won't work unless you are breathing deeply. Do three sets of ten. Set the ball and strap aside for now.

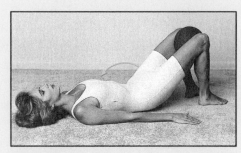

Set 2: Step 1.

Pelvic Lift and Bridge

This is a yoga exercise designed to move your energy, which has been aroused by your breathing, into your feet, creating a sense of grounding. The movement of this pelvic lift is fluid, one vertebra at a time.

Begin: Take the basic exercise position.

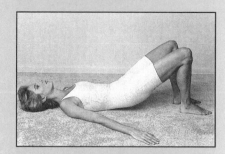

Begin.

Step 1: Start by taking a breath in and tilting your pelvis back; then as you exhale, raise your pelvis off the ground, one vertebra at a time, until you are resting on your shoulders and feet. Your body should form a straight line from your knees to your neck, forming a pelvic bridge. Use the pressure of your feet and the tightening of your buttock muscles to lift your pelvis and sustain the bridge position. Using your buttock muscles will support your spine so that you do not strain your back and will also prevent your legs from cramping.

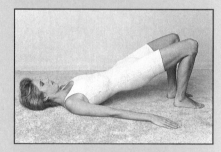

Step 1.

Step 2: Reversing the process, slowly, as you exhale, come back down, one vertebra at a time, from your neck to your tailbone. Make sure that your pelvis remains tilted forward until the last moment. When back on the floor, your stomach should be relaxed with your pelvis up and forward.

Step 3: Begin the sequence again by inhaling as you tilt your pelvis back. As you exhale, lift your pelvis one vertebra at a time. Hold this bridge position and take ten full slow breaths. On your last exhale, lower your body one vertebra at a time as you did before. Do three sets with very slow movement.

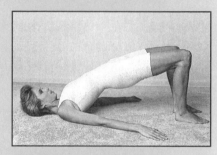

Step 2.

Step 4: This is a variation of the pelvic lift to help with grounding. Put your feet up against a wall and do the same pelvic lift. Rock your pelvis back as you inhale; now exhale, rocking it forward and lifting it off the floor, one vertebra at a time, until you're on your shoulders, feet on the wall. Take ten breaths. Hold here until you feel like coming down. You can begin to feel the muscles on the front of your thighs pulling your pelvis up and forward. This will ground your energy with your feet. Do several sets with your feet against the wall.

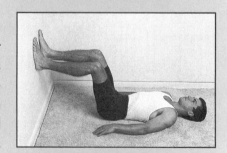

Step 4A.

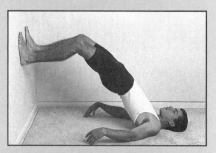

Step 4B.

Pelvic Bounce and Grounding Exercise

This exercise will help deepen and spread energy blocked in your sacrum and buttocks.

Begin: Start in the basic exercise position.

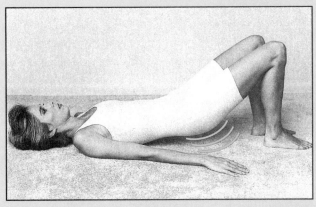

Step 1.

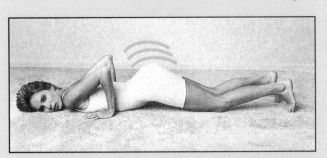

Step 2.

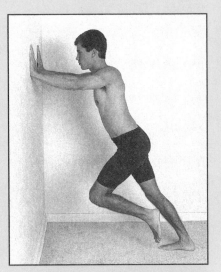

Step 3.

Step 1: Raise your hips off the ground and bounce your pelvis. Let your pelvis hit the floor gently but firmly, bouncing your buttocks vigorously at least 25 times.

Step 2: Now turn over onto your stomach and bounce the front side of your pelvis gently but firmly on the floor, bouncing vigorously at least 25 times. It is helpful to press your feet against the wall as you bounce. As it awakens the aliveness in your pelvis, this exercise may release stored anger. If this happens, write about these feelings in your journal. You don't have to work on your feelings now. But, when you do, try to find the hurt that's lying under the anger and explore that aspect.

Step 3: Grounding Exercise. Anytime you feel light headed, dizzy, unsteady during or after any of the exercises, you can do the following exercise to ground yourself and get present. Standing, place your hands against a wall at approximately shoulder height, and put one foot forward and one back. Push with both your hands and back leg as if you are trying to push the wall down. Keep your eyes open. Then change legs and push again. Do this until you feel grounded.

Fish Position and "I Am" Awareness

This position can bring your charge to a much higher level. The specific focus is to open your chest so that you can experience an interior sense of self. This is particularly helpful if your chest and heart have been closed for a while because of fear or hurt.

The deep-panting pattern of breathing in this exercise helps break through the armor of protection that keeps your love, sense of well-being, and aliveness from becoming available to you. As your chest opens, the cervical and pelvic segments can rock more freely, allowing energy to spread more easily through your body in a full orgastic pattern. With your upper chest and neck moving more freely, you will probably feel more energy in your pelvis.

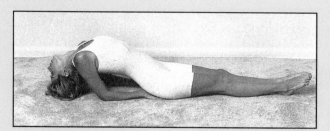

Step 1A.

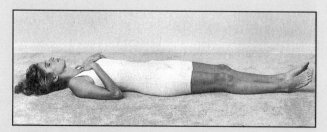

Step 4.

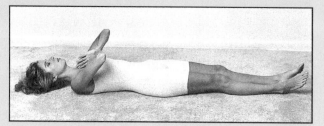

Step 6.

Begin: This exercise can be accomplished one of two ways, depending on the flexibility of your upper back and the strength in your lower back. If you have a back or neck problem, use option B.

Step 1—Option A: The fish position: Sit on the floor with your legs straight in front of you. Place your hands on the floor, palms down behind your buttocks with your fingers toward your buttocks. Lean back on your forearms so that your elbows touch the floor. Arch your back so that your head can fall back and touch the floor. Your forearms and head now form a triangle for support.

Option B. Place a large pillow on the floor. Lean back over the pillow so that your head falls back to the floor, your upper back is arched with your legs straight out in front of you.

Step 2: Draw quick, full panting breaths into your upper chest. In this way, take 50–60 breaths in a row without pausing. Make sure that your breaths emanate from high in your chest just as you have done in previous breathing practices. This type of breathing will force your chest to expand further from the inside. Don't worry if you become a little dizzy. You will very quickly be spreading the charge throughout your body.

Step 3: On your last breath, hold the inhale. Then slide down from your elbows until your body is lying flat, and let your breath all the way out—holding your breath out at the bottom of the exhale for as long as is comfortable. (You have plenty of oxygen in your body; you don't have to breathe for a few minutes.) Holding your breath out, lie quietly on the floor with your eyes closed. Notice how you feel in your body. At this point, many people feel as if their whole body is "more together," more compact, more integrated, as if all the parts are one unified whole. Pay attention to how you feel inside your body. Notice where you feel good. It may be a warmth, openness, energetic aliveness, calmness, or sense of well-being. It doesn't have to be a big feeling. Bring your focus to that place in your body of good feelings or sensations. Place your hand there. If you need to breathe at this point, take a full breath or two and again release all the breath and hold your breath out at the bottom of the exhale.

Step 4: Of course the good feelings are throughout your body, but as a primary focal point, if you haven't yet done so, bring your focus to your upper chest and see if you can feel a good feeling in this center. A few breaths may help you feel it easier. Remember, breathing can intensify your emotions and sensations.

Step 5: Next, take several full breaths through your mouth. Notice the quiet, still place at the bottom of each exhale. This is the same quiet place one experiences in meditation. Each time you exhale, feel the quiet stillness, and see if you can feel the good feeling in your chest. If you can feel the good feeling at the bottom of the exhale, acknowledge this awareness by saying the words "I am" to yourself out loud. If you can still feel the good feelings on the next exhalations, repeat "I am." If you no longer feel the "I am" experience, take five to ten breaths; then hold your breath out until you can once again feel this interior experience.

Step 6: With your palms together, place your hands at the center of your upper chest, fingers pointing toward chin. Take a big breath in and, as you let your breath out, press the palms of your hands together firmly and feel the "I am." After the pressure is released, your chest will probably feel more open, helping to heighten the "I am" well-being experience. Practice your "I am" body experience until it feels a part of you that you can take with you into your life. This is the first stage of developing the witness place in your body from which to observe yourself as you pass through life. As you continue to breathe, keeping your mouth slightly open as your breath goes in and out, let your body find its own breath rhythm without your control.

Step 7: When you are ready to get up, roll onto your side. Sit up slowly. Look at the colors and objects around you until you feel present. Close your eyes and see if you can still feel the "I am" experience in your chest. Take a few breaths to enliven the feeling if it starts to fade. Place your feet on the floor; feel that it is firm and solid. Stand up slowly and feel that the floor under you is able to support you.

Use your eyes as you begin to walk slowly around the room. Feel the floor, placing your whole foot against the floor with each step. Can you see with your eyes? Can you feel your "I am" in your chest? Can you feel your genitals? Can you feel your feet on the ground? If so, you are fully present. If you lose your "I am" experience you know how you got it, so you know how to get it back if you wish. After a while it becomes easier to sustain. The secret is not in holding onto this "I am" sense of well-being in your body but in knowing how to get it back when it goes away. (See Fragmentation, chapter 15.)

If you feel at all spacey, lightheaded, or dizzy, use the grounding exercise on page 113.

Don't forget that each time you release a tense or deadened part of your body, your breathing may diminish or stop. Reestablish your breathing pattern by repeating the part of the exercise you were doing when it stopped. By repeating any part of an exercise that is difficult, confusing, or interrupted by thoughts, emotions, or uncomfortable physical sensations, you can break through the old pattern and free your body.

Work your way through each exercise in this manner. Let your guideposts not be "progress" but your continued presence and the growing attunement between the exercises, your breathing, and the feelings in your body.

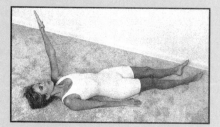

Sequence 1.

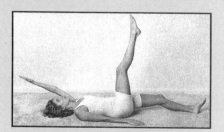

Sequence 1.

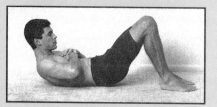

Sequence 2.

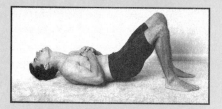

Sequence 2.

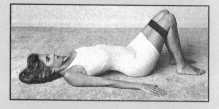

Sequence 3.

Sustaining Integration Exercise Series

After you have done the longer versions and learned the subtleties, doing the sustaining integration series below every day will help you build and sustain your sense of self and well-being.

Sequence 1: Do the cross-crawl, starting first with your upper body (arms). As you feel the rhythm take hold, add your lower body (legs). Bend your knee if raising a straight leg is too strenuous. Take full upper-chest breaths and engage your eyes by watching your hands swing up and down. Do the cross-crawl until you feel a body integration and are no longer disoriented or otherwise distant from yourself.

Sequence 2: The sit-up crunches are next. They enable your chest and pelvis to move. They start the building of a charge through movement and spread it throughout the body. Do 10–15 sit-ups each set, the first set with your head forward, the second with your head back.

Sequence 3: The strap and ball exercises integrate the pelvic lift to open your pelvis, ground your legs, and build your charge. First, coordinating your breath, do ten pelvic rocks stretching your legs against the strap. Then with the strap in place, raise your pelvis as high as you can, one vertebra at a time, into the pelvic lift. Hold this raised position ten breaths for one set. Do three sets. Follow the same procedure squeezing against the ball.

Sequence 4: The final exercise is the fish position. Take 50–60 very full, upper-body panting breaths and hold your last breath out on the exhale for a few moments. This spreads the charge through your body and expands and enlivens your chest so that you can feel your sense of well-being, your sense of self ("I am"), and loving open emotions. You may feel other emotions as well, but for this exercise, look for the good feelings, sensations, and emotions in your body. As long as you go back to the witness—your body-sense of "I am"—you will find comfort and inner strength in who you are and feel a deeper closeness with others.

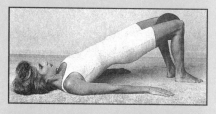

Sequence 3.

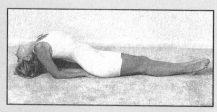

Sequence 4.

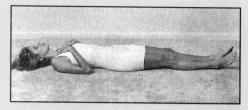

Sequence 4.

CHAPTER EIGHT

Sexual Self-Exploration and Discovery

MASTURBATION IS A WAY TO LEARN about your private sexual self, your own body, and your own erotic nature. It is a way to give yourself love and attention—to soothe and satisfy yourself. To sustain sexual satisfaction in a long-term relationship, you must be able to awaken your own sexuality and to build, contain, and release a charge on your own. Masturbation allows you to undo old emotional and physical patterns in privacy, at your own pace, and without the distraction of your partner. With the knowledge and experience you gain, you will be able to guide your partner (and yourself) into higher and higher levels of sexual excitement and, ultimately, into the realm of the total orgasm, again and again.

Source of Sexual Insights

People have many fears associated with masturbation. The most prevalent is, "I'm afraid I might enjoy it too much and never want to stop." Tolerating enjoyment is a prime message in this book. Pleasure need not be rationed; give yourself permission to experience it. Start listening to your body: hear what it wants and enjoys.

Masturbation can be a source of insight for both you and your partner. Once you know what pleases you, you can show your partner. Neither of you is a mind reader. The attitude, "If you really loved me, you would know what I need and want without my telling you," leads to anger and frustration between two adults in the bedroom. If you never ask for what you want because you are afraid to tell your partner what to do or because you have experienced rejection, you may now fear you will never get what you ask for. This is not a sexual problem, it is the psychological

body-mind awakening

arenas at play. You probably can't get what you want in other areas either.

Masturbation is a healthy way to learn about your sexual self. In fact, people who are comfortable with masturbation tend to have more satisfactory sex when with a partner. Being a good and considerate lover includes being able to know your own pathways to fulfillment. If sex isn't working as well as you would like, it is always best to start with yourself, to see your part of the problem.

By practicing the masturbation exercises, you will experience a confidence in your ability to feel sexual excitement that is not dependent on another person. You will know that you can have an orgasm when you want, and you will know that you can tolerate the excitement of a heightened orgasm.

PERHAPS NO OTHER NATURAL, normal, healthy human activity has received such condemnation throughout history as masturbation. The primary controversy is one of mind over body. In earlier times there were fears that biological erotic urgings would send people out of control, so the opponents of masturbation tried to control these urgings by controlling thoughts. *The intellectualism that became so highly regarded was just a means to distance one's self from feelings in the body.* Unfortunately, such a narrow focus on the mind suffocates the human spirit and the very urgings that bind us to one another in love, compassion, and understanding.

Throughout history, the attempt to control human sexuality, particularly masturbation, has persisted to varying degrees. In 1741, Tissot, a French physician, exerted a significant influence on the sexual attitudes of western culture. He wrote that masturbation produced "weak eyes, pimples, constipation, epilepsy, weakness of the intellectual facilities, sexual and genital disorders" and a full range of somatic and hysterical symptoms. But, this is not ancient history. In the late 1800s J. H. Kellogg suggested that parents bandage their child's genitals, tie their hands, have boys circumcised without anesthetic, their foreskins sutured shut, and pure carbolic acid applied to the girls' clitorises, all as deterrents to masturbation. Misguided attitudes caused many people to masturbate in secret, to hurry, push toward fast release, split off, limit their sound, breath, movement and contract their body, or just feel guilty, abetting many physical and psychological problems.

Whenever a person or culture successfully masks biological urges by overriding them with the mind, much is lost. The mind, without the body as a balance, can rationalize henious acts of violence and suppression against ourselves and our fellow human beings. Feelings in the body are one guide to authenticity and the human spirit. When you separate the mind and body, the essence of humanness is lost as a body experience. The more distant you become from your body, the more you will fear the surfacing of your sexuality.

Parents, religious leaders, medical professionals, as well as self-appointed moralists have used sexuality and, specifically, masturbation as a battleground for enforcing mental control of the developing child's expression and, more pertinently, his or her enjoyment of sexuality.

Fortunately, while the enforcers of "the right way" have inflicted great pain, they have never been too successful. It is a losing battle. Social and religious prohibitions have had a strong effect on the public display of erotic sexuality. Yet, our biological intuitive self wins out again and again no matter what the rules of intellect or culture may dictate.

Of course all biological urges shouldn't be acted out, but this doesn't mean that they shouldn't be felt. Many urges need to be contained for appropriate expression. Containment allows for consideration of a larger picture and the boundaries of self and others. Containment is different from suppression as the feelings are not cut off in the body. Containment is not judgmental, it does not make sex bad; it is respectful of self and others while building a capacity for tolerating intense feelings without necessarily acting upon them.

The first glimmer of sanity was seen in the late 1940s and early 1950s when Alfred Kinsey published his ground-breaking studies. Since then, much more

Discovery Through Masturbation

Through Masturbation You Can Learn

- to reawaken your sense of erotic pleasure
- what rhythm turns you on
- what parts of your body participate in your charge
- what turns you off, even when you do it yourself
- what position or stimulation helps bring you to orgasm
- how to heighten your orgasmic response with breathing and movement
- how you stop yourself or reduce your charge by pushing, splitting off, or thinking
- how to make an orgasm last longer by spreading out your charge rather than by holding back and diminishing your charge

- how to open into being multi-orgasmic by breathing, staying present, and moving in an orgastic pattern
- how to be a gentle, loving, attuned, attentive lover to yourself
- how you treat yourself in ways you would never allow others to treat you
- that you may hold your breath and race toward an orgasm, missing the fun along the way
- and most importantly, you will be able to determine if you have the same difficulties alone as you do with a partner. With masturbation, there is no one else to take blame or responsibility.

confirming data has been published. There are reliable statistics showing that masturbation activity parallels many other self-affirming activities in human life and is engaged in from infancy into very old age. At the time of its publication, the Kinsey report surprised a lot of people by confirming that masturbation was popular not only with singles but also among those who had a full sexual life with a partner.

Sex in America, the newest survey in sexual behavior today, reports: "But even the most liberal tend to see masturbation as an activity that is appropriate only for the young or those without partners. Among adults, masturbation has the taint of sexual failure, a practice engaged in by those without the social skills or desirability to find a sexual partner." Not true. Masturbation is just one natural aspect of a person's sexual expression. In fact, *Sex in America* goes on to state, "Our conclusion from this data is that masturbation is not a substitute for those who are sexually deprived, but rather it is an activity that stimulates and is stimulated by other sexual behavior." In other words, masturbation helps people have better sex with their partners.

Masturbation is probably the most frequent form of sexual activity experienced by human beings. For many people, it is their only sexual outlet. It's not only an important means of releasing tension in the body, thereby keeping the body free of destructive energetic holding patterns, but it is also essential for keeping the body alive and healthy. The pelvis, like any part of the body, when immobilized with disuse, can atrophy and cease to function adequately. Neglect can set up sites for dysfunction and disease. This is a case of use it or lose it.

Taking Charge

Your capacity to feel love and sexual desire, to be erotically charged, is within your body, your being. If you think that it is your partner's duty to make you feel sexual desire, you severely limit your capacity for sexuality. If your body or mind is closed, it is so easy to blame your partner for your apathy—for being not enough, too much, or just not doing things the "right way" to arouse your erotic interest. This feeling may be a pattern that has followed you through previous relationships.

No one can turn you on if you don't want to be turned on. But you have the capacity to drop your guard and open your body and emotions to find the hidden reserves of excitement. Your partner can be an emotional support,

but any psychological barriers you have erected are yours to overcome.

If you think it is your job to "turn your partner on," to take control of who approaches whom for sex, to take responsibility for maintaining your partner's erection, or "to give" him or her an orgasm, *sex is doomed*. Deeper excitement and orgastic states originate and are released from inside the individual. These states can be found, nurtured, and enlivened through masturbation. When you know how to arouse the sexual excitement within your body rather than wait for someone to do it for you, you will be a lover. One who keeps his or her heart and pelvis open and enlivened is a lover with courage. It is not always easy, but it brings great rewards.

BECOMING A LOVER

MANY PEOPLE MASTURBATE to relieve the longings felt in the body caused by unfulfilled needs of childhood. Unfortunately, no amount of sexuality with or without a partner can erase the past or satisfy these longings, and if you try to satisfy them through sexuality, the sexual activity is likely to feel hollow and empty. Emotionally, this can intensify any underlying sense of shame or guilt begun in childhood associated with sex. Shame is when you don't live up to your own potential or ability; guilt is when you don't live up to someone else's expectations for you.

Unfulfilled childhood needs become unfulfilled emotional longings that can haunt you the rest of your life. Attenuating and fulfilling these longings becomes part of your personal developmental journey. Paradoxically, as you fulfill these basic longings for yourself as an adult, satisfaction with others becomes more readily available; whereas, what you can't give to yourself, you are not likely to take in easily from others. If you were lucky enough, as a child, to get the love you needed, you probably have very little trouble receiving or giving love. But many learned to give love to others and not to themselves. (See primary scenario and agency, chapter 2.)

No one had a perfect childhood. Everyone has some unfulfilled longings from childhood emanating from "love" injuries. You may have been loved not enough, or too much. Getting love may have been accompanied by expectations and conditions. These wounds stay with you and create fears and mistrust along with a longing for completion, the quest for getting it right some day.

Driven by these needs and longings, you may believe that sex or love, given just the right way at just the right time by just the right person, will heal this void. This attempt to heal childhood wounds through sex is called "sexualizing your longings."

These old wounds can become so cloaked with mistrust that even the most sincerely given love, the very love you have sought so diligently and tried so hard to earn, will be viewed with suspicion and skepticism. The old wounds can keep you from being receptive to the love offered in the present. The following exercise will help you to gain a sense of your own love experience.

ACCEPTING YOUR GENITALS

YOU HAVE ALREADY READ how gender prejudice can affect your relationship (in chapter 2). Now you can learn how this prejudgment can affect your sexuality. If your prejudice is against men, you are likely to react negatively to any display of a man's erotic or masculine energy; if your prejudice is against women, displays of feminine energy or erotic energy will affect you negatively. This is true even when you are prejudiced against your own gender.

Almost everyone has some concern about their genitals: penises that are too big, too small, too thin, too fat, too crooked, long, or short; vaginas that are too tight, too loose, too hairy, not hairy enough; labia or clitoris that are too big or too small. Therefore, this is not a place to try out your humor as it will almost always seem hostile. No "smelly fish" or "little weenie" jokes. Although they may be humorous somewhere to someone, they almost always wound to the core and are never forgotten.

A prejudgment toward yourself can make you less able to experience feelings in your genitals; that is, you may tingle, vibrate, or have heightened awareness everywhere in your body except your genitals. The holding pattern may actually be in your entire pelvis, but the genitals will be the most affected.

When men who have this prejudice build a high charge, they can't feel much, if anything, in their penis or testicles. The tip of their penis is the last place they will feel the charge. Women, prejudiced against their own gender, may not feel their breasts, clitoris, labia, or vagina. After working through their prejudice, they will usually begin to feel their clitoris first, then their vagina, and then their uterus and ovaries vibrating when they have a charge.

With a self-prejudice, you may treat yourself as an object if you masturbate. You may be very hurried and distant when touching yourself and so limit your own aliveness, sexuality, and satisfaction. You may be a wonderful lover because your greatest satisfaction comes from satisfying your partner. But in the process, you may miss a whole part of yourself, the expression of your sexual identity which can be such a significant source of pride.

"Becoming a Lover" Exercise

Begin: Sit comfortably. Take two sets of five full, sighing, letting-go breaths.

Step 1: Imagine a time in your life when you loved someone or something. (It may have been for just a moment.) It may have been a parent, grandparent, lover, child, or a pet. Feel in your body the experience of giving and sending love, of being the loving one, the lover.

Identify where in your body you feel this memory of giving love. Most people feel the sending of love in their upper chest, the heart area, or down their arms. They associate sending love with nuzzling, stroking, petting, or kissing their loved one's cheek or mouth. This kind of love emanates from the heart and is expressed with arms and hands and wanting to caress the loved one. Often, tears of love are associated with sending.
Now set this experience aside for a moment. Do Step 1 before you read and do Step 2.

Step 2: Imagine a time in your life when you were the recipient of love, when you were adored by another—a time of being the loved one, the beloved. Again, you might remember this feeling more easily in relation to a parent, grandparent, lover, child, or pet. Remember their excitement at seeing you. Feel it in your body, this experience of being loved. Even though it may have just been for a moment. Identify where in your body you experience receiving love. Most people experience love as coming in from behind, as if they were being supported or cradled. Many experience being loved as being stroked on their back or forehead, or being held. *For a moment, set this experience aside. Do Step 2 before you read and do Step 3.*

Step 3: Now sit up straight, extend both arms straight out from your chest, palms up. Cross your arms. Bring them up and give yourself a hug. Embrace the back of your head, face, and cheeks gently.

Step 4: While embracing yourself, alternate your viewpoint. First be the lover and give love to yourself. Take your time so you can feel what this is like. Now be the beloved and allow yourself to receive love. Give this feeling to yourself. Now, be both the lover *and* the beloved. For a brief moment, allow yourself to experience giving love to yourself, and receiving and savoring love at the same time.

Were you able to give *and* receive love? Were you able to do either? Some people can give love better than they can receive it or vice versa. If this is true for you, notice how this may affect your sexual lovemaking, even masturbation.

From this exercise, people often realize whether they can receive love or give it, or whether they can do neither. And they realize how this struggle affects them in an intimate relationship. There is another lesson in the exercise: love is an internal, self-generated state of consciousness. If you can't give love or take it in, you will drain your lover. There are two capacities that you must learn how to arouse in your body for yourself—love and sexuality.

Many couples love each other, but not themselves. These individuals often "nice" their relationship to death—that is, they will be overly supportive, accepting, and forgiving of the other person. This doesn't keep the relationship honest and can prevent an adult sexual relationship from stabilizing and growing.

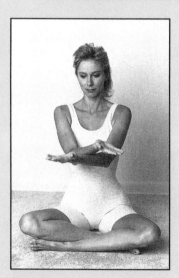

Step 3A.

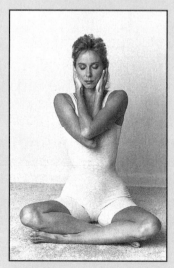

Step 3B.

Pride or Shame

For Men (and Women)

For higher sexuality, it is essential to re-own your own personal pride of gender. Many men disown their genitals; that is, they can't talk about their penis without some twinges of apology or embarrassment, even with their partners. This lack of acceptance, associated with gender prejudice, often causes a man to feel ashamed of his genitals.

Like many men, Andrew found the boys' locker room at school terrifying. He was afraid he would be exposed and laughed at because of his small penis. So he avoided embarrassment by feigning a dislike for sports. Ironically, his penis was of an average size, but he had developed his self-image by comparing his preadolescent genitals to his father's, and coming up short. After his hormones rushed in he caught up with his dad's envied size, but his childhood image was set. He never learned to like sports, and nothing that his wife, Beth, ever said could convince him to accept the reality that his penis was just fine. Perhaps the most overrated criterion for a man's ability to be a man or a good lover is the size of his penis. In general, the fascination with penile size and shape has more to do with emotional security than his sexual prowess or a woman's enjoyment. In addition, some men's penises are "showers." They look large even when they are not erect. Then there are the "growers." They look like they have small penises, but when erect they are just about as large as the showers, especially when they have a high charge of excitement.

For Women (and Men)

A woman's genitals are designed to look, feel, taste, and smell erotic. If a person has a gender prejudice against women, anything that sounds, looks, feels, tastes, or has the aroma of a woman will seem bad in some way.

Howard inherited his mother and father's gender prejudice against women. He chose Robin as his bride because her childlike femininity never failed to arouse him. He was not at all prepared when marriage released her erotic sexual restraints and she turned into a woman. Thereafter, he was always uncomfortable and didn't know why. With humor as a shield, he was able to enact his gender prejudice and keep an emotional distance from Robin. Over the years he collected all the vagina jokes he could find. When she tried patiently to explain why they weren't funny to her and hurt her feelings, he would say, "Can't you take a joke?"

Robin, subconsciously enacting her own theme of prejudice against women, scrubbed herself internally with soap every day, trying to eliminate her perfectly natural feminine aroma. Her scrubbing led to yeast infections, then to precancerous cells at the tip of her cervix. She was being treated for the third time for what was turning into a chronic condition before her doctor asked about her hygiene practices.

For some time, Claudia ruminated about taking a pair of scissors and cutting her labia so they would be small and dainty. In desperation she finally asked her doctor to perform the surgery. He refused. Therapy helped her recognize that the fullness of her labia was just a sign that she was a woman and not a little girl. Young girls did not engender her prejudice, but women, she didn't trust.

MALE AND FEMALE
GENITALS

AS YOU CAN SEE in the pictures that follow, based on a theory presented by the Federation of Feminist Women's Health Centers' book, *A New View of a Woman's Body,* the penis and clitoris are very similar. They both become erect with sexual excitement and are the primary centers of sexual stimulation and excitement. The clitoris is larger and more complex than most people realize. When adjacent parts are considered as part of the whole clitoris, it looks much like a miniature penis. And the various nerves that run through the pelvis, sending messages to the brain and other parts of the

Internal Female Genitalia

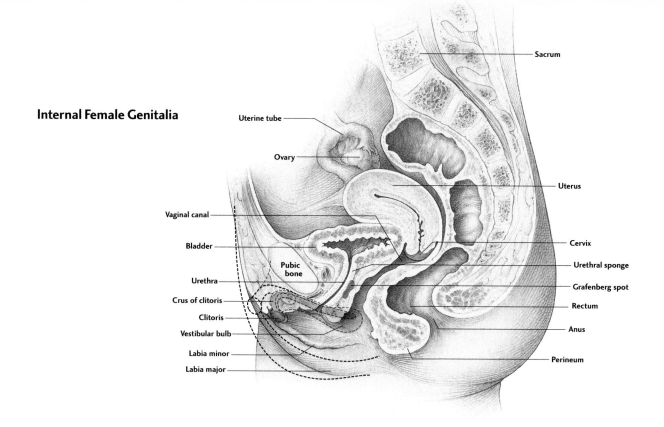

- Uterine tube
- Ovary
- Vaginal canal
- Bladder
- Pubic bone
- Urethra
- Crus of clitoris
- Clitoris
- Vestibular bulb
- Labia minor
- Labia major
- Sacrum
- Uterus
- Cervix
- Urethral sponge
- Grafenberg spot
- Rectum
- Anus
- Perineum

Internal Male Genitalia

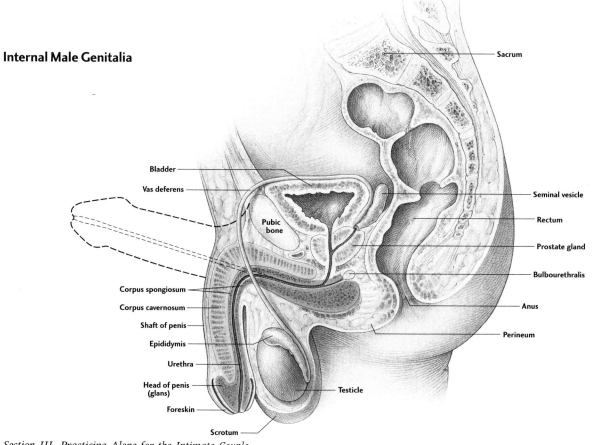

- Bladder
- Vas deferens
- Pubic bone
- Corpus spongiosum
- Corpus cavernosum
- Shaft of penis
- Epididymis
- Urethra
- Head of penis (glans)
- Foreskin
- Scrotum
- Sacrum
- Seminal vesicle
- Rectum
- Prostate gland
- Bulbourethralis
- Anus
- Perineum
- Testicle

body, explain, in part, why women's arousal and orgasm experiences vary so much. This also shows more reason for focusing less on triggers and more on the whole body charge.

THE PROSTATE GLAND
AND G SPOT

THE CLITORIS AND G SPOT for women just as the penis and prostate gland for men bring pleasurable sensations and can trigger orgasms and ejaculation. The two areas appear to be anatomically analogous, evolutionary descendants of the same tissue. The perineum, situated between the genitals and anus of both men and women is also a site that can evoke pleasure as well as act as a trigger for orgasm. Unfortunately the sensitivity of this area in women is often damaged when it is torn or cut surgically during childbirth to allow the baby's head to pass through. The loss of feeling is often revitalized as women do the excercises for opening the pelvis.

External Female Genitalia

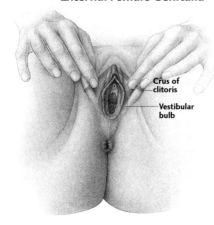

Crus of clitoris

Vestibular bulb

The clitoris and penis are both easy to reach for self-stimulation, but the G spot and prostate are more difficult.

A woman's G spot can be reached through her vagina. She can insert two fingers, feeling, pressing, and stroking the frontal wall. It is best for her pelvis to be elevated whether she is on her back or on her stomach. Pillows can be used. For some women, G spot stimulation can cause the feeling of a need to urinate.

A man's prostate can be reached only through his anus. He can find it by inserting a *well-lubricated* finger or thumb slowly into his anus and feeling, pressing, and stroking downward against the frontal rectal wall. The best position for the man is the basic exercise position, lying on his back with knees up and feet flat on the floor or bed. If he prefers, he can bring his knees up closer to his chest. The reason some men like anal intercourse is that the prostate is stimulated, creating a powerful orgasm.

When entering sensitive tissue such as the vagina or rectum, make sure that your hands are clean, fingernails not sharp, and that plenty of lubrication is used. If anything entering the rectum is to be near other parts of the body, especially if it is to be near or inserted in the vagina, it must be thoroughly washed to prevent vaginal infection.

As interesting as these erogenous areas can be, stimulating these triggers is not a substitute for building, spreading, and containing a charge of energy. When you build a heightened charge, your whole body, including these areas participate in excitement and release even if they are not directly used as triggers.

LOOK AND TOUCH:
FOR WOMEN

MEN ARE QUITE ACCUSTOMED to seeing their own genitals as well as other men's, but even when nude, women's vaginas are hidden from casual viewing. If you have never looked very closely at your own genitals, use a mirror to study this most feminine part of your body. Explore with as much curiosity and delight as you can muster. Make sure that you can see clearly. If you wear glasses, put them on. Make sure your hands are free to part the labia and clitoral folds, notice the colors, touch and feel the textures.

Can you find your clitoris? Some women are confused between the ure-thra, or bladder opening, and the clitoris. The urethra can be uncomfortable to touch and can become easily irritated, often referred to as "honeymooni-tus." The clitoris is above the urethra. You can feel the shaft of the clitoris by stroking side to side above its head.

Rock your pelvis as you touch yourself, whether you are standing, sitting, or lying. Allow your energy to move through, in, and around your pelvis. Use movement and sound to allow your energy to move.

PC MUSCLE (KEGAL) EXERCISES

THE PC MUSCLE is actually a group of muscles called pubococcygeus (pro-nounced "pew-bo-cox-uh-'gee-us") muscles. These muscles contract during orgasm and are related to sexual pleasure and thus muscle tone or lack of it affects the entire pelvic region. The PC muscle runs from the pubic bone in the front to the coccyx (the tailbone at the end of the spine) in the rear. In animals, this muscle wags the tail. In human beings, the PC muscle supports the anus and adjacent internal organs and helps to keep them from sagging. It usually lies about an inch or so beneath the surface of the skin and may vary from a half-inch to over two inches in thickness. A woman can find this muscle by inserting her fingers into her vagina, while a man can find the muscle by inserting his fin-ger inside his rectum. They can both feel their PC muscle by contracting and releasing it. This is the same muscle used to start and stop your urination.

Improvement of PC muscle tone takes consistent practice. At first, two fif-teen-minute periods a day are recommended. Exercise consists of flexing and releasing the PC muscle. Because the exercise requires concentration, it is best to begin in an environment where you will not be disturbed.

PC Muscles side view

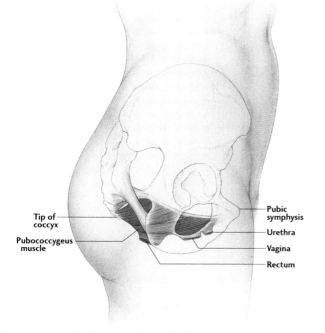

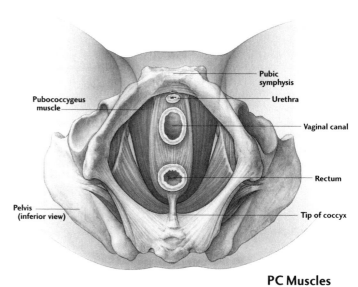

PC Muscles

Personal Hygiene

When you were courting, you probably took plenty of time to plan what to wear, shower, brush your teeth, check your breath, and prepare your body. If you were going to make love, you probably paid special attention to cleansing your genitals. Respect yourself and your long-term mate in the same way. The preparation excites your senses and stimulates erotic energy.

BUILDING AND RELEASING YOUR ORGASTIC CHARGE

YOU HAVE ALREADY LEARNED that breathing and movement will build your charge, and that presence, contact, and boundaries are necessary. Fantasy, also, can arouse your sensuality and eroticism, both of which are necessary for heightened lovemaking.

A fantasy—particularly one of the very best sex you've had, a particular position, a special moment, an erotic sight, anything that brings a rush of sensation to your body, particularly if it is about your lover—can raise your charge to the point of no return and into full orgasm. This is also the time that stimulating nipples and genitals can bring on that extra rush of energy that triggers orgasm.

The use of pornographic literature or films can sometimes turn you on, but there are drawbacks, particularly if you turn away from yourself and your partner for your source of arousal. Pornography causes a depersonalization, a separateness from the object of your desire, instead of the gain of love, compassion, and intimate contact with your partner. Often a trancelike quality pervades the viewing, and it can increase any tendency you might have to become more split off or cut off. Although pornography can initiate excitement and arousal, the external focus cannot lead to the body-mind self-awareness and exploration that are the primary benefits of masturbation initiated through your own imagery and physical sensations. Like the use of a vibrator for masturbation, pornography does not translate to loving involvement with a partner. If you find it absolutely necessary, use it to help you get turned on, but then use your aroused state for further self-exploration.

When couples mutually masturbate as they watch a pornographic film, they may have a sexual release but do not develop more intimacy or mutuality in sex. This practice can accentuate any hollowness or sadness in their relationship.

Most pornographic films are severely devoid of eroticism. Sexuality is often limited to repetitive scenes with the actor and actress hiding behind a split-off

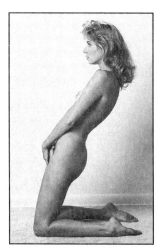

kneeling stress position

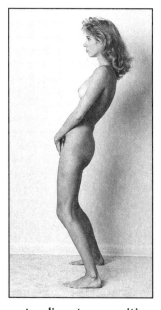

standing stress position

MASTURBATION
EXPLORATION FOR MEN
AND WOMEN

emptiness. There is little or no emotional connection between them. This is one reason why films with less explicit sex are often more erotic.

If you have a full charge and are ready for an orgastic release, it may just happen spontaneously. Other times, knowing several ways to help trigger your release into orgasm will come in handy.

Many people attempt to heighten their excitement or force an orgastic release through emotional or physical tension. To do this they are liable to create a problem, crisis, or dangerous situation, sometimes in the relationship and other times solely within their own internal world. Some people have sex at restaurants under a table, on an airplane, or in a speeding car. Others, believing, "If I really push I will be able to stay hard and get my orgasm," do create some excitement and raise adrenal input. Tension can create a faster orgasm because it constricts the body, thereby creating a smaller container to fill, but it also reduces the body's ability to expand and hold a larger charge for total orgasm. Tension often results in physical or emotional pain and can cause a crisis in the relationship.

"Stress positions," on the other hand, are designed to build and spread a charge and help with release. When you stress a particular set of muscles, they relax and let go and the charge moves more freely through the body.

Stress positions are useful for orgastic release. Stressing the quadricep muscles in your thighs, for example, is one of the best ways to help trigger an orgasm (for both men and women). First be sure that you have already built a high charge; then, while either standing or kneeling, lean back so that you feel the stress in your legs. This will force a release of the orgastic energy. If you learn how to do this while masturbating, you will find numerous ways to apply this with your partner. Choose positions that allow you to move freely while stressing your muscles.

If there is something sturdy to hold on to overhead, it is easier to balance and allows you to apply further stress to your legs. (See photograph, page 273, chapter 18) When your upper body becomes involved in the stress, it also becomes more involved in the release, adding to the pleasure.

THESE SUGGESTIONS ARE DIVIDED into three parts. The first contains general reminders useful to both men and women. The second holds specific suggestions for women, and the third contains suggestions for men. It is important that both men and women read all three sections to understand yourself and your partner.

We're not going to give you a step-by-step guide for making love to yourself. This is a self-exploration. But, to make this a new, heightened learning experience, we will give you some exercises from this and previous chapters that you can try. Make sure you have a good-sized mirror in the room when you masturbate.

Be aware of your senses, nurture them. As an adjunct to the following exercise, you can enjoy a bubble bath, massage scented lotions onto your body, or do stretches and relax. You can prepare your environment with colors, scents, lighting, and music. Create an environment that is for your pleasure and satisfies only you. Don't rush yourself. You would resent it if your partner treated you this way—with such insensitivity. Don't expect less of yourself as a lover.

Begin by just pleasuring yourself, enjoying the pleasure. Don't go for an orgasm; instead go for a charge and pleasure.

- To make sure you are present, look into your eyes in the mirror. Or look at how the colors and textures of your body change as you become aroused. Your nipples, lips, gums, labia, penis may increase in color or turn to a bright red. Your penis or labia will engorge and swell. Your eyes may shine. Parts of your body may turn pale, while a rosy flush may spread over other parts.
- Build a nice charge for yourself before you start masturbating. Use the upper chest, high-charge breathing pattern (chapter 6). Start with five sets of ten. Don't forget to pause to notice when the charge comes in like a rush. When the energy first comes in, you may feel like spacing out—don't be carried away by the energy flow. Stay present and just let the energy come in and spread throughout your body. It's just energy. See if you can welcome it.
- Use the sustaining integration series before sexual lovemaking with yourself (chapter 7) to expand your experience of sexuality.
- Try building the ball of energy between your hands by rubbing them together as you did in the energetic charge breathing exercise. Then, send that energy through your hands to the rest of your body. Stay a little distance from your skin as you stroke yourself with energy. You will find this skill useful when you are with your partner as well as alone. Make sure to keep breathing deeply to maintain a high charge.
- Your skin is a sexually-based sense organ; therefore, your whole body is basically an erogenous zone. For this reason, don't go directly to your genitals. Instead, caress yourself. Learn which areas and strokes please you while you build your charge.
- Don't touch your nipples, penis, vagina, clitoris, or anus until you feel satisfied with your level of charge, until you feel throughout your whole body the circulation of energy that comes with heightened breathing and movement. Slowly begin to stimulate and explore your whole body with your hands. Pay attention to your breathing. If you stop, start again. Please yourself.
- Continue to build your charge with the orgastic pattern: Exhale when your

For Women: Vibrators, Water, and Lubrication

Have you ever masturbated? Have you ever reached orgasm through masturbation? If you do not have orgasms, it is unfair to expect your partner, magically, to be the only one who can make you have one.

If you have had orgasms, by what means have you had them? With a partner? Through intercourse? Through manual or oral stimulation? Many women do not have orgasms with intercourse alone. But then, lovemaking is rarely intercourse without kissing, manual, and/or oral stimulation. For many women, their clitoris is not anatomically situated so that it is stimulated by intercourse. In this case, if you want to have an orgasm during intercourse, you can adjust your position or you or your partner can manually stimulate your clitoris. But again remember, the clitoris is just a trigger. Have you used your hand, a vibrator, or water for self-pleasuring? Did any of these methods bring a satisfying orgasm?

In the exercises that follow, we suggest that you use your hand and fingers rather than a vibrator. There are several reasons for this. Primarily, the mechanical intensity of the vibrator desensitizes the clitoral and genital area, causing numbness. This kind of stimulation does not increase orgastic charge or spread it throughout the body. Your body will defend itself against the onslaught of intensity, often by tensing muscles. And this concentration on the trigger, and resultant muscular tension, can teach your body to tense rather than relax during genital stimulation. Finally, over time a vibrator can create an emotional distancing from oneself, as it is far less intimate than arousal by a sensitive touch.

Another reason for using your hand is that vibrators do not translate very well to sex with a partner. You will learn more about your body using of your own hand, and you can then share this knowledge with your partner. A third reason is that when using a vibrator you are more apt to concentrate on the trigger and forget the rest of your body. Building your excitement from inside with your own breath and movement will put you more in tune with your own body rhythms and sexuality.

Having said this, vibrators can be a source of great fun and pleasure once in a while and, used alone or with your partner, it can create a different orgastic experience. Vibrators can be especially helpful for women who have never experienced an orgasm. The intensity is sure to answer the question, "Did I have an orgasm?" If you do use a vibrator, you will probably feel most comfortable if you stimulate the areas around your clitoris and are gentle with the clitoris itself. Touch lightly and back off, then touch again in a teasing fashion as energy builds up. Some women do become addicted to their vibrators. The orgasm is quick, highly intense, and doesn't require interaction with another person. But it becomes a substitute for making love with a partner. Having an orgasm with a vibrator is nothing like making love to yourself with your hand or making love with a partner. All three experiences are different.

Many women like the feel of water on their genitals. Water intensity and pressure can be varied, controlled by temperature, and where it is directed. Make sure that the water does not enter the vagina. This can upset the acid/alkaline balance of the vagina and leave the tissues susceptible to infection. The clitoris is an exquisite trigger creating a quick localized release but used in isolation from other stimulus, the tension can create an energetic block in the body.

The lubricating system in a woman's body is designed for vaginal intercourse that lasts only for a short time. The longer sexual lovemaking that we suggest requires supplementary lubrication. It is a false assumption that the amount of lubrication a woman secretes indicates how sexually aroused she is. Some women have generous amounts of lubrication even when they are not aroused and others have very little. How a woman lubricates is not a measure of level of stimulation, her femininity, her desire for sex, or her attraction to her partner. (If a man takes this to mean a diminishing interest in sex or in him, or as a negative reflection on his ability as a lover or her merit as a woman, it will create unnecessary stress in the relationship for both partners.) As a woman enters peri-menopause, the amount of her lubrication may vary and, without hormone replacement, with menopause may diminish significantly.

pelvis rocks forward, inhale as your pelvis rocks back. Remember to keep your abdominal muscles soft and loose. Use your feet for movement. Be sure that your legs are up so that you can rock your pelvis. The best way to do this is to put your feet up against a wall as you did in the grounding pelvic lift (chapter 7). Let your neck move freely with an easy flowing movement.

- Move to your genitals, slowly and with plenty of lubricant (women, although you may lubricate well, try using an additional lubricant). Men, even if you are not accustomed to it, use a lubricant. Become aware of what lubrications feel good on your body. Refined, natural oils such as olive, almond, or coconut are good. Plain baby oil is excellent. Stay away from anything that contains chemicals, perfumes, or alcohol; they can irritate delicate mucous tissue.

- Stay open, sensitive, curious, and accepting with your senses: your sight, smell, taste, sound, and touch. Allow yourself to make soft sexual sounds in your throat as you breathe out. Pay attention to sensations: tingling, heat, vibrations, streaming energy, and pulsation. Notice where these sensations spread throughout your body. Notice whether your emotions and thoughts interrupt or support your enjoyment, your sexuality, and your aliveness.

- Stimulate more than just your genitals. Throughout this exercise keep breathing, stay present, keep moving, keep your abdominal muscles soft, don't push, keep your feet grounded solidly on the floor or against a wall. When you play with any of the triggers, try teasing rather than heavy rubbing. When you touch your nipples, notice if you can feel the sensations in your genitals. Women, don't forget to touch all your vaginal areas, not just your clitoris. Men, slow down, focus on the charge, not the trigger.

- Notice if you start to have longings in your pelvis, chest, mouth. Try sucking your thumb, a finger, or fingers while masturbating. When you do, suck hard, keep breathing (through your nose), keep your pelvis rocking and your stomach muscles soft.

- Experiment with the stress positions, both standing and kneeling. Keep breathing while you orgasm. Do not hold your breath.

After your orgasm, pay attention to your body's experience of satisfaction:
- Stay awake, take 10–30 charging breaths, then hold your breath as you did in the "I am" exercise (chapter 7). Meditate on the "I am" experience. Notice if it feels more pronounced or different after an orgasm.

- Touch your skin all over your body. See how different it feels. To spread your release and well-being, lightly massage any part of your body that still feels tense.

- Watch how quickly the outer world seems to come rushing in after your orgasm. Notice if you begin resolving unfinished business from the past or planning for the future before you savor your peaceful mood. Notice if you can retain your sense of well-being twenty to thirty minutes after your orgasm.

- Look at yourself in the mirror to see how different you look after a release. See how your facial expression has changed, notice your openness and glow of aliveness. Look at other alive things, such as plants and pets. What do you notice?

EXPLORING YOUR SEXUALITY: WOMEN

TAKE TIME TO BUILD a charge of energy throughout your body before you begin to touch your genitals. Use the sustaining integration exercise in chapter 7. Above all, maintain your breathing, pelvic movement, and presence throughout your masturbation.

Stroke your breasts, touch your body, look at your body in the mirror. Look into your eyes in the mirror. See if you are present. Breathe fully to load your body with energy.

Explore your clitoris. It isn't just the button tip that sticks out. Feel its stem or root by rubbing its side through the skin. This is less intense and allows for the energy to spread, warm, and excite you. If there is a hood-like fold of skin covering the tip, gently pull it back with your other hand, uncovering the clitoris. Try different motions, circular, across the top or sides, pressing or light pinching. Don't stay too long with clitoral stimulation without pleasuring other parts of your body. Find out what feels good to you from moment to moment. It will continue to change. Keep breathing.

Stroke and massage your labia and inner thighs to spread energy. Try stroking over your clitoris, toward your vagina and back, using the vaginal juices to lubricate your clitoris. Try extra lubrication with a light, unscented oil. Stroke your face and head in loving, nurturing ways. Massage your feet for grounding. All this will help to spread the charge and encourage your whole vaginal region to become engorged with blood and energy. Keep breathing fully.

Find your G spot; feel around inside your vagina and locate your cervix. Get to know yourself inside. You can squat, or lie on your back with legs apart or knees up. Be curious. Bringing your attention to an area will enliven it, and it may begin to tingle with energy.

How do you like your breasts touched? Touch your genitals with one hand and your nipples with the other. Can you feel the energy moving from nipples to clitoris? Keep breathing.

Touch your perineum, the area between your vagina and anus, pressing and stroking to enliven the area. Touch your anus, running your finger around the anal ring. Surrounding your anus are pressure points that release energy as you press. Many women enjoy a penis or finger inside of their anus. If you wish to try this, make sure that your finger and anus are well lubricated and be careful of fingernails. Insert your finger slowly, a little at a time, pausing along the way. Once inside you can press gently but firmly against the walls to loosen the orifice for further release. After any anal contact, always make sure that you clean your fingers and fingernails well before touching your vagina or other parts of your body.

Experiment with what turns you on. Practice using your PC muscles. This will help stimulate lubrication, bringing a rush of blood and erotic sensations to your vagina. Squeeze as you rock and breathe. Check to make sure that you aren't holding your stomach muscles tightly. Keep them soft by using your feet or knees to rock and move your body. Try different positions, sitting, kneeling, standing, or lying on your back, stomach, or side.

As you approach orgasm, no matter what the method, the sensations may feel too much, too intense. But if you want to have an orgasm, you will need to learn to tolerate this feeling. If you back off completely each time the intensity builds, you will never reach orgasm. So back off slightly, keep breathing and moving, then, in a gentle way, restimulate the clitoris or trigger you have been focusing on. If your entire body energy is building at the same rate, the intensity won't feel so uncomfortable. Spreading means moving and breathing, letting go of blocks that are in the way.

If you are uncomfortable with the intensity, try bringing yourself to a small, quick orgasm—you will then feel more comfortable. Then do long, slow pleasuring that builds to a larger orgasm. When you feel you have a high charge and are ready for orgasm, practice stressing your quadriceps (see page 128). Try kneeling with your knees slightly apart. As you continue to breathe and rock your pelvis while masturbating, lean back so that you stress your thighs. Maintain the stress. Continue as the intensity mounts and you will find yourself bursting into orgasm. If orgasm remains difficult, it is probably your character style (chapter 12). Try using a vibrator. It's difficult *not* to have an orgasm with one. But once you know you can have an orgasm, go back to using your hand.

EXPLORING YOUR OWN SEXUALITY: MEN

IT IS VERY RARE that a man does not know how to bring himself to ejaculation. The exercise that follows does not teach masturbation for ejaculation but how to use it as a means for learning and integrating other skills.

The first task of masturbation is to teach you to *build a high charge,* spread it out, *open your heart,* and add this to sexual feeling. The second is for you to learn *ejaculatory control;* to have an orgastic release when you wish, without splitting off or cutting off your excitement. The third task is to learn to have an *orgasm separate from ejaculation* so that if you wish, you can have multiple orgasms without ejaculation. The fourth is to learn how to *heighten your ejaculation and orgastic release by stressing your legs and body.*

Men who participate in masturbation wholeheartedly will find it can do much more than just relieve sexual tension. Excess sexual tension can hinder a man's ability to tolerate excitement with a partner, often leading to ejaculation that is premature for him, meaning before a complete charge has been built. Masturbation teaches how to stay present during sex, develop an ability to tolerate a heightened charge, and any need to please or perform is eliminated.

Take time to build a charge of energy throughout your whole body before you begin to touch your genitals. Use the sustaining integration exercises (chapter 7). Don't go into a trance when you masturbate. Notice how tempting it is to just go away. Stay aware of how splitting off lowers your charge. Always come back to the sensations in your body. If you notice you have split off, take two sets of five upper-chest breaths, then use your eyes; in this case, look around the room or at yourself in the mirror. Become fully present.

Bring an awareness to your whole body. Give yourself a light massage, stroke to awaken your body. Make sure you are breathing fully as you bring your awareness to your pelvis; stroke your buttocks, your legs, all around your groin, pubic area, your lower belly. Use the pelvic bounce to awaken and spread the energy. These masturbation suggestions are to help you enliven your whole body, especially your pelvis, rather than just going directly to your penis. Building a full body charge is completely defeated if you hold your pelvis immobile and just rub your penis. Keep your hands still. Use your pelvic motion to provide friction against your hands, rather than moving your hands up and down your penis. Keep your feet grounded, using them to create a rocking motion as you did in the orgastic pattern. It is the movement of your pelvis and full charge breathing that creates your charge.

Try the Japanese Testi-pull massage technique if your testes and penis are held up tight most of the time. It is a means of bringing relaxation and awareness to the scrotum and testes, and it helps loosen genital tension. It can be done in any position and any time tension is present. Take one testicle in each hand and gently pull down. Hold until there is a reflex that pulls the testicle back up. Resist gently against this pull. Repeat this three or four times. If you don't get the pull-reflex, you probably don't need this exercise. This exercise is not recommended for those men whose testes hang quite freely.

EJACULATORY CONTROL

THIS IS A TIME FOR YOU to practice ejaculatory control. If you are approaching the urge to ejaculate, stop stimulating your genitals. Keep your abdominal muscles relaxed to help spread out your charge. Rock your pelvis *slowly* (rapid movement can increase the need to ejaculate). Increase your upper-chest breathing, take about 30–50 breaths. Focus on your breathing, not on your penis. Move slowly so that your charge spreads. If you hold still you will probably have an ejaculation. After your charge has spread, go back and build it again. If you are having difficulty with this procedure, you are probably not spreading your charge and are building it by rubbing your penis. Back off of your genital stimulation or go ahead and have an orgasm. The next time around, slow down to half your previous pace. Focus on the charge, not the trigger. Squeezing the tip of your penis will also help you stop an ejaculation, but is not as useful as learning ejaculatory control from the inside by spreading the charge with breathing and movement techniques.

ORGASM WITHOUT EJACULATION

ONCE YOU HAVE good ejaculatory control, you can practice having an orgasm without ejaculation. Remember, once you have reached a high level of charge and feel the urge to ejaculate, stop stimulating your genitals. Then start to breathe with full charging breaths from your upper chest. Lying on your back with your feet grounded against the wall, move your pelvis in an orgastic pattern. Do *not* yet touch your penis. Suck on your thumb, finger, or the web of your hand between the thumb and fingers. Suck very hard. Accentuate the orgastic pattern movements, pushing with your feet to rock your pelvis forward. Keep breathing charging breaths and rocking. Don't hold your breath.

With a little practice, you will be able to build and release an orgasm without ejaculating. Orgasm is a release of energy and does not feel like an ejaculation. It has its own pleasure and joy. You may feel a tremendous calm or a surge of love or closeness, sometimes accompanied by a feeling of oneness with nature similar to the "I am" experience. Keep breathing to enhance this feeling, otherwise it will not last long.

Stay with this feeling or, if you wish continue to masturbate to have an ejaculation with another orgasm, you will have to build your charge again by taking full upper-chest breaths. Notice that you have not lost all of your high charge. Just a few breaths (10–30) will have you right back to your former excitement level. Some men become alarmed if the firmness of their erection is in part lost after an orgasm. Don't worry. That, too, can return at only a moment's notice or with some slight stimulation, becoming present and heightening charge through breath and movement.

This exercise is difficult if your only experience is orgasm with an ejaculation, so you will need a little practice before you easily separate the two. You needn't be upset if it takes some time to learn. Remember, sex is about pleasure and loving, not about sexual tricks.

PRACTICING TOGETHER
for the
INTIMATE COUPLE

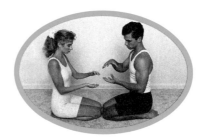

C H A P T E R   N I N E

Building Mutuality and Trust

PRACTICING TOGETHER WITH YOUR PARTNER is an opportunity for adventure—exploration leading to new and exciting shared sexual experiences. You've learned to enliven, arouse, and understand yourself sexually. Now is the time to join with your partner to increase your charge, mutuality, and intimacy.

SUSTAINING MUTUALITY

MOST COUPLES LOOKING for intimacy never establish the mutuality and trust that supports it. Mutuality implies a state of reciprocity: sharing an equality of participation in giving and taking, receiving and offering positive intention and love. Yet, many couples care about one another, share beliefs and tastes in common, have plenty of give and take, but they live lives that function more on a parallel track than in mutual participation. Parallel activities do not provide a feeling of attunement. There is little or no contact, emotional or physical touching, or joining. It is the communion of mutuality, the ability to join in spirit and body with volition, attunement, and equal commitment, in work and play, that heightens intimacy and erotic sexuality.

Working in close contact with one another's body, as in sexuality, is inevitably bound to bring your internalized issues of intimacy to the surface. As you open your body, these somatic memories are likely to be released,

A Guide for Responsibility and Respect

Don't forget that the responsibility for initiating and maintaining erotic sexual excitement remains with each partner. If you try to teach your partner to build or tolerate excitement, the volition, motivation, and energy will be coming from you, from outside, rather than from within your partner. You can facilitate the adventure, but you can't *make* anybody else enjoy anything, not even sex. Each of you should set your own pace and respect each other's boundaries.

Don't forget, by doing these exercises with you, your partner is inviting you into a deeper, more vulnerable joining. These exercises are a guide to opening and relaxing the body. If they are successful, you and your partner are liable to feel exposed, laid open, more sensitive to words, tone, touch, and physical closeness. This means that respect is imperative. Any hostile joke or remark will be felt at a much deeper level than usual, and is likely to make your partner's body close more deeply and tighter than ever before. Likewise any supportive and loving gesture is likely to be greeted with a greater appreciation than usual, as long as it is genuine. When a person's body is open, he or she is more apt to be aware of what does and does not ring true. A subtle and slow attentive pace is the guideline. Pay attention to new rhythms and boundaries.

- Some people think everything is their fault; others think all their problems emanate from outside themselves. When either stance is impenetrable, sex is doomed, and practicing together becomes just a new battleground for old familiar skirmishes. It is important to be responsive and to stay self-aware.

- As you practice together, you may become acutely aware of your partner's disruptive character style behavior or attitude. First, look to yourself to see if it is actually the acting out of *your* character style that is triggering your partner. No relationship can tolerate a high level of character style traits acted out. If either partner is withholding, not reasonably affectionate or emotionally available, the other partner may feel emotionally starved. These stances are nonrelational and both are due to character style.

- Learn to identify your disruptive patterns from the psychological chapters. Locate the ways you might be eroding the hope, trust, and bond in your relationship. With a little consciousness, these patterns will no longer have the power to affect your thoughts and emotions in secret or control your behavior. With a little practice, you can work through, tolerate, or overcome these obstacles. Or, at least, you can develop a sense of humor about the nature of being human.

- Beyond reading the directions for the exercises, *avoid telling your partner what to do.* With heightened sensitivity, even silent judgments may be felt and can inhibit progress. Because you will be working with your body and its energy, your character styles will probably be very active, and you may both find yourselves unable to do or say anything right, no matter how hard you try. Don't make a crisis out of this.

- Being this close to someone you care about has the potential for triggering agency, and nothing lowers excitement like agency. These old patterns, learned in the nursery, tend to inhibit new patterns you are trying to develop. Agency prevents you from focusing your attention inward on self-awareness, self-pleasuring, and change. Those who feel it their duty to overly help their partners do not realize that they often rob them of their right to use their own volition and develop their own excitement.

projected, and played out through your scenario, agency, and character style. Suspicion, mistrust, anxiety, caution, hesitation, and defensiveness can sabotage sex as well as the work of opening and enlivening yourselves. When anything seems uncomfortable or difficult, it is typical to place blame on how your partner helps or does not help enough or in the right way, or how your own physical or perceptual limitations stymie your success, or how the exercises are written. The ability of you and your partner to work together in an intimate environment, each of you with a positive intention toward the other, is essential to working at higher charges. It's even more important when making erotic sexual love.

LIVING WITH CHANGE

TO ENHANCE THE JOY of making love, people in long-term relationships need to allow a paradigm that embraces change, continual change *within the same relationship*. Just as a person changes continually, so do alive relationships. A relationship is a living entity rather than an object or thing. It must be cared for and nurtured. Change in our intimate and sexual relationship is normal as well as inevitable, and we must not allow it to disturb the trust and mutuality between partners.

So, to heighten sexuality, you must focus on change as a necessary part of your sexual relationship. Couples that don't know how to do this become set in a pattern. Sex then becomes routine and boring. Within your relationship new experiences, exploration, or experimentation help keep it alive.

Distractions

Anything that distracts you from being present and comfortable with yourself or with your partner has to be dealt with. (See chapter 5 for the guide to working with interruptions.) To heighten sexuality, learning to deal with emotional distress is just as important as doing the physical exercises. An upset won't simply go away. Unattended, even little upsets collect and grow into betrayals.

Look first toward your patterns of trust, intention, and vulnerability. Do you, through gender prejudice or your character style, hear everything as a criticism? Through an assumption of negative intent, do you feel that your partner is trying to hurt you or put you down? If one partner is bent on hearing everything either as assertions that he or she is bad or defective, how can either partner talk about anything they don't like? Interpreting everything that is said to you by those who care about you as a criticism is an effective way to keep them at a distance.

Can you maintain the larger picture of a loving and healthy relationship while hearing and discussing a small problem? Smaller, more subtle issues need to be kept in perspective. Can your partner say, "Pardon me, you are standing on my toe," without your hearing "You are bad,

mental health aids

you are clumsy, the relationship is terrible, and, furthermore, I am leaving"? Remember, no matter whose idea it is to do the exercises, the fact that your partner is doing them with you means that he or she wants to create something new and more loving and sexual with you.

Your partner need only remain silent and present while *you* figure out what is keeping you from continuing your practice. You can usually identify the problem by identifying which arena pattern is acting up. The good mother messages, agency mantras, and the character style reality check inside/outside exercise will usually restabilize you rather quickly.

If you have to say something to your partner in order to feel comfortable enough to continue, keep it simple. If you make your partner feel bad or wrong, you will probably receive a defensive reaction. Your partner's response back to you also has to be kept short and simple: "You're not bad." "I hear you." "I love you." "I'm sorry." "I understand." "That's not my experience." "Of course." "This is not a crisis." "I'm not upset." "Thank you for telling me." Silence is not an acceptable answer.

Anything that is alive is continually changing, especially sex. Partners tend to see each other as static. An image or reputation once established is hard to shake, no matter how dated it has become. When you miss noticing your partner's growth, you miss knowing the person.

MUTUALITY PRACTICES

THE MUTUALITY EXERCISES that follow will help you to feel close to your partner and will bring you in tune with one another. This all takes time, focus, attention, and positive intention. You needn't do all of the exercises at once, but because you will experience something new with each exercise, make sure that you do all of them before moving on to the next chapter—Awakening Your Bodies Together. Repeat the ones that are your favorites. You can use them as a way of establishing mutuality before you go on, and as a preparation for lovemaking.

Decide with your partner on a set of times to practice. Allow an average of once to three times per week. If you do all of the exercises in the first session, you are working too fast and need to spend more time on each exercise. If you can, imagine yourself moving in slow motion. That's the best way to integrate this work. Any time you begin to feel a bit distant from yourself, do a little breathing, look around, focus your eyes, and get present; then find the "I am" feeling in your body. The more you practice centering yourself, the easier it becomes. When you are not in jeopardy of losing yourself, you will find that you can allow a deeper, more intense joining experience when you make love.

From time to time we refer you to the psychological section to clarify or elaborate upon the subject at hand. We sometimes suggest that you stop what you're doing and write in your journal. This is a helpful tool in many ways. It brings you out of the past and into the present. It helps you see the dynamics of your relationship and the respective contributions of each partner. It can also help you get out of the sometimes paralyzing state of fragmentation.

Energetic Charge Breathing Exercise—with Mutuality

This is an extension of the exercise you learned in chapter 6. This time, in addition to building and moving the energy within yourself, you will also be moving the energy between you and your partner.

Begin: Sit upright, face each other, about one foot apart. You may sit either in chairs or on the floor. If you choose the floor, place a pillow, blanket, or rolled towel under your tailbone so your torso is slightly lifted. This will relieve back strain and help you remain upright. If you are on chairs, make sure your feet are flat on the floor. Synchronize your breathing.

Step 1: As you did in chapter 6, take five sets of five breaths, and then rub your hands together in a quick back-and-forth motion to create friction. Then hold your hands apart to feel the ball of energy between your hands.

Step 2: Once you can feel the ball of energy between your hands, place your hands on your knees. Begin to rotate the energy in a triangle—right hand, left hand, heart—as you did before. But this time, complete the energy cycle with you and your partner looking at each other, fully present, "sending" the energy out to your partner through your eyes. The energy moves right hand, left hand, heart, and up and out through your eyes. The most aliveness will be sparked by energetically meeting halfway between the two of you. Let your partner come half way to you. Feel the energy in your heart and then let it be expressed through your eyes. Synchronize this movement of energy by one partner speaking the words, "right hand...left hand...heart...eyes," as you do the exercise.

Step 3: Take five sets of five breaths and rotate the energy in a triangle—right hand, left hand, genitals—back up through the heart and again out through the eyes. "Send" the energy out to your partner through your eyes. This time the other partner can speak the words to synchronize the movement of energy.

This is an exercise, once learned, that you can silently use any time you are together, especially when making love. This exercise is very effective in helping you move past psychological-emotional irritations and hurt feelings.

Presence Eye-alogue and Shuttling

This is a silent presence exercise—a dialogue with your eyes. Many people get the idea that presence means constant contact. This is not natural, possible, or authentic. It is, however, important to know in your body the difference between emotional and energetic presence and absence. It is also important to know how to "show up." This is a time to stabilize your internal presence and make energetic contact with your partner without words. Do not talk.

Begin: Start with one to three sets of ten breaths.

Step 1: Sit up, facing each other. Decide which person will practice first. That person will be called Partner One, the other person Partner A.

Step 2: Look into each other's eyes for a few moments. Are you still breathing freely? Are you present? What do you notice? Does it feel like your partner is present? Close your eyes for a few moments. Being present means being alert and in contact with one's self. Can you feel the "I am" feeling in your chest? It is possible to be physically present in the room but not emotionally or energetically present with your whole being. Open your eyes again. Do your partner's eyes pull you in, push you out, blur you out, or do they meet you? Now, both of you close your eyes. Bring your attention to your interior "I am" experience. Did it feel better making eye contact, or do you feel calmer and less anxious or inundated with your eyes closed? Open your eyes.

Step 3: Partner A, with your eyes open and looking at Partner One, say your multiplication tables (use the 7's) to yourself, silently.

Step 4: Partner One, look into A's eyes. What do you notice? Is A present? How can you tell? When A is not present, what do you feel in your body? Where do you feel it? What has happened to the energy coming from A's eyes? Are A's eyes clear or spacey? Hard? Fogged over? Do you feel better or worse than when you simply made eye contact? Do you feel abandoned or relieved when A is "gone"? Are you paying attention to blinking or eye movements rather than to the energy in A's eyes?

   Note: This is all information for you—to help you recognize whether or not your partner is present. Of course, if you are not present yourself, you may not be able to tell if anyone else is present. Sometimes just being present with another person is enough to cause you to become nervous, to turn off, go away, close up, or even alter your breathing. Are you going away? Remember, don't talk up to this point, just look and be present.

Step 5: Partner One, describe your experience to A. Tell A what you feel when A is "gone." Remember, this is not about your partner, it is about your response. Shuttling between contact with your partner and your own internal experience can trigger your primary scenario, character style, and agency reactions (See the boundary-pillow and emotional pie exercises, respectively, for review.) What do you feel like doing when your partner goes away? Does separation trigger abandonment or relief? Some people emotionally leave when their partners leave. Some want to shake them back to their senses. Some just get hurt, angry, or depressed. Some want to join with the absent person. Others want to physically leave. If your agency is high, you might want to go after and fix your partner. This process of energetically shuttling between contact and separation is the underlying struggle that happens unconsciously and triggers most hurt feelings, emotional upsets, and arguments in intimate relationships—especially in the bedroom. We must become conscious that our responses are our own and not due to our partner or the relationship.

Step 6: Partner A, now it is your turn to look into your partner's eyes while Partner One silently recites the alphabet backwards. Partner A, ask yourself the same questions from step 4; then tell your partner about your experience. Now that you know what presence is, figure out what you have to do to become present in the moment, then look at your partner.

Step 7: Join hands in such a way that you hold each other equally. Don't hold your partner's hands any more or less than he or she is holding yours.

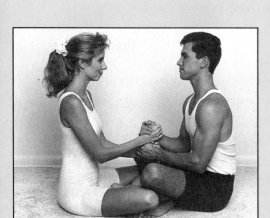

Step 7.

Step 8: Take three sets of five charging breaths. Now each of you close your eyes and focus your attention within yourself. At the bottom of your breath, try to find your "I am" sense of well-being, the place of calmness in your upper chest. Experience this for at least a minute. Come back, open your eyes, and make contact with your partner. How do you feel when in contact? Compare your inner presence with your outer contact by shuttling inside, then outside. Go inside again and experience your inner presence more fully—find the "I Am" experience. Then come back, open your eyes, and again make contact with your partner.

Shuttling: Moving back and forth between internal and external contact can be very useful. If you don't engage in enough contact, it is difficult to form or sustain a relationship. If you give yourself away to the relationship, there is no one for your partner to engage with.

The "I am" feeling of well-being in your body, combined with a willingness to make an honest connection, will help you to stay present and then build and contain a charge within yourself and when you are with your partner. You will each have to face certain parts of your character style, such as, "Nobody can tell me what to do"; your fear of commitment; or attachment to, "My way is always right."

Shuttling brings you closer to your own body, your own authenticity, and lessens your character style. Your lovemaking will be more fluid and natural when you feel who you are as a body experience.

"I-Thou"

Your partner will receive the nonverbal message that comes from within you whether this is the same as the words you speak or not. In fact, unwittingly, you are communicating more than you think you are. Body-to-body communication is more authentic than words. To do these exercises with your partner successfully, find a generosity of spirit within yourself.

Begin: Kneel upright facing each other. Put your hands on both sides of your partner's head while your partner places his or her hands in the same way on your head.

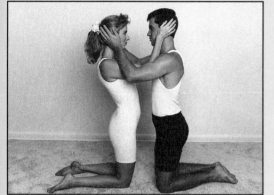

Begin.

Step 1: Now each of you in turn describe to the other what you hold between your hands. ***Do this part before reading any further.***

   Note: Many people describe the physical entity between their hands but don't feel the person who is there or their energy. They refer to their partner's head as an "it"—an object: ears, hair, bones. If you described what you held as an "it," that's how you held your partner. This also is how your partner probably felt when you held him or her. This may well represent your general attitude and how your partner usually experiences it.

Step 2: Still holding each other's heads, look into each other's eyes and, in turn, shuttle your attention first to yourself and then to your partner by saying the following aloud: Partner One, say, "I-it"; then Partner A repeat, "I-it." This will give you a feeling for what it's like to treat a person as an object. Notice what it feels like in your body when you are treated like an "it."

Step 3: Now Partner A, say, "I am–you are" aloud to your partner several times. Then Partner One repeat the same words, "I am–you are." This will give you a different feeling—what it's like to treat a person not as an object but as a human being. What does it feel like in your body when you are now treated like a human being? "I am–you are" identifies separateness: "I" here, "you" out there. It is still not intimate.

Step 4: Now say, "I-Thou," alternating each phrase as in steps 2 and 3. Does this give you a different feeling? This implies, "We are separate....We are one."

"I-Thou"—A Relational Process

Martin Buber wrote in his book *I-Thou* that when "Thou" is spoken, a person is no longer treated like a thing or an object. When "Thou" is spoken, it implies a different level of consciousness and most people feel a more caring, soulful, and human connection. With this level of consciousness you cannot treat another person like an object.

The phrase, "I am—you are" acknowledges separateness and boundaries. In the I-Thou feeling, there is a relational process: the flowing back and forth of the individual self and the other—a little of you is in me and a little of me is in you, and there is a sharing in this encounter.

Silent Conversation

Now practice being with your partner and bring your attention to your hands and your partner's. Find out more about yourself and your partner by communicating without words. Let your imagined "hand-voice" speak without words to your partner; then allow your partner's hands to "answer."

Begin: Sit facing each other and hold hands. Take about ten full letting-go breaths.

Step 1: Both partners, at the same time, imagine that your hands can speak, that you can give them a voice through subtle movement. Without either person speaking out loud, send your communication through your hands. An internal conversation could go like this: "I'm holding you tightly because I feel nervous and I feel your calmness reassuring me." You may guess that your partner is answering, "Please don't be afraid; I will not hurt you," or, "I too am tense and am holding on to you."

Step 2: Continue this hand inner-dialogue for two to three minutes; then talk about this experience. Tell each other about your thoughts, feelings, and insights and what you each thought your partner's hands "said" during your silent hand conversation.

Note: Some people can feel a tremendous amount of trust when they touch and feel close in silence. They actually are good at sensing communication, both in sending and receiving. But often with the silent conversation, we find that couples become blatantly aware that they can't read their partner's mind, and they feel totally off-track. It is always best not to expect your partner to guess what you are feeling or what you want. If you are hurt or angry, check with your partner to find out his or her intentions. Just remember that your assumptions may be wrong. Approach with positive intention to work out any misunderstanding. If you want something, speak up. If something is troubling you, it can get worse with silence. In silence you invite people to fill in the blanks with their worst fears, sorrows, and beliefs. This exercise is to help you become more comfortable with communicating through your bodies—it is not meant to replace verbal communication, which is essential but not the focus of this exercise.

Dancing with Energy

If you're like most couples, you would like your relationship to be egalitarian—mutually respectful, with room for individual and mutual attunement. Most people know what they want but don't have a body-feel for how to bring it about. This exercise will help you develop a body-feel for a new relationship pattern—one that fits the two of you and your individual identities as well.

In relationships today, no one wants to be a follower, at least not for long. Most want to be the one in charge, but not of everything all the time. Unfortunately, to accomplish this, many people emotionally or psychologically push against their mate with their character style. Others become dependent or behave like defensive victims. Neither reaction can bring about a sense of self, mutuality, or reciprocity. Some couples give up on mutuality and seek parallel lives, not really interacting very much. Others just drift, not even realizing that no one is in charge.

It is common to mistake being in charge with being in control. See how the two of you function together in this exercise. Practice being present with your partner and bring your attention to your ability to arouse and increase energy. Remain silent during the exercise; talking will only distract you. If you wish this exercise to reveal the nature of your interaction with mutuality, follow the notation that advises you to stop reading until you have completed the suggested experiment. If you go on and read the explanations, you will be led by them and not identify the issues to focus on in your relationship.

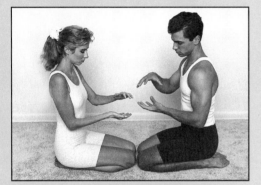

Step 1.

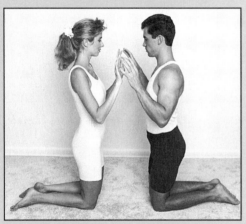

Step 2.

Begin: Sit facing each other on the floor. Take three sets of ten breaths through your mouth, high in your upper chest, with an emphasis on the inhale. With each set, look around, use your eyes, stay present. Don't allow the rush of energy to cause you to split off.

Step 1: Rub your own hands together rapidly for a minute to generate the ball of energy. Feel the energy by placing your hands about six to ten inches apart.

Step 2: When you can feel the ball of energy, place the palms of your hands up in front of you, an inch or two from your partner's hands. Stay just close enough to feel each other's energetic presence without touching hands. Move your hands toward or away or pass your partner's hand back and forth across his or her energy field. Make sure you are not holding your breath as this will cut down on the flow of energy.

Step 3: Take one or two sets of ten breaths. Now, with your hands still almost together but not touching, move them as in a dance. Do this for a few minutes. See what rhythms you create together. Don't forget to keep breathing. *Do this part before reading the next step.*

Step 4: Notice who was leading. Can you agree on who was leading? Is it obvious? Or did you automatically take turns leading? Was there any struggle, was there any giving in?

Step 5: This time make the leader-follower relationship explicit—decide who will start out as leader. Both positions are important in relationships. *Decide before reading on.*

Note: *If a person is told he or she should be or can be the leader, who is in charge? The person who decides who should be in charge—even if they give leadership away—is really the one in charge. Or, do you force your partner to take charge by not taking charge yourself? Some people are hesitant to take charge because they don't want to be wrong or responsible for the outcome.*

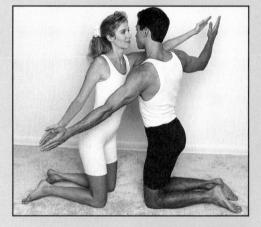

Step 3.

Step 6: The person who has decided to be in charge, please say out loud to your partner, "I'm in charge." The one who is to follow, please say, "I'm going to be the best follower you have ever seen." A leader needs a follower or there is only self and no relationship. Take ten breaths, then begin the dance once again with your hands a few inches apart. Leader, move your hands so that you can tell if your partner is really following you.

Step 7: After a few minutes stop and discuss how both positions felt. Next, take one or two sets of ten breaths and shift so that the other partner is the leader and says, "I'm in charge." The other says, "I'll be the best follower you have ever seen." *Do this part before reading on.*

Note: *Which position feels the most comfortable to you? Which feels most natural? Which turns you on and makes you feel more alive? Which do you like the best? A leader must pay attention to where his or her partner is and how he or she is doing. Some people try to maintain leadership when they are the follower by giving directions or complaining. Others just split off when they are the follower so that the leader never feels joined. Both follower and leader must show up fully. The body feeling of mutuality doesn't take place unless both people show up and pay attention to the other.*

Step 8: Take one or two sets of ten breaths. This time, without hand motions, take turns sending and receiving the following messages. Slowly, pausing between statements to allow for experience, one partner send these messages by saying the words, "I'm in charge." Then, "I'm in control." Then again, "I'm in charge."

Note: When you are the receiver of these messages, do the words control and charge feel the same or different? When you are the sender, do they feel differently? Do you take leadership by telling your partner what to do and how to do it? This is a sure way to sabotage leadership.

Find another way to lead, such as by realizing your internal rhythm and expressing it in movement and tempo. When you lead or follow, do you space out, tune out, or do it grudgingly? If you are having trouble in this department, it is not an intimacy issue, it is one of character style. When you lead, do you try to do what will please or feel good to your partner rather than taking the opportunity to express your rhythms? This is more an agency issue.

Step 9: Now take turns being leader and follower. Take two sets of ten breaths. Shift leadership by one person saying, "I'm in charge," and the other answering, "I'll be the best follower you have ever seen." Without additional words, let the lead come from one of you. Then pay attention to when the energy shifts and it is time for the other to lead. Don't space out or get into a rut and miss the beat for your cue to lead. Switch leadership back and forth until you feel a sense of attunement and well-being flowing between you. *This is the body equivalent of mutuality.* Move slowly from a kneeling to a standing position. Allow this movement to just happen. Continue to switch off leadership when the time is right. Have you found a timing or rhythm that works for both people? Observe your partner's sensitivity to you, and yours to your partner.

Step 10: Talk about what you each discovered about yourself and each other. Share how it felt to be the follower and the leader. How did character style, agency, or gender prejudice surface?

Ongoing Mutuality
Don't stop dancing just because the practice session is over. This shifting from being the follower to being the leader and back is applicable to everything from making dinner, driving the car, going on vacation, taking care of the kids, and, of course, to making love. Practice makes mutuality. With mutuality, heightened lovemaking is just around the corner.

Sensing Each Other

This last joining is a simple, quiet, physical attunement. It enhances a feeling of being close and an awareness of one another's body—without involving sexuality. It allows you to feel each other's rhythm of breathing and physical connection.

Begin: Sit next to each other, facing in opposite directions. Lie back on the floor so you are next to each other, and place one hand on the other's belly, close to the solar plexus.

Step 1: Take a few full sighing, letting-go breaths. Allow the full weight of your body to sink into the floor with each breath. As you lie quietly together, check your body. Notice if there are any tight places. If so, take a few more breaths and let the tension go with each letting-go breath.

Step 2: Once you feel at ease in your body, turn your attention to feel your partner's body. You may first notice the temperature and texture of his or her skin. Touching and being touched may cause you to feel more calm and/or more stimulated. You may notice your partner's body vibrating slightly with excitement or nervousness. In this position, you can also feel your partner's heartbeat. Tap into this vital lifeline and feel your lover's rhythm. Lie this way for a few minutes.

Step 3: Again, pay attention to your own inner rhythms. Can you feel your heartbeat? With your breath, release any tense places. See if you can find the place of well-being in your body.

Step 4: Notice the rhythm of your partner's breath. Feel his or her energy. Feel the closeness. Notice your passing thoughts and emotions. Set them aside and, shuttling, focus on your body rhythms and on your partner. If thoughts continue to interrupt, stop and write them down in your journal to work on at a later time. Your breathing rhythms may become the same, but don't make any effort to have this happen. Just lie quietly and be aware of your breath and your partner's.

Step 5: Silently alternate between sending love, being the lover; and receiving love, being the beloved. (If, after you feel present and in contact, you wish to build a charge together before engaging in sex, bring your legs up as in the basic breathing position.)

In a relationship you can't make everything perfect. But then again, you don't need to. You don't need to change who you are. You don't even have to fix or change your partner. You need to shift your focus to sustaining your sense of self while wholeheartedly and authentically being present with your partner. Remain conscious of your own psychological patterns and put them to rest within, or note them in your journal. Contain your impulse to act them out when everything is going well just to interrupt the growing closeness. Remember, your partner is feeling just as vulnerable as you are.

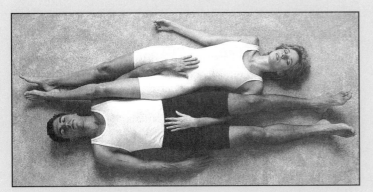

Begin.

CHAPTER TEN

Awakening Your Bodies Together

AS YOU BEGIN:
SEGMENTAL BODY
RELEASES

IN THIS SECTION, you will have the opportunity to open your senses, your body, and your relationship to higher levels of awareness and sensitivity with mutuality. These exercises are a way of joining and touching in a manner of prolonged foreplay, but they are not a prelude to sex. This way of being together is a joy unto itself.

These exercises are designed to help you develop new habits for building, containing, and releasing charge.

Overcharge

It doesn't do any good to build a higher charge than you can comfortably contain. You must remember to give yourself time to acclimate to these heights. Ground your excitement and support it; don't dissipate it. In this way, you'll learn to tolerate it. (For more about overcharge see page 88 in chapter 6.) If the heightened energy becomes so strong that you feel you just can't contain it, stand up and push against a wall. See grounding exercise in chapter 7. Then use your eyes and look at the other person.

Calming

If your muscular vibrations become so strong that you feel overwhelmed, roll onto your side and curl up into a fetal position. Your partner can put his or her arms around you. Lie quietly, breathing slowly with belly breathing. All the uncomfortable sensations will fade in a couple of minutes. Don't worry, you are in charge. You have a safety valve; you can always slow down or stop for a while.

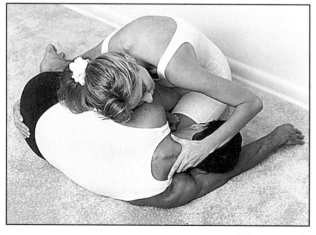

Calming Male

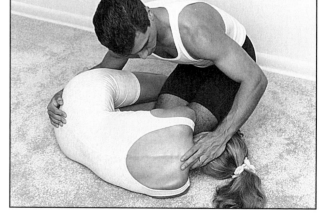

Calming Female

Undercharge

What if these exercises don't work? You might say, "I've done all of the breathing and pelvic movements, and I don't feel any charge, I don't feel any change." If you are undercharging, this is unusual, so check any medications you are taking. Even simple antihistamines will decrease your ability to build a charge. If you are using any drugs, particularly marijuana, tranquilizers, or downers, it is virtually impossible to build a charge.

Look next at your character style. If you think you are "supposed" to build a charge, your rebellious, "Don't tell me what to do" attitude may be hindering you. Next, check to see if you are doing these exercises for yourself or to please someone else. If you are doing them for someone else, it may be agency, and you are not acting from your own volition. Another possibility is that there is a lie. Any inauthenticity in your relationship, or forced performance (trying to look good or do it right) will greatly compromise your ability to build a charge. Use your journal to identify your part in undercharging.

SEGMENTAL BODY
RELEASES

The best explanation for what body work is about comes from a friend and teacher, Robert Hall, the founder of the Lomi School: "When we die, something leaves the body. It is that something that we are working with."

TO BE ABLE TO BUILD and contain a heightened full-body charge, each body segment must be as free of holding patterns as possible to enable energy to build, flow, and spread. Some holding patterns remain the same, while others change. When you are successful in releasing, enlivening, or freeing one segment of the body, another segment you previously opened may start to close down. We will point out where closures are most likely to occur. The most easily recognized symptom of closure is a change or restriction in breathing pattern.

Holding patterns in the body can be released in a number of ways. Bringing your awareness to the area is sometimes sufficient to allow letting go, but often you will need more know-how. When you have a holding pattern in your body, it can be very helpful if your partner touches the held muscle, enabling you to feel it and let it go more easily. If your partner encourages the muscle to move in a full natural way, the body begins to remember and relearn its most natural rhythm. This happens when pressure is applied to the muscle with vibration, stretching, shaking, or stroking. A light lubricant may be applied to avoid any pinching or stretching to the skin. You can also, of course, use movement and breathing, as we have done already.

These body opening techniques are different from massage, which is usually received rather passively. In these exercises, the practicing partner is an active participant. The intention here is for both people to open from the *inside out*—through breath, movement, energy, and awareness—while working together.

One partner is the Guiding Partner who assists the other partner as he or she attempts to release holding patterns and build a charge through breathing and movement. As the Active Partner is learning to release and build a charge, the guide is learning how to be comfortable being exposed to the higher energy and intimacy levels.

Begin by choosing which of you wishes to practice first; you'll switch roles after finishing the complete set of exercises. The instructions are primarily for the Guiding Partner, who is in a better position to glance at the book, but excitement and arousal are contagious. Physical sensations and all the psychological issues will be affected by the interactions. Guiding Partner, watch your presence and breathing patterns as your partner's charge rises. Most importantly, notice when your psychological issues—the arenas—are activated.

Remember, If Problems Arise...

mental health aid

- *Don't get stuck by over-discussing the problem.* Try not to interrupt your practice every time you feel an upset or interruption. Stay with the body release you are working on and use it for relief. Remember, the function of many of these upsets is to stop a release or to prevent your comfort with a higher charge or feeling of well-being. Don't make a crisis out of it. If upsets persist, set aside a time, separate from these exercises and lovemaking, to process these issues together, but only after you have worked on your part of the problem in your journal.

- *Become aware of how the problem is affecting your body and mind.* Every upset has both physical and mental components. You can work on the content of the upset: "You didn't look at me....You touched me too roughly," etc. Or, you can focus on the physical holding in the body that results from the upset: a restriction in the chest, splitting off in the eyes, a pain in the gut, etc. It is hard to tell if your body has become tense and

then you look for a problem, or if a problem has caused your body to become tense. Finding a problem with your partner, however, does give you a good excuse to shut your body down. Add a little gender prejudice to the mix, and you can see how very complicated relationships, mutuality, and sex can become. This is the incentive for you to learn about all your underlying bodymind secrets.

- *Notice if each time your body opens, it closes again.* One segment may close just because another has opened in the body's attempt to maintain the status quo. You may find that a segment closes due to the physical and emotional closeness and interactions; just repeat the exercise for that segment.

- *Don't worry if your charge suddenly diminishes.* Use this as an opportunity to find out what causes you to lose your charge. By now you both know how to breathe and move to reestablish your charge.

Each time you begin your exercises together, start with the sustaining integration exercise (chapter 7) to assure that each person begins by being present, open, and alive. Because you are charged and open, you will be able to see where your partner's body can use more help, and, more importantly, to feel the impact on your own body. It is not difficult to build a charge; *the difficulty is in sustaining it* in an intimate relationship.

When exercising with your partner, it is best not to work in the nude.

This is too distracting. You may feel sexually aroused as you do the exercises no matter what you wear, but try not to slip into sex. These are exercises for body-opening, body-charging, and energy-spreading. Don't shortchange yourself by moving too quickly into sex.

Do not try to force an opening of the body for yourself or your partner. It is very tempting to try to break through holding patterns, especially when someone is heavily armored, but you should go slowly and open from the inside at your own pace. When it feels right, energetic holding patterns will diminish and you will feel more open and alive. Body holding patterns are protections and are there for a reason. It is not a good idea to throw defenses away without knowing their function or before developing better skills for self-care.

If at any time you feel uncomfortable, do a little breathing, look around, focus your eyes, and get present. Find the "I am" feeling in your body. As this becomes a habit, it will become easier to do. When you are not in jeopardy of losing your sense of self, you will find that you can allow deeper, more intense joining experiences when you make love.

Make sure Active Partner keeps his or her eyes open throughout the exercises, as this helps maintain presence. Closed eyes encourage splitting off. Also, holding one's breath or reversing breath-movement patterns indicate some discomfort—physical, emotional, or psychological—and this can inhibit the charge.

Remember, these are far more than just physical exercises. Join with your partner in heart and spirit. By now you have learned that you have the power to transform yourself from within, to turn your irritations into excitement, to empower yourself. Focus on your well-being; ready yourself to be a witness to aliveness; relish and delight in your shared existence.

Approaching Body Contact

In this exercise, notice how sensitive your body becomes when you have a charge. With a charge, your emotional body boundaries become more important. It may take both partners some time to adjust to the closeness.

Begin: Active Partner, lie flat on the floor in the basic exercise position with knees up. Take about ten full, sighing, letting-go breaths. Now, with the high-charge breathing pattern (chapter 7), take one to three sets of ten charging breaths. Let the rush come in and spread. Continue full letting-go breaths throughout the sequence of exercises.

Step 1: Guiding Partner, check first to see if your partner is in the basic exercise position as described in chapter 7 on page 99. If not, tell your partner what adjustments are needed.

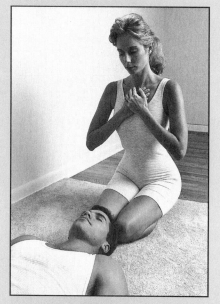

Step 2: Kneel behind your partner and take two to three sets of ten charging breaths for yourself. Let the rush come in and spread. Take a moment, place your hands at the center of your own chest, and find the "I am" sense of well-being in your chest.

Step 2.

Step 3: Rub your hands together to create the ball of energy. When you feel present, put your energized hands next to Active Partner's ears—*but do not touch.* Just allow Active Partner to feel the energetic presence of your hands. To send energy with your hands, imagine that you are still holding the ball of energy. Notice how your partner responds when you do not send energy, and then when you do. Keep your hands near your partner's ears for a minute or so. Notice that your partner can feel your presence without your touch. *Be aware that your energy actually does the touching.* This will be useful knowledge when you are making love. You bring something special to a relationship in the form of your own personal energy that you can transmit to another person.

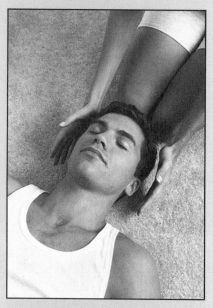

Make sure you are both breathing easily and feel comfortable. Take a moment to *shuttle,* going inside to find the place where you have a sense of well-being, then back to your partner. Be aware of your partner with all your senses. Be aware of your partner past your expectations, judgments, longings, and what he or she looks like or does in the world. When you do

Step 3. this, notice the feelings this generates in your body.

Step 4: Guiding Partner, gently and slowly slip your hands under Active Partner's head from behind and hold it in your hands. Rest the backs of your hands on the floor so that you are comfortable. Embrace your partner's head gently and tenderly. You will both sense the care this touch implies. This is the physical ambiance for doing these exercises and for making love: caring and a sensitive touch.

As you hold Active Partner's head, synchronize your breath to his or her breathing pattern. Remind your partner to breathe through the mouth normally but fully. Watch your partner's chest move. Notice any tension in your own body as you are breathing. Let go of the tightness in your own neck, shoulders, etc. You may find that you can feel in your own body where Active Partner is holding tightly. Find a loving feeling toward your partner, be a lover, and send this loving energy through your hands.

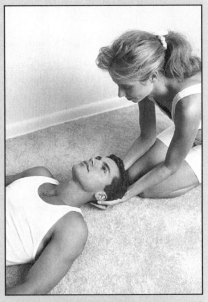

Step 4.

Step 5: Active Partner, be the beloved and receive the love. See what you have to do in your body to let the love in, awakening in yourself the feeling of being loved. Go back in time: remember again in your body the feeling of being loved. Now, let your lover's caring join your own feeling of being loved.

Now that you have worked on contact and have become comfortable working together, it is time to begin more specific exercises to release segments of the body. (Refer to the chart in chapter 7, page 97.)

Ocular Segment: Head and Neck

By watching your hands in the cross-crawl exercise, you mobilize your eyes and break up the fixed pattern. Using your eyes to look at colors will also bring presence. To work with the eyes, we usually work with the back of the head because holding in the ocular segment often comes from a tightness in the back of the head, neck, and shoulders.

The ocular segment is divided into two bands: band 1, the top of the head and forehead; band 2, the eyes. There is a fascial sheath that connects the forehead frontalis muscle with the occipitalis muscles in the back of the head. Thus, they act as one band running across the top of the head and are used to move your scalp. Emotions associated with this band are worry, complexity, despair, and tense forms of thinking and feeling.

Another muscle in this band is the temporalis, which fans up the side of the head. It is one of five muscles used to close the jaw. It is possible to keep this muscle tight even when the jaw is relaxed, making the eyes look hard even if one doesn't feel angry. Anger or resentment may be felt with the release of the temporalis.

As you relieve both bands, pent-up emotions are also released, and the eyes become more open for expression, including erotic expression and aliveness. Communication of the eyes functions two ways: They take in what they see and send out feelings from within. Certain blockages are deeper and more chronic; others are more superficial. A glazed look is usually more temporary and superficial, and a deadened, flat look is often deeper. The eyes are where the soul shines through and are very private.

Begin: Active Partner, in the basic exercise position, take about ten full sighing, letting-go breaths. Now, with the high-charge breathing pattern, take one to three sets of ten charging breaths. Let the rush come in and spread. Continue full letting-go breaths throughout the sequence of exercises (no pelvic rocking during the head and neck releases).

Guiding Partner, an interruption to this breathing pattern usually indicates that a distracting thought, sensation, or emotion has occurred.

Step 1: Neck-Occipital Ridge Massage-Stretch: Guiding Partner, *place your hands at the back of Active Partner's neck,* just where it meets with the skull. This is called the occipital ridge. It is a site of major holding in the eyes. Massage this area well. It may be tender but can tolerate firm pressure. Use your hands, not just your fingers, to massage the back of the neck, lifting up with each stroke. Hold, pull up, and let go; and hold, pull up, and let go. Then move your hands up a bit, to the lower ridge of the skull and repeat massage.

Step 2: Neck Lift-Stretch: The long muscle across the shoulders and up the neck, used to raise the shoulders, is called the trapezius. This muscle tends to hold a lot of tension and is apt to keep you "in your head" or split off. Guiding Partner, start at the base of the neck and with a long, firm, slow movement, lift and stretch as Active Partner breathes fully. As your hands reach the skull, pull the head to create a slight pressure or traction. As you do this, match your breath to Active Partner's. Inhale before you begin and exhale as you apply pressure, lifting and stretching the neck. Do this six or eight times.

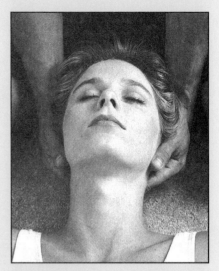

Step 1.

Step 3: Head-Neck Rock: With the back of one hand resting on the floor, cradle your partner's head at the base of the skull. Begin to move Active Partner's head slowly, back and forth, by closing and opening the palm of your hand. Active Partner will have to let go, stop thinking, and trust. Remind her or him to soften and not help you—to let you create the movement.

Step 4: Head-Neck Stretch: Keeping the same hand behind your partner's head, place the other hand on your partner's shoulder. Use your hands to stretch the trapezius muscle that runs from the base of the skull, down the neck and across the shoulder.

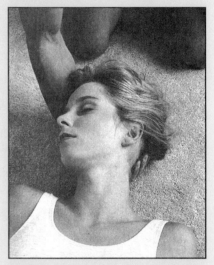

Step 3.

If your partner is holding his or her breath, this may be an indication that your partner's tolerance for intimacy, for being touched, or for having an open body has momentarily been reached.

Sometimes a brief check with your partner—asking what is going on— will banish the tension. If not, suggest he or she take a breath or two. Once the breathing pattern has been reestablished and your partner is present, move again to the neck and repeat the steps to loosen it up.

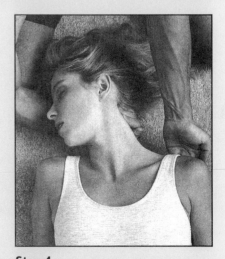

Step 4.

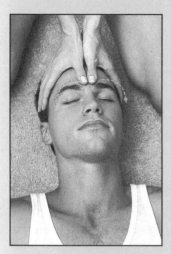

Step 1A.

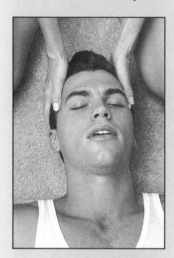

Step 1B.

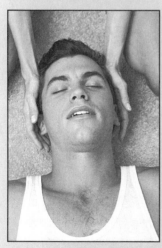

Step 2.

Ocular and Oral Segments: Head and Face

Touching the face stimulates the brain, directly arousing emotional response. This is why kissing and sucking are felt so powerfully on the face. So be aware of feelings that emerge as you work in this area. Also, be careful not to press or rub hard on the face because the skin is very delicate and can become stretched. When massaging the face, use a little lubricant and don't pull the skin—baby oil or face cream is fine. Unlike other parts of the body, the muscles are attached directly to the skin without a fascial layer for protection.

Begin: Active Partner, lie flat on the floor in the basic exercise position with knees up. Take about ten full sighing, letting-go breaths. Take one to three sets of ten charging breaths. Let the rush come in and spread. Continue full letting-go breaths. Guiding Partner, sit behind partner's head.

Step 1: Guiding Partner, place your thumbs together in the middle of Active Partner's forehead with your fingers resting on the temples. Stroke his or her forehead by rubbing your thumbs across it and over the eyebrows.

Step 2: Use the heel of your hand to massage along the temple and the sides of the head above the ears. This muscle, the temporalis, is used when you bite down, and a great deal of holding takes place here. Just in front of the ears, there is an area with many nerves close to the surface. *Use caution not to press hard in this area.*

Step 3: Eyes: Gently cover your partner's eyes with the palms of your hands. Both partners breathe and let go.

Step 4: Place your thumbs below the eyes, starting at the sides of the nose. Press with your thumbs. Circle and lift. Move about a quarter of an inch, press and circle again. Do this all the way around to the sides of the face. Remember to press lightly, rather than stretch or pull.

Note: Guiding Partner, find out how your partner feels about the pressure you are using. The mouth and jaw, the oral segment, *is very important as it participates in respiration, nourishment, aggression, and sexuality, as well as biting, spitting, smiling, talking, crying, laughing, gagging, swallowing, and sucking. The mouth is considered a sexual organ, and releasing the mouth or jaw, such as in kissing or sucking, can be used to release the pelvis.*

The major muscle circling the mouth is the orbicularis oris. This muscle and several attached smaller ones are responsible for moving your mouth. Like other sphincter muscles, it may contract somewhat in the breathing process. Sucking is one of the best ways of relieving this holding pattern, and yet may produce a number of aggressive, sexual, longing, soothing, or comforting feelings.

The muscles of the floor of the mouth and throat often block "swallowing" or hold expressions of sadness or hurt. Working with facial muscles helps to break down the "mask" of emotional holding and, as a result, many feelings may surface. As feelings come through, your partner's breathing may again become inhibited.

Step 5: Upper lip, jaw: Place your thumbs above the lip on the muscle just at the bottom of the cheeks. Beginning at the center, massage along the sides of the maxilla, or upper jaw. Again, pressing lightly against the bone, circle and lift in the same way across to the side of the face.

Step 6: Lower jaw: Do the lower jaw the same way, going around the chin to the muscles of the mandible or jawbone. The masseter muscle is a thick and heavy muscle in the jaw. To find it ask Active Partner to bite down and it will flex. Do not use hard pressure because it can be quite sensitive.

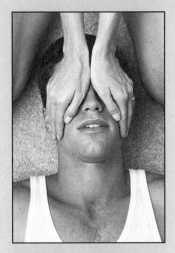

Step 3.

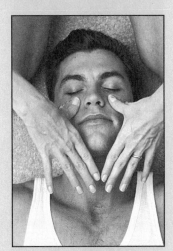

Step 4.

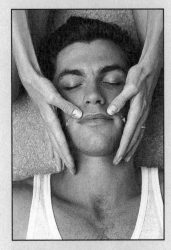

Step 5.

A BLOCK IN THE *CERVICAL SEGMENT,* or throat, can often be heard in the sound of the voice or the quality of the breath. The muscles of the throat are important in their correlation to pelvic blocks. It is best not to do muscular releases in the front part of the neck, because the throat and neck hold many vital and sensitive structures, including the jugular vein, the carotid artery, the parathyroids, and the carotid sinus that regulates blood pressure. You can, however, use a firm pressure on the back of the neck.

The *thoracic segment,* or chest, is known as the home of the heart—the doorway to the sense of self, the witness "I am" experience, the place of well-being and compassion, love and empathy. The thoracic segment extends from the diaphragm to the clavicles. It includes the lungs, heart, and rib cage. The arms and the hands are extensions and are used for reaching out and holding.

In opening the body, we often focus on the eyes first, but the heart is of equal importance. This opens the way for trust. It is always a good idea for this trust to be firmly established before any opening of the pelvis. This softening of the heart allows the other segments to open more easily. Once a sense of well-being and the "I am" experience is established, it can always be found again when you are with your lover.

An injured or "broken" heart might engender sadness, longings, pity, pain, and sorrow. People who hold in their chest tend to lack energy. Remember, as in other segments, the holding goes all the way around, so the back must also be worked on. Muscle spasms or knots in the back can be released through breathing, movement, and massage.

The *diaphragm* is a broad, flat, sheetlike muscle that originates at the rib cage and attaches to the spinal column. It functionally divides the top and bottom halves of the body. The diaphragm is directly related to breathing and is relatively resistant to change. Deep diaphragmatic blocks are very common. Certain types of yoga and breathing techniques, such as those taught to professional wind instrument musicians, can armor the diaphragm.

Because its function is both automatic and controllable, the diaphragm is the best access for influencing the autonomic nervous system through breath and movement.

The diaphragm holds down "gut" feelings in the belly and sexual feelings in the pelvis, creating the split between the heart and pelvis (loving and sexual feelings) so they are not felt at the same time. With anxiety, people often hold their breath and tighten their diaphragm lowering or eliminating these uncomfortable feelings, but causing others such as pain and nausea. The emotions that are not dealt with become internalized and create stress.

Massaging under the rib cage during exhalation, and working on the intercostal muscles between the ribs and the gag reflex help to release the diaphragm. (The fish position, chapter 7, is especially useful.)

Many people hold their breath during sexual excitement, thereby lowering their charge. They push down with their diaphragm to force an orgasm, or they pull their diaphragm up, trying to refrain from releasing into orgasm. This holding cuts off feelings in the pelvis. These ways of reducing your support for aliveness are freed when the diaphragm moves without restriction.

The *abdominal segment* runs from the diaphragm to the pelvis. It is a very vulnerable and unprotected segment. Many emotions are stored here, and to avoid feeling uncomfortable in times of stress, people often tighten these muscles. The primary muscle, the rectus abdominus, should be released in a kneading manner rather than with deep pressure, because of the vital organs beneath. Don't forget that the other side of the abdomen is the back. Tightening in one side will affect the other.

Don't lean over your partner. In your eagerness to be helpful or intimate you may be tempted to say something or just to be closer, but this may impart a feeling of smothering, being pinned down or invaded in some way. This goes for women as well as for men; it has nothing to do with relative size, weight, or caring. Remember how feelings of inundation were aroused when a pillow was pushed in each person's space in the boundary exercise (chapter 3).

Cervical, Chest, Diaphragm, Abdominal Segments

Begin: Active Partner, in the basic exercise position, take a few full sighing, letting-go breaths. Now take one to three sets of ten charging breaths while rocking your pelvis. Inhale; then as you exhale, push with your feet and rock your pelvis forward. Do this breathing and rocking pattern very slowly and rhythmically. Let the rush of energy come in and spread. Continue the full letting-go breaths and rocking movements throughout the exercise.

Step 1: Guiding Partner, kneeling behind your partner's head, watch as your partner does the pelvic rock in the orgastic patterns. See if you can tell which areas of his or her body are not moving fully and easily. Watch your partner's breathing. Is there a full inhale and exhale through the mouth? Does the breath originate high in the chest? Does the pelvis move in a full rock: forward with an exhalation and back with inhalation? Are the abdominal muscles kept soft? Do your partner's feet remain firmly planted? Is your partner's upper body relaxed and flexible so that it is set in motion by the lower body movement? Does your partner's neck and head move as he or she rocks?

Note: If your partner is having a very difficult time with the orgastic pattern, the cross-crawl will help overall coordination. However, if all that is needed is further work on coordination or on enhancing the charge, movement, or openness in the segment, proceed to the next step.

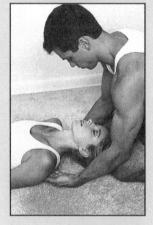

Step 3.

Step 2: Gently put your hand on any tight area you see in your partner's body to bring his or her awareness to that area. Active Partner will feel your touch and the energy from your hand. This alone may relax the tightness.

Note: This is also true when making love and dealing with the subtle and sensuous energy of the body. This energetic level, rather than the grosser physical level of actual touch, is felt even more dramatically in lovemaking.

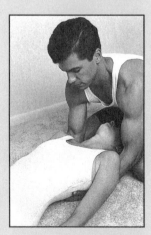

Step 4.

Step 3: Upper chest: Since a block goes all the way around the body, freeing the back releases the chest. For some people, their major holding is in their back. Place your hands under the V of your partner's armpits. At the base of the V press your fingers against the body where you will find the teres major muscle. This muscle is often tender to the touch. Ask your partner to breathe to expand his or her back. Active Partner, breathe against the pressure of your partner's fingers several times until your back begins to move freely with your breath.

Step 4: Upper chest: Guiding Partner, shift your hands to the center upper back of your partner, just between the shoulder blades. These rhomboid muscles are the ones that are often in knots. Active Partner, again use your sense of your partner's hands as a focus to breathe into your back.

Step 5: Upper chest: Guiding Partner, massage the upper chest just above the breasts, remembering that these pectoralis muscles, which are often quite tense, may be tender as well. This will help your partner feel where to let go. You can't force anyone to let go, so don't try. Just massage enough to help him or her become aware of the tension and holding there. As you work on these tight areas, notice if Active Partner's breathing becomes deeper and the body becomes more relaxed. A rocking motion on the whole shoulder or intermittent pressure works better than forcing your way through the muscle.

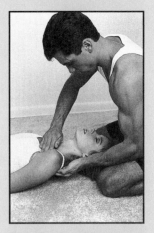

Step 5.

Note: If you are working with a woman, be careful of mammary tissues. Not only might they be tender and the tissues subject to damage, but, without an agreement to be sexual, it can feel invasive.

If you're working with a man, remember that these are very heavy muscles. Even if you are nearly the same size, you might have to add quite a bit of pressure to be effective. By working firmly on these muscles, you will assist him in beginning to use his chest better in his breathing pattern and in loving.

Step 6: Upper chest: Rest two hands, palms flat, on Active Partner's upper chest just below the clavicle bone. Again, avoid the mammary tissue. Start by moving your hands easily, following the inhalation and exhalation rhythm of your partner.
a) After you get a sense of your partner's breathing pattern, inhale, then wait for your partner's exhale. As you and your partner exhale together, press with your hands to the bottom of the breath. Use just enough pressure to give your partner a feeling of wanting to express more air for a longer period than usual. Encourage Active Partner to let go in this area, expelling the air completely and allowing the tension to release with it. Don't try to break through the holding pattern; if you push too hard your partner will just have to tighten more to protect from injury. Do this three times.

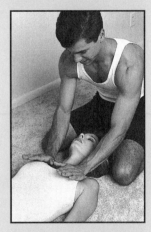

Step 6.

b) Switch to pressing with your hands each time your partner *inhales*. This gives your partner resistance to push his or her breath against. Do this three times.
c) Follow your partner's breath with the pressure of your hands to the bottom of the exhale and *maintain the pressure* for *two* inhalation breaths. Release the pressure *quickly* at the beginning of the third inhalation. As the muscles for breathing are still straining against imagined pressure, it will cause your partner to take a fuller breath. Repeat this series two or three times. Active partner will probably feel greatly relieved in her or his chest—freer, lighter, able to take fuller breaths—and find it easier to breathe.

Step 7: Shoulder: Move to Active Partner's side. Sit or kneel. When you complete this series, you will be reminded to move to the other side.

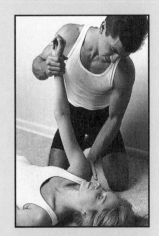

Step 7.

Place your left hand firmly under your partner's shoulder. Then take hold of your partner's arm with two hands. Shake the arm so that the shoulder moves. Move the arm up and down and in circles. See if, with movement, you can break up the rigid holding patterns of the shoulder and upper back and chest. Active Partner, see if you can become totally passive and relaxed, allowing your partner to move your arm for you. At the beginning, the arm may move as if all the muscles were one solid mass. By shaking, the muscles can individuate, let go, and become more alive and flexible.

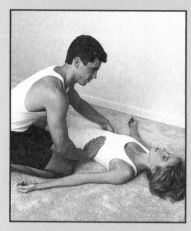

Step 8.

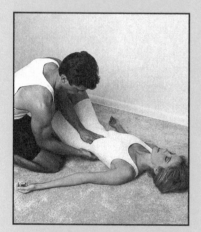

Step 9.

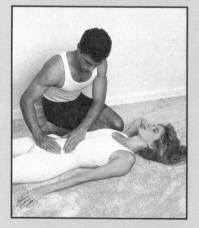

Step 11.

Step 8: Lower Chest: Next, place your left hand under partner's back and rib cage, and your right hand on top of the lower-chest and rib cage. This area is constricted in many people and doesn't move easily. As Active Partner exhales, pull and press up with the left hand and push away and press down with the right. Release pressure on inhalation. On each exhale, add a little pressure through your hands, encouraging her or him to let go, to let the air out completely. Think of your hands as holding a ball of energy. As you continue, add more motion, rock, shake, and bounce to free the rigidity of the holding pattern.

Step 9: Diaphragm: Now bring the side of your left hand to the bottom of the rib cage. Use your right hand under your partner's ribs to support and hold the area. Again, feel the ball of energy between your hands. With each exhale, press down gently but firmly under the ribs with your right hand. From the outer perimeter of the body to the center and back, press just enough for Active Partner to feel the tight muscles; then let go. Press with each exhale and, easing the pressure with each inhale, continue to move your hand to find the tight spots. Active Partner, with each exhalation, see if you can let go of the tight muscles. Guiding Partner, as the muscles loosen, you will be able to press your fingers further under the ribs. This is a good way to relieve tension in the diaphragm. Once open, the chest may close again and breathing patterns may become constricted. You might have to come back to portions of this exercise.

Step 10: Abdomen: The abdomen holds many delicate organs and is the seat of many emotions, and tightness can result in distress and physical disorders. Move in slowly with your hands, and massage with clockwise circular motions. If you feel tight, hard spots, hold your fingers still against them to heighten your partner's awareness. Ask your partner to breathe and to try to let go of the holding by relaxing from the inside with each exhalation.

Step 11: Abdomen in orgastic pattern: For those who have difficulty moving their pelvis without using abdominal muscles, this exercise may help. With both hands take hold of the two long muscles that run up and down the abdomen from under the rib cage to the pelvis, the rectus abdominus muscles. Holding them firmly, slightly lift and then shake them back and forth. The Active Partner can then try rocking his or her pelvis while you immobilize these muscles by holding them. Although this can be very effective in the letting go of a pelvic holding pattern, it is not a particularly easy technique to do. Fortunately, the bodies that usually need this release the most are those with highly developed rectus abdominus muscles. With this muscled abdomen, the muscles are easier to feel, handle, and manipulate.

Step 12: Move to active partner's other side and repeat steps 7, 8, and 9.

THE LAST SEGMENT to work with is the pelvis. All the segments of the body are directly associated with psychological and emotional patterns, but none compares in intensity to those stored in the pelvis: sexuality, eroticism, desire, trust, vitality, empowerment, and freedom. The holding in the pelvic region is intricately entwined with all the other segments and subject to our moment-to-moment emotional body-mind state. No amount of physical or emotional prodding, begging, or force can sustain the openness of the pelvis. If any of the other segments of the body are shut down, the risk of the pelvis closing is inevitable. Yet, the body can be made malleable again given the proper conditions such as are set in *The Intimate Couple* exercises. Like with the other segments, pelvic holding has a reason. Opening the pelvis is not difficult. But, keeping it that way is, unless you also deal with the cause of the holding.

Actually, you have been working with pelvic release from the beginning of the first exercises. The breathing and movement work, developing the "I am" sense of well-being and mutuality, working with all the previous segments, the psychological issues of self and relationship—all provide a foundation for sustaining pelvic opening and sexual awakening.

Pelvic blocks are caused by emotional and/or physical trauma. Sexual abuse at any age can cause the pelvis to close, while lesser known body-mind traumas are due to childhood enemas, early toilet training, and almost any continual boundary infringement. Toilet training before the sphincter control is attained at about eighteen months of age, requires the contraction of contiguous muscles of the thighs, buttocks, a pulling up of the pelvic floor as well as respiratory inhibition. Punishment for sexual curiosity or masturbation as a child often creates a similar holding pattern as the child tries to avoid feeling sexual desire or turns to secrecy. For women, the primary site for holding emotional tension is in the uterus. This can cause a block and the resulting lack of desire. For both men and women, a fear of pregnancy or a previous abortion (no matter how long ago), an inability to sustain comfortable limits sexual or otherwise with a partner, a lie in the relationship, either partner having an affair, gender prejudice, are all examples of themes that can cause pelvic blocks and an array of sexual dysfunctions. Blocks successfully diminish natural emotional and erotic sensations in the pelvis and expression. There are an infinite number of causes for why our bodies become inhibited as we grow up. Almost everyone has some holding in their pelvis. Yet, we most surely did not come into the world holding back our aliveness or our sexuality. Nor do we have to stay that way.

Pelvic Segment: Moving Energy

When you've gotten this far with the exercises and your partner is breathing fully, you are ready to begin the pelvic movements. With the breathing and movement patterns going easily, you are probably feeling tingling sensations.

Begin: Active Partner, lie on your back in the basic exercise position. Keep your knees up and arms along the sides of your body, palms down.

Step 1: Guiding Partner, check your partner's position; then, kneeling between his or her legs, place your knees so that they press slightly against the buttocks.

Note: If this position makes either person uncomfortable, deal with the interruption. Most likely there is an intimacy problem. It may have to do with an old injury, speed limits, boundaries, or character style. Whatever the origin, you must be able to trust and be close to one another or you can't really go any further. If you can continue exercising, find time later to read the psychological chapters and write in your journal about the discomfort. Talk to your partner about it later.

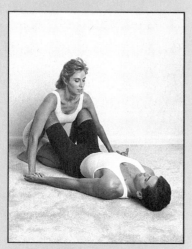

Step 2.

Step 2: Knees: Guiding Partner, make contact by placing the palms of your hands on your partner's knees and take about three sets of ten full charging breaths. Shuttle back to yourself. Allow both your own and your partner's breathing patterns to settle. Make eye contact and pay attention to your own feelings. Close your eyes. At the bottom of your breath, in your body, find your sense of well-being and the "I am" body experience. When you find it, from this feeling, be the lover and send love to your partner for a moment or two.

Step 3.

Step 3: Hands, Radial Pulse: Turn Active Partner's hands over and place your fingertips on the radial pulse of each wrist. You may have to place your arms either around or through your partner's legs. Do not lean over your partner's body any more than necessary, as this can feel very inundating. Shift slightly forward so your body weight places some pressure through your hands. Take your time until you can feel the throbbing of Active Partner's pulse. Take ten more breaths. Find your "I am" feeling.

Step 4: When you can detect the throbbing of the life force in both wrists, allow yourself to experience this energy. Then, breathe and *silently* send love to your partner through your fingertips. Notice whether your character style is interfering with your ability to feel the love or to send it. If you find that you are willing to send the love, let your partner know by saying, "Sending."

Step 5: Active Partner, when your partner sends love, see if you can find a way to take it in. How does your character style or agency deal with love coming toward you? If you are willing to take in the love, say "Receiving."

Step 6: Feet: Guiding Partner, firmly place the palms of your hands on the top of the feet of Active Partner. Use some of your body weight to place pressure. Hold for a few minutes. Then again, if you are willing to send love, let your partner know by saying, "Sending." Your partner can respond by saying, "Receiving."

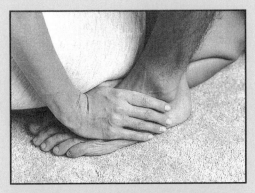

Step 6.

Step 7: Heels: Cup your hands around both heels, thumb on one side and fingers on the other. Squeeze and hold. Again, if you are willing, send and receive love.

Note: Any difficulty with your partner's breathing pattern may be due to this new position. Just sit comfortably and wait for a few moments. Remember, there is no hurry. Usually the breathing will just start again.

If your partner continues to have difficulty breathing, have him or her do about one to three sets of ten of high-charge breathing. This is one of the best ways to increase energy flow rapidly. Then pause for a moment and repeat.

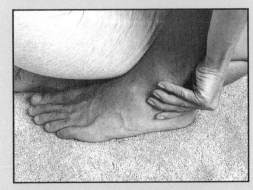

Step 7.

Pelvic Segment: Freeing the Orgastic Pattern

Guiding Partner remains in kneeling position between the legs of Active Partner, who remains in the basic exercise position. Because mastering the pelvic rotation is imperative for improving sex and aliveness, a number of exercises are provided for your use. Try them all; they each have something additional for your pelvic opening. See which helps you most and use that one for future release.

Step 1: Thigh-Pull Rock: Place your hands on Active Partner's knees. Now slip your hands down to the top of his or her thighs.

Step 2: Pull back toward yourself and release, causing your partner to feel an assisted and exaggerated pelvic rock. Continue the assisted rock until your partner gets a good feel of the rocking motion.

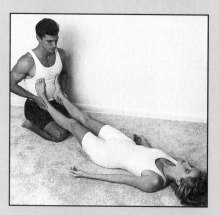

Step 1.

Step 3: Active Partner, continue this rocking motion on your own by pushing with your feet. See if you can "let go." (Guiding Partner, don't help.) Keeping your body loose, feel how easily your pelvis rocks when you are not being psychologically or habitually resistant. This gives your body new knowledge, a new memory. If you are having difficulty, most likely it's your character style keeping you stuck. Try telling your partner, "I'm going to learn this even if you want me to," or "even if I want to," whichever feels most true.

Step 4: Straight-Leg Rock: If Active Partner can't continue this rocking motion on his or her own, stand up or kneel, and pick Active Partner's legs up by the ankles. (Be careful of your own back.) Keeping your partner's legs straight, place his or her feet against your chest, stomach, or thighs and push-pull with both your hands and body motion to create a full-body rock. This will impart the body feeling and memory of a naturally synchronized upper and lower body orgastic pattern.

Step 4.

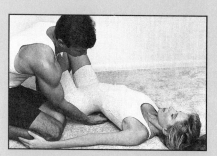

Step 6A.

Step 5: Active Partner, practice the pelvic rock on your own with full breaths, staying present and in contact. Because the charge has the potential for going much higher at this point, expect interruptions: physiological, relational, and emotional. Remember to elongate the inhale for a fuller rotation of your pelvis. Then elongate the exhale or the letting-go breath while pushing with the feet, causing the pelvis to tip forward more toward the head.

Step 6: Pelvic-Guide from Side for Fuller Rotation: Guiding Partner, move to Active Partner's side, the right side if you are right-handed, the left side if you are left-handed. Place your hand under the small of your partner's back, at the waist. **(a)** Instruct Active Partner to press her or his back against your hand with each exhale. **(b)** As he or she inhales, apply pressure to the back by lifting your hand and causing the back to arch. Doing this greatly enhances the full rotation of movement, which in turn enhances erotic feelings during sex.

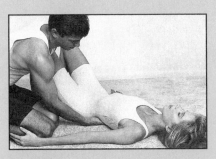

Step 6B.

Step 7: Buttocks: An aspect that hasn't yet been discussed is the common holding pattern in the buttocks and anus. Place your hand directly under the coccyx or tailbone. You will feel muscles around and just below this point. Squeeze these muscles by pressing your fingers toward the palm of your hand. As you squeeze and shake your hand a bit, encourage Active Partner to let go in the anus as he or she rocks and breathes. Don't try to force the muscles to let go. Just bring the awareness of the muscles to your partner.

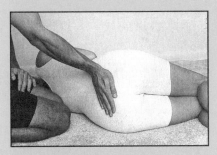

Step 7 (hand placement).

Step 8: To encourage a letting-go in the buttocks, touch any tight muscles to bring awareness to them. You can also shake or rock the tight muscle. Again, encourage partner to let go.

Note: The movement in this series is slow and is to be done very smoothly. Concentrate on it for three to five minutes, doing the movement and the breathing, and with Active Partner making an almost inaudible sound on the exhale…back and forth…keeping the stomach soft, breathing out as the pelvis comes forward toward the head and the lumbar area of the spine presses into the floor. As the energy rises you'll find that your partner's breathing pattern may change again.

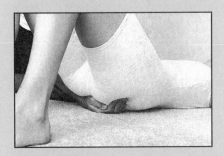

Step 7.

Step 9: Both of you should be breathing in unison at this time. If you feel as though your breath is tightening, your partner's probably is, too. Concentrate on getting your partner's breath going fully and easily again. The pelvis should move easily each time a breath is taken—back with the inhalation and forward with the exhalation.

Step 10: After a while you can begin to encourage your partner to emphasize and accentuate this movement, elongating and deepening the breath, elongating the rock of the pelvis so that it swings in a fuller arch. Keep in mind that no one can bring energy into the body from the outside; the actual energy and movement has to originate from within.

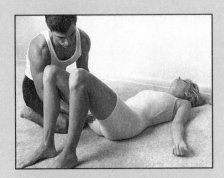

Step 8.

Pelvic Segment: Freeing the Orgastic Pattern (continuation of 6)

Begin: Active Partner begins the orgastic pattern, moving pelvis with feet, keeping the stomach soft and the breath synchronized with pelvic movement. Guiding Partner, return to kneeling between your partner's legs and place your hands on his or her thighs near the knees.

Step 1: Guiding Partner, to assist the pelvic movement, apply a pulling-back pressure to Active Partner's legs.

Step 2: Pelvic Bridge: Active Partner, breathe in and, with the exhale, lift or "bridge" your pelvis off the floor slowly, one vertebra at a time, as you did in chapter 7. Use your feet, legs, and buttock muscles to lift your body, not your stomach muscles. Focus on your feet, making sure that your full foot, toe to heel, is firmly planted and pressing on the floor as you lift your pelvis. Make sure your feet are parallel. Raise your hips as high as possible and hold your pelvis in this position for a few moments while taking ten full charging breaths.

Guiding Partner, maintain pressure on Active Partner's thighs as he or she inhales and lifts; ease pressure with the exhale. Watch to see if breaths originate in the upper chest. Make sure the abdominal muscles are soft and relaxed. If they are not, use your body to put more pressure on your partner's feet and legs.

On the last breath, lower pelvis down one vertebra at a time. Do this lift series three times. If you have a high enough charge, you will feel the energy from your pelvis go down your legs to your feet and back up again.

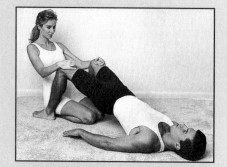

Step 2.

Step 3: A more advanced position is to rock your pelvis while in the raised position, without tightening abdominal muscles. Don't do this if you are not in excellent physical condition. It can cause strain. In this raised position, see if you can do the pelvic rock with your breath synchronized. Shift the "origin" of your breath down to your genital area as you did in the original exercise. Imagine that your breath is drawn in and expelled through your genitals as you move. Take two sets of five breaths, exhaling when your pelvis rocks forward toward your head and inhaling when it rocks back. Then just hold the up position.

While holding the up position, your pelvis may vibrate or bounce. Allow this to happen. It is merely a natural reaction to muscles letting go. When you are ready to roll down, do so slowly, one vertebra at a time, starting at your neck. All this time, your partner can encourage the feeling of grounding by pulling back and pushing down on your legs.

Step 4: Active Partner, if you don't feel a high charge in your pelvis—one that streams to your legs and feet—do the strap and ball exercise from chapter 7 with your partner putting pressure on your legs. Your charge must be high to feel the streaming. If your charge is not very high in your chest, also do the fish position from chapter 7. Then go back and do the pelvic lift again.

Step 5: Towel Rock: Guiding Partner, move to your partner's head. Roll up a small, thin towel lengthwise, placing the center behind Active Partner's head. Bring the ends of the towel up around the head, being careful of the ears. Overlap the ends to create a handle.

With your hands on the towel, use a gentle, intermittent, pull-release motion to cause your partner's whole body to rock. The rock originates with the head but, if Active Partner is relaxed, his or her whole body will follow. Active Partner, allow your partner to create the rocking motion. Don't assist. Soften your jaw and the back of your throat. Just let yourself feel the freeing motion.

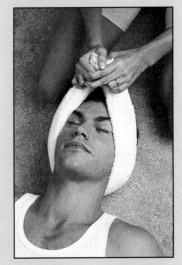

Step 6.

Step 6: Active Partner, once your body moves freely for a minute or two, begin to add to the rocking motion by pushing with your feet. Use your feet to activate your pelvis while your partner continues to assist with the intermittent pull-release motion.

Active Partner, it is best not to talk about your experience right away as this can interfere with the somatic presence and integration that is taking place. See how long you can maintain your newfound openness and charge. When you lose it, you now know a number of ways to get it back. The releases in your body and new insights will continue well after you have completed this series of exercises. You may also find that your dream life is far more active. Write about these experiences in your journal.

Set a later time for you to guide your partner through these body-opening, enlivening exercises.

PSYCHOLOGICAL INTERRUPTIONS
for the
INTIMATE COUPLE

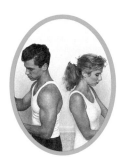

CHAPTER ELEVEN
Arena 1: Primary Scenario

THE PRIMARY
SCENARIO ARENA

SO POWERFUL IS THE IMPRINT of your childhood experience that throughout your lifetime you carry its lessons, which are inextricably locked into your body and manifested in unconscious habitual patterns of behavior. These aspects of yourself, long kept in the shadows, are so closely identified as self that you may not be aware of them. Yet others see your repetitive patterns only too well because they continually have to contend with them. They are not just replications of childhood, but distant echoes, distorted reflections, and metaphorical paraphrases. As Louise Kaplan has so perceptively put it, "The maturing adult is continually reliving and revising his memories of childhood, refinding his identity, reforging the shape of his selfhood, discovering new facets of his being." (Kaplan, *Oneness and Separateness*, 1987)

No one has survived childhood—no matter how loving and supportive, or how damaging their family life—without some emotional injury, habitual patterns or themes, beliefs and assumptions, and unsatisfied longings that can affect their sexual relationships. No matter how committed and long-term the relationship, both you and your partner are bound to have old wounds that bleed through into the present, especially in the bedroom.

SECRET THEMES

FROM YOUR CHILDHOOD whole primary scenario motifs can emerge as "secret" themes that haunt you like ghosts from the past. They drift through your feelings, beliefs, and assumptions about yourself and your world. Particularly when you are vulnerable—as you are in love, intimacy, and when your body is open for erotic sexuality—undermining themes can show up in the form of uncomfortable thoughts and body feelings such as panic, anxiety, fear, anger, humiliation, shame, a sense of inadequacy or danger, or just disinterest, doubt, sadness, or betrayal.

We each have certain personal themes that we use to understand our experiences. They are based upon prior experience that forms beliefs about ourselves, about others, or about life and are used to shape and create our assumptions and to explain feelings and experiences. Unconsciously, these themes can obscure reality and lead you to the same false conclusions over and over again. The dogged, incessant quality of these themes makes them feel so akin to what you think is true that you are not likely to question their validity.

Because the same conclusions are reached so often they seem like profound personal truths. *They are not*. The conclusions reached are based on badly skewed, matrix-forming lessons held in the body rather than on the truth. If you were raised by a mother who didn't trust men, the matrix for mistrust was set up in your body before you were old enough to question it. As an adult, when you are in the presence of a man, you will most likely feel a warning sensation in your body reminding you to reserve trust. This will surely alter your experience of the man. Wherever you go, a feeling in your body will constantly remind you to distrust men. These body feelings shape each relationship encounter, job, or social situation.

When themes that are the result of childhood emotional injury are evoked, they only serve to cloud our experiences and cause further emotional injury. These "themes" that follow, when left unconscious, are a consistent source of interference to your sexuality. The older you get, the louder they speak.

Some themes may have originated through your own experience, but others were inherited like unwanted heirlooms from long-forgotten relatives. Themes can even skip generations. Some are particularly destructive to intimacy and descend upon your bed to dampen your passion, rendering sexual lovemaking impossible.

This section presents common themes that can disturb anyone's sense of self and relationship. Your personal themes may be somewhat different, but part of establishing an ongoing sense of self is being aware of your own themes and how they affect you and others. If any of these themes are part of your primary scenario you probably are resurrecting fears, emotions, beliefs, and longings from old injuries and tacking them onto current life situations or people—most likely your mate. The bond of your relationship can be destroyed if you unconsciously act these themes out, project them onto another, or make them the responsibility of others. Secret themes are a threat to your sense of self, and they obscure the authenticity of your experiences.

Generational Secret Themes

These themes are passed on in families from generation to generation, since parents unconsciously do to their children what was done to them, often at exactly the same stage of development. In their own lives, children compulsively repeat their parents' prejudices, injuries, relationship blunders, and unresolved issues, interests, assumptions, and beliefs without recognizing their origins.

These inherited themes will be difficult to work through unless they are first identified and recognized as not having developed from one's own life experience. Unfortunately, once they become integrated into your perspective, you find evidence to validate the adopted themes everywhere you look. Nowhere is this more true than with gender prejudice (see chapters 2 and 8).

MY HEART BELONGS TO DADDY (MOMMY) THEME

Even to enter a relationship with someone other than a parent—much less give your heart or body to another person—is often enough to cause severe guilt and fear of hurting the parent, even if the beloved parent is deceased. If you have sex, particularly if you enjoy it, you may feel unfaithful to your parent.

When your heart belongs to Daddy or Mommy, you often glorify that parent, and everyone else pales by comparison. Childhood idealizations are often godlike, whereas in adulthood we must be able to accept the human fallibilities of those we love.

PHANTOM LOVER THEME

The origin often obscure even to the carrier, a person with this theme may carry a feeling in their body that something is wrong, which starts them thinking, "This is not the right person....I'm such a fool....I've made another mistake....I shouldn't get too close to this person because the right one will come along someday." This will certainly promote emotional and sexual distance from any current partner.

Usually initiated by the loss of a first idealized love who died, left, or was given up for a "wiser" choice—perhaps someone your parents favored—for those hexed by the theme, the fantasy of the lost love and the "perfect fit" is never relinquished. Because this idealized relationship did not last long enough for realities to emerge, the fantasy persists, assuring that no subsequent partner would ever measure up.

It is hard to build the security necessary for heightened sexuality with your current lover while actively waiting for the phantom-lover to come along. The decision to leave the relationship may always be churning just beneath the surface, or, as a victim or martyr, you may tolerate your partner. Neither allows you to commit fully to the relationship.

VICTIM-MARTYR THEME

In adopting the victim-martyr stance, a person carries a body experience of being "done to," of not being in control of situations. It is a powerful theme because it makes other people feel guilty, and they tend to give in. A victim physically must embody the symptom of weakness to be believable; thus the stance becomes a self-fulfilling prophecy. This prevents the victim from feeling empowered and from taking charge of his or her life and sexual essence. A martyr is really a victim who is proud of it.

This scenario often results in somatic symptoms, such as a depressive-like collapse of the body. Have you ever noticed that a person who acts like a victim looks like one? If you assume this stance, you probably are not the only one in your family who knows how to play this game. If you are a victim, everyone and everything in life is a perpetrator. To break the bonds of this theme and empower yourself, you must simply ask yourself, "How else can I look at this situation so that I am not a victim?" This process may take a little diligence and practice, but the results can be life altering.

OUT OF CONTROL THEME

When you have been raised in a household plagued with alcoholism, drug abuse, bizarre or out-of-control behavior, severe depression, suicide, near-death experience, physical or emotional illness or abuse, or in wartime, you will often carry in your body a sense of impending crisis. To compensate for this body feeling, you may have become overly controlled and controlling, particularly around sex and, explicitly, orgasm—a paradox since orgasm is a letting go of control. The body experience keeps people from realizing that their problem, rather than lack of control, *is one of over-control*. People who are over-controlled often have very "tight" bodies, which decreases the amount of excitement that can be generated. The tight body makes you afraid of letting go, and the fear of letting go makes your body tight. It is a circular, closed experience.

Being in control is an illusion. You can be in charge of your life but rarely in control. When you try to be in control, your attention is drawn away from your core body sense of self and you may become in reaction to everything in your environment. Use the sustaining integration exercises in chapter 7, along with the steps out of fragmentation in chapter 15, to calm the physical and emotional feelings of crisis in your body and sustain a sense of well-being.

Birth Secret Themes

Some themes are formed surrounding issues of our birth and infancy, sometimes even in the womb. Formed at such an early, preverbal time, they are like a background voice in your unconscious, a hum in your body. They are rarely specific to one area of life and are usually generalized feelings of self that extend to one's body and sexuality. These themes are less likely to go away than generational themes, and it is best to learn how to live with them.

The first step is in realizing that these themes reveal what happened to you through your parents, i.e., *they* didn't want a child. The next step is to remember that the recurrent feeling you have about yourself is just a memory of a past emotional injury, not a statement of your worth. Each time the feeling recurs, you can remind yourself that it is natural for your body to remind you of how you felt as a child when you sustained the emotional injury. Witnessing your feelings in this way allows you to make a conscious decision to spare yourself from indulging in the old negative emotions still one more time.

Unwanted Child Theme

Being wanted is a feeling in your body. If you pay attention you always know whether you were wanted, who wanted you, and why. It registers as a truth in your body and is sometimes different from what you were told.

When a baby is not planned, when there are financial difficulties, when the timing is wrong, when the parents are too young or not married or already have too many children, an unwanted child theme may result. If you were unwanted at conception or at birth—even if your parents loved you and gave you a good home—you may be uncomfortable in social situations and, particularly, in intimate relationships. You may wonder, "Am I really part of this relationship, team, or organization?" People who were not wanted at birth can become leaders and yet feel unaccepted. With an ardent lover who cherishes you, you may find false "evidence" of rejection.

Wrong Gender Theme

If your parents or grandparents desperately hoped that you would be a boy and you turned out to be a girl, or vice versa, you have probably spent a lifetime not feeling quite good enough, no matter how much you excelled or how much you were loved by your family. This perceived rejection of the core of your being can cause you to feel defective and be critical of yourself, and it can lead you, in part, to mimic culturally defined characteristics of the opposite gender. If you are trying to be other than who you are, no matter what you try or how successful you are or how good sex is, you will not feel a sense of satisfaction. You can't get rid of the uncomfortable feeling in your body by behavioral change. This does not necessarily have to do with sexual orientation.

Defective Product Theme

If something happened to you at birth or as a result of a childhood illness or injury, and your family treated it as a defect, you may carry the feeling that there is something wrong with you. Often the original "defect" is healed or long forgotten, but a vague discomfort remains that something about you is embarrassing and must be hidden or fixed. Since the "defective product" is an ongoing body feeling, it can get channeled to your sexuality as, for example, a feeling that your genitals are defective. You can always find evidence to match your body feeling. And because of this you may feel unworthy and unlovable when someone loves you and test their love to the breaking point.

More Early Abandonment Themes

Any separation or loss of a birth parent, particularly birth mother, can cause a severe breach in the building of a continuous feeling of security (constancy) in a child. When abandoned, children always think that they caused the problem—that they did something bad or that they are inherently defective or unworthy—which may result in a person prone to severe anxiety around any form of separation. (See appendix for Living with Abandonment Anxiety.) Those that carry the vague feeling in their body that they are bad, often compensate by being overly giving and caretaking.

ILLNESS THEME

A severe illness or hospitalization of either parent or the child can cause severe abandonment anxiety if it occurs during the first months or years of a child's life. In adulthood, new upsets can bring back all the fears and emotions of this early experience, which can cause regression to infantile states such as staring at your fingers or hands, sleeping in a fetal position and pulling up the covers to simulate the womb, making preverbal sounds, feeling you are going to die, or clinging to people or things. Releasing into orgasm can liberate these feelings and feel terrifying if not understood. The fear is of dropping into these early feelings of loss or annihilation that you once lived through.

ADOPTION THEME

Adopted children, or children otherwise not with their birth-parents, often describe a lifelong theme of searching for "the right one," "the right thing," always searching, longing—even if it was not until they were adults that they learned they were adopted. A child spends nine months with the birth mother's rhythm and energy and, once born, is comforted most readily by the familiarity of this rhythm and energy. If the birth mother is not available a substitute will have to do, but the longing remains, at least unconsciously, even if the adoptive parents are wonderful, very loving, and desperately want the child. A child has a strong link to the birth-father as well, even if he never participates in any way other than conception. These early separations cause longings in the body for completion, which repeat throughout life. Like others afraid of abandonment, adopted children often crave consistent sexuality even if satisfaction is not there.

DEATH OF A PARENT THEME

Children who lose one or both parents at birth or during early childhood suffer profound loss and grief. If no one helped them deal with their loss, they will usually, unconsciously, feel that they did something wrong to cause abandonment. This leads them to be excessively careful for the rest of their lives for fear of hurting yet another person and being abandoned again. The loss of self that often accompanies this level of abandonment fear can severely inhibit the sense of security needed for heightened states of sexuality.

SEXUAL SECRET THEMES:
INCEST, RAPE,
MOLESTATION

THESE INJURIES ARE SEVERE violations and, of course, can profoundly affect the lives of both men and women in many ways. The actual event is often a travesty against our morals, our body, our core sense of self, our spiritual sense of equality and humanity. The pain of the event and its lessons are carved indelibly into our body memory.

A sexual molestation perpetrated by parents or others who were loved or trusted is more emotionally injurious than if it were done by a stranger. The questions forever held in the body are: If I could not trust someone who should have been most concerned for my well-being, can I ever trust anyone I am close to again? Do I have the right to boundaries with others? Does my body belong to me? Can I ever feel love and be sexual without having to relive the feelings of abuse? Am I always supposed to comply and give everything to be loved? Am I bad or soiled? Am I bad when I feel sexual, and will this feeling get me into trouble? These questions and many others always become associated with intimacy and sexuality and lead to constant nagging fears of yet another emotional betrayal.

Surrounding the event are other implied questions: Was there anyone trustworthy you could talk to or did you have to keep your pain and fears a secret? Did you receive comfort, protection, or help to express your feelings and put them in some perspective? If you told about the molestation, were you believed? Were you made to feel bad about yourself or blamed in any way? Where were your parents or guardians? Were they more concerned about what other people would think than about you?

When there is any type of emotional injury in childhood, particularly when it is of a sexual nature, your primary task is to come to terms emotionally with this past injury so that it does not interfere with your sense of well-being and the ability to live a full and healthy life. With this task in mind, *it is imperative to deal with any underlying themes that were reactivated separate from the sexual nature of the trauma.* Shifting your focus to the underlying themes allows more possibility for resolution and frees sexuality so that this special joining can be reserved for the joy of true lovers.

We each bring our own set of unresolved childhood wounds and issues to any trauma. That is why the experience and resolution is unique to the individual.

These underlying themes hark back to the earliest patterns of emotional betrayal by caretakers. Our earliest childhood experiences scream in our bodies for understanding and resolution with every altercation, developmental transition, and trauma experienced later. The early injury may seem quite different from the current dilemma; *yet its themes provide clues and the possibility for resolution. Difficulties in adult sexual relationships are usually caused more by the fragmenting reenactment of the early emotional wounds than by the molestation itself.* If you couldn't tell or be supported or saved by your caretakers, then the molestation was yet another example of nonsupport or lack of caring, safety, and respect for your physical and emotional boundaries.

Therefore, it is important for you to identify the themes you carry from childhood and consciously come to terms with them. You will find the clues for identifying these themes throughout the psychological chapters and, more specifically, in the secret themes. Reviewing your history using the questions supplied in the appendix will help you to clarify and organize your themes. The scars of a molestation can best be addressed by simultaneously working with the event, your psychological family themes, and your body.

When trust is undermined because of underlying molestation themes, it can continue to haunt loving sexual relationships. This is because when the body opens with love and sexuality, old body memories come to the surface. Sometimes these memories are projected onto a partner and may cause you to feel that old injustices are once again happening. Other times these memories may cause you to feel so badly about yourself that you fail to stop new injuries from happening. Once you establish a somatic sense of yourself by doing the exercises in chapter 7, you will be more aware of the difference between past and present experience. The body is the main source for making sense of it, letting it go, and most importantly for renewing your sense of self.

Work in your journal. You don't necessarily have to forgive, but you must be able to come to terms with any childhood injury. You may not eliminate the scar, but the old event can lose enough of its power that the associations no longer define current reality. Remember, it is not what happens to you, but what you do with what happens to you, that determines your sense of self and your ability to be in a trusting, loving, erotically sexual relationship. If the old injury continues to interfere with your current life, you may need a competent body psychotherapist who is trained to work with all three components: the early primary scenario injury themes; your physical, energetic holding patterns; and the actual sexual molestation itself.

Although more young girls are molested than young boys, we are less aware of the scars to males. An inappropriate "sexual introduction," made with the intention of providing a passage into masculinity, can introduce a boy to sexuality far beyond his ability to handle it. Sex can never be a badge of masculinity.

These frustrating secret themes are body examples of a closed circular system that perpetuates itself. It is important not to identify overly with any trauma, for it is not who you are; it is part of the picture. These themes may originate in the nursery, but once established they are locked in the body as a belief, attitude, or assumption and can easily result in withdrawal, either from the mutuality of a relationship or from one's core sense of self. However, people can make peace with these secret themes if they realize that they are just ghosts from the past, that they can end their torturing effects in the present by dealing with them.

We have given you many things to think about concerning your personal history and its ramifications. It is now time to put all of this into some sort of context or format that will enable you to see yourself and your history in a new light. "The Narrative History of Your Primary Scenario" in the appendix will help you in coming to terms with your interior world.

Themes for Emotional Maturity

To feel mature emotionally, you must be able to feel yourself as separate and whole: become conscious of the themes your parents have passed on to you; not expect your parents (or anyone else for that matter) to "parent" you; come to terms with your issues from the nursery so that they no longer haunt you in the present; and refrain from using what happened to you as a child as an excuse for your behavior today.

Individuation is a body-mind experience of adult emotional health and maturity. It does not mean leaving town and never seeing your parents again; it means seeing them with a life of their own, as people who were living and coping with their own dilemmas during your upbringing. With individuation you can be close to others—parents, lovers, friends—without a childlike dependency or fear of loss of self. Here are ways you can explore the experience of separateness and wholeness. Use your journal.

1. Become separate from your parents.

Identify what happened to you in childhood, both positively and negatively, and update your story. Become aware of your parents' story and see them as people separate from your needs.

Realize that they no longer have the power over you they once had. Realize that you are the one who now makes the choices in your life, even when you choose not to choose.

body-mind awakening

2. Forgive your parents or come to terms with that which is unforgivable.

Realize your parents did the best they could do, given their personal limitations. Recast your story so that you are no longer a victim. Express your resentments in your journal. Then turn your resentments into appreciations, i.e., "I resent that you were never around. . . . I appreciate that, because you were never around, I was able to learn how to take care of myself and become independent."

3. Admit that what was once done to you, you are probably now doing to yourself and to others.

In your journal, identify what you now do to others and/or yourself that was once done to you by your parents. If what you are doing is abusive, stop. There is no excuse for abusive behavior, especially to yourself.

4. Accept that there is pain in life and in the world that you cannot avoid or change.

There are parts of yourself that you are uncomfortable with and embarrassed to admit. There are some things you cannot change that you just have to learn to live with. Life is not always fair. Your childhood memories and longings are held in your body and will never completely go away. Pain and painful experiences are an inevitable part of life.

CHAPTER TWELVE

Arena 2: Character Style

IF YOU HAVE A HIGH LEVEL of abandonment anxiety, moving closer to someone you care about will temporarily relieve any fears and discomfort felt in your body. If you have a high level of inundation anxiety, creating distance will temporarily relieve the distress. But if you have a high level of both anxieties, you are liable to feel immobilized, unable to move either way without triggering one anxiety or the other. Whether you feel both anxieties or you alternate between them, together they create more anxious feelings in the body than most people can tolerate and still remain present.

To cope with these anxieties, we create character styles, or protective ways of being. To the degree that you act out the traits of your character style, you build a facade or barrier to core self-experience and intimacy. And, when a couple plays tug of war—one battling for closeness and the other for breathing room—attunement and mutuality are nowhere to be found.

Your character style, developed in childhood as a protection for the core body self, now acts as a mask worn to face the world. Thus your character style is displayed for all to see, while your core self yearns to be known and touched.

As If Character Style

People who struggle with both abandonment and inundation anxieties—the *As If* character style—can usually remember a time in childhood when they first realized that being who they were was not gaining them the love, respect, and nurturing that they needed. To hide their presumed flaws they acted as if they were their adopted pseudo-personality. Some simply rebelled; others went along with their parents' picture of how they ought to be, borrowed a fantasy character from the screen, a storybook, television, or any image that they thought would enhance their desirability.

After a while they could no longer tell the difference between acting and just being themselves. Now, no matter how well they do, their *As If* facade keeps them distant from themselves and everyone else, and they don't feel real. When they are loved, they don't truly believe it because, after all, it is only their facade that is loved.

If you never dare let anyone see who you are behind

body-mind awakening

your facade, you may vehemently defend your right to do everything your way—even when it doesn't work—for fear that others will discover that you don't know who you are. Thus, you may find yourself defending who you aren't and never were, against who you are and want so much to be. Without an inner somatic sense of self for support, a person is left forever trying to figure out how to be. A false self always feels precarious. Like a balloon, it might burst or deflate if anyone comes too close with a sharp word or offers an authentic touch that breaches the protective coating and reveals the real self. Without a body commitment to authenticity there is little hope for sustaining a heightened body experience of aliveness and sexuality.

As one brilliant attorney said, "I feel as if I live in a double-walled glass bubble. I rarely allow information to come through the second wall, so I never have to respond with my emotions or being. The problem is I rarely touch others or feel touched. Most of the time I feel isolated and alone."

CHARACTER STYLES are not pathological, but are ordinary human behaviors. To help you identify parts of yourself that would otherwise take years of soul searching or therapy, Jerry, Lena, and Harold will provide examples. Their character styles are quite high and yours may be more subtle. After each story, you will find a self-survey for identifying your own characteristics. Remember, any style can disrupt or even destroy intimacy, and even one's life. You can use the examples and surveys to identify ways of being that cause difficulty in your intimate relationship. Only your body knows which traits and examples are important and true for you. As you read the profiles, you may feel seen and understood for the first time in your life.

Styles vary both in terms of *range,* whether you veer more toward fears of abandonment or toward inundation, and level of *intensity,* the degree your style is felt and acted out. Your range is fairly permanent, but the intensity, the variable that creates the barrier, can change.

Fill out all three character style profiles as all have traits that will be familiar to you and no one completely fits any style. They are meant, not to categorize or label, but to help you discover parts of yourself that are so automatic you don't notice them. When you read about a hidden part of yourself that is difficult to accept you may feel excited, anxious, angry, hungry, sleepy, bored, or spacey. No one style is better or worse than another.

With recognition, acceptance, a reawakening of authenticity in your body, and by learning skills for lowering your character style, you will have less need to act out your defensive barrier. When you can muster a little humor toward your and your partner's character styles, attunement will grow.

BECAUSE HE DID NOT HAVE a close bond with his parents, Jerry has a typical "high abandonment" frailty about him and feels that nothing is ever quite enough. Forming and maintaining a bond is his major focus in relationships.

"Although I don't always act on my feelings, I get so upset when Dolly won't let me know where she is, what she is thinking, feeling, wanting, or doing. Or if she is late or changes her mind, I feel devastated, as if she has gone away forever, and I wonder 'What's the use?' I will do almost anything so Dolly won't leave me."

Jerry spends an inordinate amount of time, energy, thought, and work focusing on their relationship trying to get Dolly to reassure him of her love. "I like a lot of sex and making love for long periods of time. It's never too much. Is there anything wrong with that? I really like the second and third orgasms in a day. But it's not as good for me if we're not really making love. If Dolly isn't fully present I can't feel satisfied, no matter how much sex we have. I need her to really look at me, get in close, be with me. Even when I get what I want, it never seems quite enough."

Jerry sexualizes his emotional longings and tries to get them fulfilled by Dolly. As this is impossible, it is a setup for disappointment. This childlike quality he brings to sex doesn't sustain adult sexual excitement. He has a sense of urgency that creates anxiety around sexuality: if, when, and how he is going to get it. As his body opens with sex, it only heightens his feelings of abandonment. He then worries that Dolly won't be close again, or that she will leave or die.

The sexual-lovemaking positions he prefers are those that provide the most body and eye contact. He likes kissing, sucking, and caressing. Sex provides a sense of wholeness in his body for a short time. Hence he finds sex most pleasurable and most frustrating.

Jerry must take responsibility for his own abandonment anxiety and stop interpreting every act of God or of his partner as an abandonment. This inappropriate, self-perpetuating stance is guaranteed to erode the bond and the erotic feelings, thus making his worst fears come true.

Because his longings and emotions are on the surface, he may look more like an emotional wreck than those with other character styles, but he need not apologize for his high abandonment anxiety. Like both Lena and Harold, given the choice, Jerry would not exchange his style for another.

He has an abundance of flowing, changeable emotions. He can get close, find his own excitement, and make commitments. The psychological work he needs is primarily with boundaries, containment, tolerating his longings, building his capacity for satisfaction, and appreciating how well his personal qualities and behavior actually work for him. The Good Mother Messages and body exercises will help establish an internal base for his somatic sense of self, which he will never find in the approval of others or through accomplishments alone.

Abandonment anxiety can develop in a number of ways. Most likely Jerry received love, affection, and body-to-body contact at an early age. Then he may have been either physically, emotionally, or energetically abandoned by his birth parents. Most often abandonment is more subtle—the parent is split off and the child can't feel an energetic connection, even though the parent is doing and saying all the right things. A loss must take place very early in life to leave a person with a high abandonment anxiety, forever in fear of being left once again.

The following is the first of three surveys. The others follow Lena's and Harold's stories.

These surveys list several traits of each character style and then give examples of how each trait is commonly acted out. Cross out the *examples* that do not pertain to you. Then go back and review those that do fit, giving each a number value from one to ten: One means "this hardly pertains to me" and ten means "right on target." To average your intensity level for each trait, add the number values you have given. Then divide by the number of examples that pertained to you for that trait. This will give you a total number value for each trait. Remember, we are describing extremes; your traits may be more subtle. And keep in mind, most people rate themselves much lower than their partner rates them.

Because each example has a unique, separate body experience, take time to be aware of where and how each feels in your body. Do not believe or accept anything that you do not identify with or feel is true for you. Remember, when you look for truth, you will find it as a feeling in your body, not as a thought.

ABANDONMENT
CHARACTER STYLE
PROFILE

Trait 1. Abandoned: I Will Do Anything, Just Don't Leave Me
If you didn't get enough closeness as a child, you will:

☐ ☐ intensely focus on forming and maintaining a bond in relationship;

☐ ☐ feel abandoned, rejected, or unwanted, more often than you want to admit;

☐ ☐ get emotionally hooked by people who won't let you know where they are, what they are thinking, feeling, wanting, doing;

☐ ☐ hold on to poor relationships forever, feeling there is just one more little thing to do and then it will be perfect;

☐ ☐ get sick on vacation when you don't have your familiar pillow, pictures, toilet, or usual things to do;

☐ ☐ not be able to tolerate unfinished situations like open drawers and cupboards, or not knowing when your mate will call or the next time you will have sex;

☐ ☐ feel devastated if you have to move to another job or task, especially if you have to move to another location.

Trait 2. Eternal Longings: No Matter What, It's Never Enough
Because your longings are closer to the surface than other styles you will:

☐ ☐ always be in search of something, yet you won't know exactly for what or whom;

☐ ☐ always feel hungry or sexual. If you get the right quantity, you'll be upset about the quality;

☐ ☐ have very flowing changeable emotions, are big hearted and sensitive;

☐ ☐ have eyes that are always seeking, hoping to draw others in.

Trait 3. Few Boundaries: There's No Such Thing as Too Close
Your idea of being close is to become one, therefore you will:

☐ ☐ believe, "Because I love you, you are mine. We are one; what's yours is ours; if you really loved me you'd think and want everything I do;"

☐ ☐ interpret healthy natural separation as abandonment;

☐ ☐ not notice other people's boundaries, and if you do, you don't take them seriously; boundaries make you feel locked out, distant, and alone;

☐ ☐ without boundaries have an inability to contain thoughts, secrets, sexual energy, feelings of well-being, aliveness, or private information for long. Everything about you just seems to "leak out;"

☐ ☐ have difficulty setting limits on yourself, sometimes eat, drink, and smoke to excess. You can get addicted to things like chocolate or a lover at the drop of a hat;

☐ ☐ feel entitled to know your partner's every passing feeling, thought, movement, or fantasy. But you just have to know. Once told, you often feel betrayed by their "thought crimes," the old "…you what?" response;

☐ ☐ usually let others use you and then feel hurt or betrayed.

Trait 4. *Constellate Around Someone or Something*
Hoping to calm your longings and fear of abandonment, like a moth around a light bulb, you attach yourself. You will:

☐ ☐ throw yourself completely into anything you do; work, play, sex, or relationships;

☐ ☐ be a good support system to others, a good joiner, and work hard for other people; be easily counted on when someone needs you.

☐ ☐ usually have more than one constellation (addiction) going at a time: food, sex, love, drink, drugs, work, children, hobbies, etc.; start out on another project simultaneously, or as soon as one is finished;

☐ ☐ with sex you can wear out even the most eager of partners, or you may excessively masturbate to rawness, yet still not feel satisfied;

☐ ☐ feel like life is hopeless when your spouse doesn't want to have sex when you want to.

Trait 5. *I'm Hyper-Vulnerable and Aware of My Body*
You are so aware of everything that goes on in your body that you will:

☐ ☐ often get a stomachache, headache, cold, or other body (somatic) symptom;

☐ ☐ feel an empty sensation of rejection in your body even if you miss an elevator or your partner doesn't call or come home on time;

☐ ☐ focus on symptoms, therefore be led from one health practitioner to another to feel better.

INUNDATION
(SUPER TROUPER)
CHARACTER STYLE

LENA'S CHARACTER STYLE is based on a defense against invasion. Breathing room does not have to be fought for, it just is.

"I feel a little detached from people. I like being independent, running my life and doing as I please. I only make relationships with people like my husband, Richard, who know and respect my limits. I like to work alone, be alone. I don't care much about being emotionally close. I don't even like to be around Richard for long periods of time.

"Feelings don't seem to get in my way as they do for some people. I'm very clear about what I believe and stick with my decisions. I don't like when people are dancing around and not saying directly what they mean."

Lena often sees life in black and white and thinks concretely. If people feel hurt by her unavailability and rigid stance she thinks something is wrong with them, not with her. Lack of containment is not her problem; she holds too much inside.

Some children are born preferring more breathing room. Others build a body fortress of safety against physical abuse, being ignored, or being treated as an object. Then, closeness becomes a warning that danger is near. Children raised well, but in families that were not physically or emotionally expressive, either do not develop a comfort level with emotional closeness or just do not feel the need.

Lena acknowledges, "I can have a good orgasm, although sometimes it takes me a while, but I don't have a lot of emotion with it." It also takes her a long time to open her heart to loving feelings. If she chooses a lover with a nature similar to hers, she will find satisfaction. If, however, she chooses someone who is warm, loving, and gregarious, hoping that the association will open and soften her, make her feel more alive, she is doomed to struggle. If she wants closeness she will have to open to a deeper experience of self.

Lena's excitement comes from pushing her body to open and trying to break through to her feelings. She can learn new body opening and release positions, but the problem is really in learning to build internal sexual excitement, and that comes from softening the heart, falling in love, and opening the body. All the techniques in the world can't give Lena the courage to feel; she just has to be brave.

Fill out this survey using the same procedure you followed with the abandonment profile.

INUNDATION
CHARACTER STYLE
PROFILE

Trait 1. Separate and Removed: I Am What I Am
It's not that you dislike people, but because relationships are just not a big deal to you, you will:

☐ ☐ run your own life and do as you please. You're very independent and don't feel that you "need" others in order to feel complete;

☐ ☐ be the one others count on in an emergency to keep your head, be solid, courageous, steadfast, honest, and trusted to be who you say you are;

☐ ☐ be a team player, a good soldier, a super trouper—only sometimes doing things with others: mountain climbing, canoeing, getting projects done.

Trait 2. Cut Off from Feelings and Emotions
Emotions are just not part of your awareness, nor do they draw you towards intimacy. So you will:

□ □ not feel longings from childhood. The past is the past;

□ □ not have a lot of joy, but you also don't have a lot of sadness;

□ □ not try to get in too close or talk a lot, especially about intimate relationships;

□ □ not like to say, "I love you," because you're afraid the other person will think you want to get close.

Trait 3. Defined, Rigid Boundaries and Assumptions

Because breathing room is just your way of life, you will:

□ □ set boundaries rather rigidly and firmly;

□ □ be unconscious of the effect you have on others and often startle or offend other people;

□ □ be remarkably consistent and reliable and yet be emotionally distant and isolated;

□ □ feel like an isolated soldier as you age, fighting all the wars alone.

Trait 4. Literal, Right or Wrong, Black and White Assumptions

There is no such thing as indecision or duality. You will:

□ □ think concretely with rather rigid parameters. See everything, including people and relationships, as either good or bad. There is no in-between;

□ □ not have feelings get in the way of your thinking as they do for some people. Think, "Therapy? What's to work on? Besides, intimacy isn't important;"

□ □ like stability in your life. It turns you off when people have up-and-down mood swings;

□ □ feel betrayed when someone changes his or her mind. Once you make a decision you usually stick with it, not bothered by the burdens of abstraction, internal conflict, brooding, and rumination.

Trait 5. Physically Cut Off and Emotionally Armored

Because you cut off your emotions in your body you will:

□ □ find your emotional affect is generally flat and even;

□ □ protect yourself with a coat of armor. You can "fat," "thin," or "muscle" feelings or people out. You like the strength that comes from muscles;

□ □ hardly ever get sick, and if you do, you cut off the feelings and don't give in to weakness;

□ □ have eyes that look present yet don't let anyone in. In fact, they push others away;

□ □ build a high charge during sex without feeling much. It may take a long time to release or even have an orgasm;

□ □ not let go in your heart. There will always be a part of you that holds back. You may have sex without making love.

THE ABANDONMENT-
INUNDATION (AS IF)
CHARACTER STYLE

HAROLD HAS JERRY'S abandonment and Lena's inundation character styles, plus the special problems that the combination creates. These six additional traits establish a much greater barrier for love, intimacy, and erotic sexuality to penetrate. *Although your range and intensity may differ, Harold's dilemma is the one that most of us are faced with.*

Harold is bright, successful, good looking, witty, and charming. He looks, to others, as if he has everything going for him. However, his confusion between his character style and sense of self undermines his foundation for aliveness and interpersonal attunement.

"I want to be in a relationship, but if I get close to Felicia, I feel like she is trying to control me. Even when it feels good to be close, it doesn't last for long. I get overwhelmed by emotions; then I always seem to do something that makes Felicia angry, and she turns away from me. Then I feel unloved and try to make up. She takes everything so personally. She gets hurt all the time. She's so sensitive." Harold blames Felicia for his own problems.

He splits off, becomes intellectual, or changes the subject when he or anyone around him shows emotions, especially in sex. "When things get emotional, I get busy, change the subject, or fall asleep."

During different periods of their ten-year marriage, he and Felicia have taken turns playing the "not too close" and the "not too far away" roles. Either way, they never seem to want to be close when the other is available, so they never get together and the struggle goes on.

"I can pretend that I'm listening" says Harold, "but most of the time I can't take in what others say, particularly if the information is of an emotional, intimate nature or someone acts like an authority. It seems like they are telling me who I am, how I should be, or how I should look." Felicia complains that Harold always has a good reason why he can't or won't do whatever it is she asks.

No amount of rebellion, accomplishment, or validation fulfills Harold's search for an experience of self. He tries to calculate and control the nonrational, nonquantifiable imperfections of life. He is impatient with human frailties, feelings, suffering, softness, longings, and limitations, his own or anyone else's. He pushes himself beyond healthy limits and expects the same of others. He expects others to fulfill his requests and longings and is resentful when they don't. He consistently sees his problems as emanating from others. "What's yours is ours; what's mine is mine." Harold wonders why people get upset with his expectations and entitlement. "We're married, so I have a right to your body and money and expect my needs to be fulfilled."

Like a battery that easily loses its charge, Harold does not feel very alive in his body, and is always trying to plug into someone else to get a charge of excitement or understand himself. "If only she had larger breasts I'd be able to maintain my erection." He tries to get others to make sense of his internal confusion for him. Unfortunately, because of his closed way of being, it is impossible for anyone to help. He desperately wants to know who he is, but with only his character style as an internal reference, he doesn't know how to know. In an attempt to make up for the absence of internal body validation, he can turn to fame, money, or position, or defiantly reject them all.

As a child, Harold may have had parents who were caught in the same abandonment-inundation dilemma themselves. Although, he could have had one parent who was abandoning and the other inundating.

Harold enjoys sex but has a struggle feeling loving and sexual at the same time. He can't tolerate higher levels of emotions and excitement. So, he splits off and then can't contain, heighten, or enjoy sexuality. He is sensitive, but often attunement with another is impossible without a deep attunement within.

To compensate, he often has to be in control down to the most minute detail. "In the sexual realm, I have to be the one who initiates. If my wife tells me what she likes, I can't do it that way at that time. If I try to get myself to do something, get turned on, have an erection, maintain excitement, it becomes the one thing I can't do." His rebellious stance can get so strong that he can't have sex if Felicia wants to, no matter how turned on he is.

In sex, until Harold can stay present with a high charge and tolerate some intimacy, he can't even begin the first steps of heightened intimacy. The good news is that with awareness and the courage to know who he is, his somatic core sense of self, Harold can open his heart and temper the expression of these primitive defenses.

Ironically, society often supports the acting out of character style by mistaking it for strength of character, individuality, or masculinity. Although this style often leads to success in terms of power, control, and independence in the work world, when brought home it destroys intimacy, erotic sexuality, and an internal sense of well-being.

If Harold uses his character style to intimidate or to gain power over others, like the "emperor without clothes," they may never let him know how his behavior affects them. They will just leave, and he will feel isolated. His protective fortress pushes others away and isolates him from everyone, even his true nature. If Harold never learns how to modify his character style, especially his sense of entitlement and primitive rage, he will find himself isolated, emotionally shallow, and spiritually empty.

ABANDONMENT-INUNDATION CHARACTER STYLE PROFILE	*Trait 1. Automatic No: Nobody Can Tell Me What to Do* You don't like to be told what to do or who you are. You will:

☐ ☐ be relatively closed to outside information, opinions, and instructions, and have difficulty letting others in emotionally;

☐ ☐ have to do it your way; often present a *fait accompli* or unilateral decision;

☐ ☐ make your own rules. "I want to do what I want to do when I want to do it;"

☐ ☐ have difficulty with any kind of closure: making or following through on commitments, receiving or giving gifts, being on time, or expressing appreciation and saying good-bye;

☐ ☐ be very sensitive to being told who you are or what you are feeling; may interpret any comment as critical or controlling;

☐ ☐ reword and change your statements when others try to repeat what you have said. For example: "I hate my father." "You hate your father?" "Well, I wouldn't say hate. He just wasn't there." "He wasn't there?" "No, I hate my father;"

☐ ☐ always have a good reason for not taking information in: "If only you had said it in a different way, in a different tone of voice, at a different time; or that you didn't look at me, or if you had only said this before you said that. . . ."

☐ ☐ have a difficult time working for someone else, therefore tend to be your own boss;

☐ ☐ sometimes feel compelled to enter the exit door, drive in the opposite direction of the arrows in a parking lot, see stop signs as only suggestions. You may collect traffic tickets and fight authority in secret little ways;

☐ ☐ not be able to tell yourself what to do; finish paperwork, theses, or assignments; pick up the clothes at the cleaners or stay on a diet or exercise program;

☐ ☐ have had difficulty learning to read, spell, or do math in school as a child;

☐ ☐ tend to take an adversarial position and find excitement in sparring.

Trait 2. Have an Idea of How Things Should Be and Cling to It

You are attached to your picture of how things are. You will:

☐ ☐ do whatever it takes to prove your idea (or bring it about). You have to be right;

☐ ☐ try to calculate life, thinking more than responding from your somatic core emotions or sensations;

☐ ☐ have difficulty living in the moment, constantly turning to the past and planning the future;

☐ ☐ rarely learn from new experiences as you only focus on whether an experience matches your picture or not. So you keep making the same mistakes over and over;

☐ ☐ live life according to "when, then," that is, "when (something) is complete, then I'll (something)."

Trait 3. Treat Myself and Others as Objects

Because you do not accept your human frailties, you will:

☐ ☐ push yourself beyond your healthy limits and expect the same of others;

☐ ☐ be unconscious of your effect on others, miss or misjudge human emotions and wonder why people get upset;

☐ ☐ see your problems as emanating from others;

☐ ☐ overestimate your emotional or physical capacity.

Trait 4. Authenticity Gap: Tend to Lie Up or Lie Down

You exaggerate and consistently miss the mark for authenticity. Because you don't tell the truth, particularly to yourself, you will:

☐ ☐ lie *up* about yourself, presenting a better picture than is true;

☐☐ lie *down,* modestly making yourself less and not getting pleasure or satisfaction from life or your successes (lying down is as much a lie as lying up);

☐☐ feel like a phony because you present yourself to the world outside differently from how you feel on the inside;

☐☐ feel alienated from your partner, or, more likely, your partner will feel alienated from you (no matter where or what the lie is);

☐☐ perpetuate your inauthenticity by trying to get people to accept your false front so they will think well of you;

☐☐ though you may be perfectly innocent, engender mistrust in others.

Trait 5. Intimate Relationships: Not Too Close, Not Too Far Away

Partners may take opposite sides of the struggle between closeness and separation. You may do both alternately or simultaneously. You will:

☐☐ find that closeness triggers fears of inundation, distance triggers fears of abandonment;

☐☐ perceive separation as abandonment, or friendliness as inundation;

☐☐ when you feel close, say or do something hurtful that creates distance;

☐☐ miss the feelings of mutuality and of being understood, and miss the human essence of your partner and the relationship;

☐☐ fail to recognize or accept the constant dance you impose on any intimate relationship you are in.

Trait 6. Feel Split Off from Self, Body, Emotions, and Aliveness.

Overwhelmed by feelings, you disassociate from your body and will:

☐☐ not be present and not have a full range of your mental, sensory, and emotional capacities available;

☐☐ deaden your aliveness and heighten your sense of aloneness by self-abandonment;

☐☐ have blank spots in your memory because you were split off and not really there;

☐☐ seek excitement, validation, and support for who you are from outside sources;

☐☐ with little interiority, not identify illness early, or recognize when you become hungry or tired;

☐☐ have a shield that keeps you from really making contact with others and others with you. "It's as if I have a glass bubble around me;"

☐☐ make quick responses from intellectual rather than emotional or body feelings;

☐☐ avoid emotions and feelings of excitement or well-being; have a limited ability to contain feelings and energy. You will probably either discharge or split off, especially during sex;

☐☐ become intellectual or change the subject when you or others show emotions or have body sensations;

☐☐ heighten split-off sensations by using drugs, alcohol, or other substances. Favorite drug of choice is marijuana.

WHAT IF YOUR CHARACTER STYLE, the emotional feelings in your body from past injuries, and your impulse to act out these traits of your style were never going away? Just as you can't erase your history, you can't get rid of your character style, but you can learn to live with it. With acceptance, what would you have to do differently?

The first step is to identify and acknowledge the one that most closely describes your experience. Any trait in your style that you have identified as active at a range of four or higher can cause problems in your relationship. If you are still unclear as to which character style is yours, you are probably struggling with a combination of abandonment and inundation.

Notice how much easier it is to identify your partner's style. Most people can accept physical aspects of their partner that can't be changed, like their height and color of their eyes, yet they are unwilling to accept those that are psychological.

Second, observe yourself as you interact with people, and notice if you act your character style out more with your partner than with others. Pay attention to the responses you elicit and your own body reactions. You can't just simply make a resolution to stop your character style as this only causes it to exaggerate and become more entrenched.

Notice how the issues of abandonment, inundation, and the combination of the two influence you throughout the day. Awareness does not come with a flash of enlightenment. It is composed of little knowings felt in the body. Eventually you will see that your body is speaking to you and you will learn how to listen.

Guides for living with abandonment anxiety and inundation anxiety are found in the appendix. The rest of this chapter will deal with the most common and difficult character style to accept and live with, the As If. With this style you have to deal not only with the first two anxieties, abandonment and inundation, but also with the perplexing six additional traits the combining of these two anxieties create.

LIVING WITH THE SIX
TRAITS OF THE AS IF
CHARACTER STYLE

MANY WHO LIVE with this style at a high level, or have spouses who do, shed tears of relief when their problem is identified and the description fits their experience. They finally see a way out of their despair, isolation, and frustration.

Florence said, "At times I found myself hoping that Arnie was an alcoholic or an addict, something he could stop or could get help for. At other times, I thought I was the problem, if I could just say it right or do it right or be right, he would be different. I've almost killed myself in the effort."

Florence's mistake was in thinking that Arnie's character style was just a communication problem that could be solved through her agency. The more accurate she became, the more exacting her disappointment. She tried so hard to figure out how to deliver the simplest message and became exhausted from trying to say it the right way, at the right time, in the right tone, only to be wrong and disappointed again.

Character style is an automatic reactive way of being that developed in childhood, and it will not significantly differ, no matter what a partner does or does not do or say. Only you can break your cycle of inflexibility and can lower the degree to which you act out your own character style traits. You are in charge.

AUTOMATIC NO: "NO ONE CAN TELL ME WHAT TO DO"

THE AS IF CHARACTER STYLE is a rebellious stance originated to gain a sense of self by separating from parents. As an adult, you can't gain a sense of yourself by opposing others, all you'll get is separation.

In sexuality, it comes out as, "I've got a headache, upset stomach; it's too late, too early; something else is more urgent." This "no" stance can be acted out by the body in the form of a vaginal infection, an inability to maintain an erection, premature or retarded ejaculation, or an orgasm that is unsatisfactory or nonexistent.

Alan could readily admit to and was vehemently proud of his "no one can tell me what to do" stance when it came to his very successful business, but now he was bemoaning his inability to sustain intimacy in relationships. He brought his current girlfriend into therapy because she was ready to leave. He adamantly denied that his business stance had anything to do with his sex life. When asked if she had anything to say, Ruth shyly and reluctantly said, "There's one little thing. You know that I have difficulty having an orgasm unless I can be on top, and you never, never will do that position."

He answered, "That has nothing to do with being told what to do. I lose my erection when you are on top." The therapist asked him, "Do you lose your erection in any other position?" He answered, "No. Strange that I have never had a problem in that position with any of my other girlfriends. Although I have had trouble with other women in different positions." Then he paused, "Come to think of it, it was always in the position that they liked best." His "my way or no way" was sinking the ship again.

Anyone really caught in an automatic "no" is forever vigilant. In the bedroom everything looks like a sign they are being asked for sex.

Ruby sighed, "When I wake up in the morning, even before I open my eyes, I start to worry that Al will want sex. I just know that he is lying there watching me, waiting for me to open my eyes so he can grab my breast or crotch and then jump on me for sex. I try not to move so he won't know I am awake yet.

"Yesterday, I woke up wondering what excuse I could use this time. With my plan set, I opened my eyes only to remember that Al was in Chicago.

"I wonder how many other times that I awaken upset, my body tight, looking for a problem, and it is just my automatic 'No.' Al is so handy, if I can pin my irritability and stomachache on him and his wanting sex, then I don't have to face my own character style."

Judy and Fred were just back from their honeymoon when she prepared a

Manifestations of the Automatic No:

A closed system: Although Gloria never seems to take in information from Sam, weeks later she repeats it back to him as though it were her idea, "I was listening to the radio and had this great insight...." When asked to take out the trash, Phil will conveniently forget or leave some part of it undone, like dropping papers along the way, leaving the last slimy remnants stuck to the bottom, or forgetting the lid in the alley.

Psychological deafness: Harriet is not deaf or hard of hearing, but she literally can't hear a man, especially an authority figure, if he is imparting information she doesn't want to deal with. Whether man or woman, you might have this "deafness" with either gender.

Spite: "Cutting off his nose to spite his face," Richard will actually harm himself to torture Joan, who cares about him, to prove she is wrong or that he can't be told what to do. When Joan returned from the hardware store, she saw Richard changing the blade of the saw without unplugging it. In panic she shouted, "Stop! Unplug the saw before you change the blade." Defiantly he thrust his hand in the air. Thoroughly enraged, he yelled, "See these fingers. They are mine and I'll cut them off if I want to." And he continued to change the blade his way.

Any deadline is spitefully seen as a command: writers who can't write; composers unable to compose the moment they get a grant; Ph.D. candidates who do everything but finish their dissertations. Even the most mundane tasks become impossible to fulfill: paying bills on time, flushing the toilet.

beautiful meal. The lovely dinner ended in a bewildering argument. Fred said, "It's all your fault. I was looking forward to sex all day, but because you are so demanding, I don't feel like it anymore." Stunned, Judy said, "I don't understand." He shouted, "Well, you put candles on the table. That is just like telling me to be romantic and have sex with you. I'm not going to perform for anyone." That incident was the beginning of many years of Fred teaching Judy not to ask for sex or in any way show interest or excitement. She eventually learned to act reserved and indifferent.

HAVING AN IDEA OF HOW THINGS SHOULD BE AND CLINGING TO IT

A MAJOR PART OF MENTAL HEALTH is the ability to learn from experience and new information, being willing to change your mind, and recognizing that your ideas are not your identity. Buddhists speak of attachment as the source of pain in life. In a similar way, the attachment to an idea, not the idea itself, causes pain and rigidity. Life is constant change; if it rains, you may have to cancel the picnic. If you get an idea of what love is, or how sex should be, and your experience deviates even slightly, you are liable to feel indignant and betrayed.

Diane and Sam's sex life consists of mostly arguing over when and how. She complains that Sam always seems to approach her late at night and this makes her feel like an old sock; yet, she rarely initiates sex unless it is between two and three in the afternoon. This is clearly a character style battle.

Couples get an idea of who their partner is, how they should be, what they want from them, the kind of longings they want to have fulfilled—on and on—and keep a vigilant eye to see if their partner matches up. This causes distance, disappointment, ongoing fragmentations and hurt feelings.

The obvious solution to holding rigid ideas is being able to change your mind. Accept that you might occasionally be wrong and that being wrong doesn't mean you're sick, defective, or stupid. Those who lead with an automatic no usually find a partner who leads with getting an idea, and vice versa. There is an element of unreality to both: a lack of body experience, but a stance of nonquestionability.

TREAT MYSELF AND OTHERS AS OBJECTS

IF YOU WORK fifteen hours a day, put aside your feelings, you don't go to the bathroom when you need to, don't feed yourself properly or get enough sleep or take care of basic health needs, you are ignoring your body, your interiority, and your humanness. In short, you treat yourself as an object. You probably treat others the same way, as oblivious to their feelings and needs as you are to your own. The people closest to you suffer the most; while people at a distance may find you warm and generous.

Larry's range for closeness looks like a target. The bull's-eye in the center represents Larry; next are those to whom he is most related, such as his immediate family. The ever-widening circles represent friends, acquaintances, strangers, and distant communities. The closer someone comes to the center of his target, the more he acts out his character style. The more distant someone is, the safer Larry feels, and the more open and magnanimous he is. As he grew older, Larry began to feel the isolation he had created from those who loved him the most. He knew he felt uncomfortable with closeness and was missing a human element, a spiritual connection, that others seemed to feel, but he didn't know why.

AUTHENTICITY GAP: TENDING TO LIE UP OR LIE DOWN

MOST OF YOUR LIES are to yourself, and nobody else knows of them or cares. Any sort of lie, false modesty, or exaggeration creates a feeling of inauthenticity, engenders a lack of trust from others, and an absence of personal competence and satisfaction within. In a relationship, if you do not tell the truth, your partner will feel your inauthenticity. Lies create emotional walls between people. When you tell a lie, notice the sensation in your body.

Can you simply tell the absolute truth? Try it. Start with age, weight, height, net worth, number of sexual partners in your lifetime up until now, etc. Notice how you miss the mark. Do you exaggerate or diminish the truth?

INTIMATE RELATIONSHIP: NOT TOO CLOSE, NOT TOO FAR AWAY

THE NOT TOO FAR AWAY aspect of relationships is easy enough for most couples to cope with. When a couple feels too distant they can kiss and make up. Separation brings out feelings of abandonment, then emotions flow, softening the body, and the desire for closeness naturally comes to the surface. It's the not too close aspect that causes trouble. When a person's speed limits are reached or they have just had enough, they usually do not know how to graciously take a little breathing room. Instead, hurtful things are said and done precisely when they are feeling the most loving. Familiar with their partner's vulnerabilities, they know just what to say to hurt or infuriate, they employ hostile humor or sarcasm, belittle and embarrass, start an argument, or act out any of their other five character style traits.

It is normal and healthy to feel the underlying flux. There is no right, fixed amount of closeness or breathing room for all couples. People and relationships are different. Become aware of what is right for you and your relationship. Neither clinging nor avoiding contact will support the bond of the relationship. Be willing to ask for time alone and time to be close without doing it defensively and without insult or injury.

SPLITTING OFF FROM SELF, BODY, EMOTIONS, AND ALIVENESS

MANY PEOPLE SPLIT OFF and yet continue to talk, losing their excitement and focus as they ramble and repeat themselves. Some just cut off or split off from their ability to feel.

Spencer, a businessman, confessed, "People sit across the desk from me. They sometimes tell me very tragic or meaningful things about their lives. I know that I should be having feelings, but I never do. I try to figure out what emotion I should be having so I can appropriately respond to them. Then I feel shallow. It feels like something is missing in me that other people have."

Some people disown or energetically cut off from different parts of their body: ears, not hearing; genitals, not feeling sexual; heart, not feeling loving; feet and legs, not feeling grounded or supported. Parts of your body that we are embarrassed about or do not accept will not maintain their vitality for long.

As you do the breathing and movement exercises and are able to sustain the witness "I am" body experience, the necessity to split off or cut off will rapidly change.

Those who are unwilling to embody who they are beneath their character style are stuck, unable to unite with their core body voice which would provide them support, wisdom, and access to spirituality. They are just as stuck if they cannot accept their human fallibility which can lead to compassion with others and companionship on their life journey.

So they are left struggling with neither God nor humanity—alone. Joining with their authentic body-voice is their only salvation and means to discover a deeper, true knowing. Childbirth often helps women through this dilemma through the physical-emotional opening of her body, especially her heart. In this wondrous event she cannot avoid her body. Whereas men are often rewarded for a lack of feeling, enduring pain, and splitting-off from their bodies. Some men defiantly assert their As If character style, mistaking it for the body experience of masculinity.

To find meaning in life or even just relief from their interior struggle, the As If adult often embarks on a quest, usually a spiritual, a business, love, or occupational quest or a wondering journey. Their search is an external journey looking for the meaning of life. But, in truth, they are looking for the experience of being alive, and the only place they can find this truth is in their body.

This is the essence of the lost soul, the seeker, not truly connected to a higher force or deity, whose feelings are alienated from humanity. Because we can all identify with this dilemma, our hearts cry out to such a person and the injured child they once were.

Much as we empathize and try to help, they must do the work for themselves. No matter how much loving, caring, and insight people offer, they will not see it, or will see it as controlling, telling them what to do. Even leaving them alone may be seen as manipulation. Any interaction can increase their defensive character style, heightening their aloneness and life's dilemma. To be in relationship with an As If, who acts out these character traits full blown either as a lover, a parent, or friend, can be maddening and painful. But there is hope.

It is often through a profound opening of the heart that the As If can momentarily awaken his or her body and thereby make an authentic connection to the interior self that leads to a core experience with another. *With this emotional-physical opening to self, there is hope for seeing his or her character style for what it is, an outmoded defense against phantoms from the nursery.*

If we then accept our character style without pride or remorse, we open ourselves to an awesome opportunity to know ourselves in depth. To do this, we must risk looking at our own being in a new way, as through new eyes.

Arena 3: Emotional Agency

SELF-AGENCY IS THE CAPACITY for self-illumination. Like an inner light, it helps you see yourself from the inside, to experience what you do and what you feel, need, and desire. It allows you to see who you are as a separate and unique being rather than who you are in response to others, their needs, or their view of you. It is the body experience of feeling that you are the author of your own life.

But if, in the first years of life, a child feels that its survival and ability to gain love depend on its ability to focus on the parent, to be or do what the parent wants, to please and stabilize the parent, then its self-agency is diverted to satisfy this more urgent requirement. Assessing the parent's emotional state and needs becomes at least a prerequisite, if not a substitute for self-awareness. With agency, the subtle shuttling from self to other becomes locked in an outward focus, and the agent is left to see his or her self only as a reflection.

AGENCY IS A BODY EXPERIENCE

IF YOU TURN YOUR ATTENTION inside you will notice that if you have sex when you don't want to, a place in your body "shrinks," as a part of yourself is lost. The relationship suffers as well because both people know, deep down, the difference between sincere participation and mere compliance. Lovers always know.

You can certainly have sex sometimes when you are not particularly in the mood, but you still have to find your own volition. You can make love when you aren't feeling sexual. If you are feeling loving, you can at times, participate strictly to please your partner but, if this is your only way of being, you are both in trouble.

People ask, "How do I know whether I'm doing something in agency or just because I care about someone and I want to be loving?" The answer is, you can't know by behavior alone. You have to find out in your body.

Long before a behavior is initiated, your body shifts into preparation for agency. If you pay attention, even exaggerate your desire to be helpful, you will be able to feel the tightness, shrinking, and numbing loss of awareness in your body, as if you are physically and emotionally being diminished. You will find that, sometimes, this body reaction is triggered with the slightest hint that someone wants or "needs" you. It is only by becoming aware of these internal symptoms that you can tell whether any particular action is taken in agency.

This means you must pay attention to your body signals. Don't be fooled by the short-term gratification you might feel as a successful agent. Look for the energetic holding pattern in your body and the feelings of anger, deadness, confusion, or inundation it causes.

Agency, then, is a physical, energetic, and emotional self-perpetuated experience, and a warning signal that you are not listening to your own inner voice. As long as you think agency is about other people, you will remain stuck with it.

When asked what she wanted, Sherry faltered. "I—I—don't know," she stammered in her confusion as if this information were not accessible to her.

Your body knows, though. It knows whether your inner voice speaks for yourself or in service of other people, old rules, beliefs, or themes. It doesn't matter whether you are in agency to your boss, kids, mother, or yoga teacher. The rage from a lifetime of self-abandonment, fueled by the lack of hope, will eventually turn toward your partner. Its outcome, anger or indifference, squelches sexual excitement. Electing yourself to be in charge of another's well-being in exchange for love or support puts your health, relationship, and sense of self in serious danger.

When agency causes your body to contract, it extinguishes your feelings of vitality and well-being. It can kill your loving and leave you always wanting. It further suppresses desire, which is expressed by the body as boredom and shows up in the relationship as sexual indifference.

Agents rarely make first-order decisions, ones in which a desire emanates from their own volition. A second-order decision is one in which someone else initiates the idea, but you can make a yes or no decision. If you perceive your partner as always wanting sex, you may feel the despair that comes when first-order decisions are made impossible. In an attempt to exercise your volition, you may add something to the other person's suggestion, but it will still be a second-order decision. A third-order decision is when you just go along with the other person's idea without choice.

If you consistently make second- or third-order decisions, you will eventually feel like a victim. Your self-agency voice will remain mute, unheard, undiscovered, unknown. If you make too many third-order decisions, you may feel like a martyr or get sick. If you only make first-order decisions, your character style is getting in the way and you are not really part of a relationship. If you are not initiating, on your own volition, at least 50 percent of the time, you are stuck in agency.

Agency is like a blanket that covers your core self and your character style, leaving you feeling like a nonentity. Because of this, agency prevents you from actually working on yourself or in your own behalf. Feeling and acting through your own volition is an important aspect of core self-experience.

This begins when you can feel your own core desires in your body—desires that are about you. Without this, there is little hope or excitement felt in your body. You must also be able to act on your desires, for instance, initiating when making love. If you always follow your partner's feelings, desires, and sensations instead of your own, your pleasure can only come from your partner's pleasure. You must use your volition to act on your own behalf in a predictable, consistent manner, in bed and out, and to allow the body experience of self-satisfaction. You can't satisfy your needs or inner longings by trying to fulfill them in others, hoping that they will then return the favor. Agents, taught to put the needs of others first, do for others what they want or need for themselves.

Agents are so focused on pleasing people that they rarely notice when they are being taken advantage of or even conned. They don't want to make waves; then later they feel foolish to find out how naive they have been.

EARLY ADAPTATION TO AGENCY

AGENCY TAKES ON different forms depending on whether it began in infancy or in later childhood. If, in the first years of life—probably before you could talk—you were taught to put someone else's needs and feelings before your own, your feelings of self will automatically go numb or find it impossible to access self experience when the person you feel responsible for is nearby. *Because agency produces an ongoing feeling in your body of being bad—as though you have done something wrong—you may do almost anything to be loved but will settle for just not being abandoned.*

You may misinterpret your partner's needs and the satisfaction of those needs as your own: "If it makes you happy, I'm happy." You may spend a wealth of time and energy defending and explaining yourself, trying to prove that you are good, that you haven't done anything wrong, that you have done a good job, that others should be as kind and considerate as you. You may describe your needs endlessly, but then find yourself once again just going along with your partner.

If your self-agency was relegated to a back shelf in the first years of life you may draw a blank screen when asked directly what you, yourself, feel or want—unless of course there is someone else for you to consider. When asked to go to a movie, for example, you may not know what you want until you hear the other person's choice. You may not make the same choice, but once the other's decision is made, the agent often finds it easier to access a sense of their own desires.

EARLY AGENCY SEXUAL TRAPS

• At first it will be a turn-on to make your partner happy and satisfied. You will delight in the wonder and excitement of how good it makes you feel to please someone. It's quite a thrill because the results of being a good agent show up immediately with sex.

- You will be a wonderful lover for your partner, but you may not feel much erotic-sexual satisfaction for yourself.
- You may never think of having sex for your own pleasure, separate from the pleasure you can give.
- Eventually you will get tired of having sex for someone else and then you probably won't want to have sex very often or at all.
- Sex with a stranger, especially one you think you will never see again, is not a relationship and therefore is not apt to be a call to agency. Consequently, agents can find overwhelming freedom and excitement in a passing affair. But as soon as the stranger becomes familiar, agency returns and reaches out with its tentacles once again to engulf sexuality.
- Inundated by agency, you may have sex as "just another duty." Trying to get sex "done and over" leads to disappointment and anger because it won't stay done. A "good job" just whets the appetite, and your partner, of course, will want more. On the other hand, your own lack of desire may leave your partner feeling empty, hungry for more and more sex to fill the emptiness from not feeling joined. If you don't participate through your own volition, desire and excitement, sex doesn't work.

When Joyce first met Stewart, she wanted to make love all the time, to let him know how much he was loved. She liked how excited he was and loved feeling so close and special to him.

Now when he reaches toward her sexually, her body tightens and she feels she is being asked for something, to do something in order to be loved. Joyce has lost her sexual desire and thinks, "Why can't Stewart just love me instead of asking for sex?" Her mind knows that he is not using her. But her stomach, speaking in an archaic somatic language, tightens with hopelessness and says, "Just love me. Don't ask for anything in return."

More accurately, Joyce hardly ever initiates sex with Stewart because she is never sure whether he is in the mood. So she watches him. If he initiates sex, then she can decide if she wants it or not. Because she doesn't act directly from her own body feelings, she doesn't exercise her own volition and feels that, "Stewart is always pulling on me, asking for sex." A more telling truth is that she never asks. "I thought I was such a sexual person. What has happened to my excitement? Does this mean that I don't love Stewart any more?"

LATER ADAPTATION
TO AGENCY

YOUR AGENCY RESPONSE may have developed after your first few years of life as a result of a crisis in the family, an illness, a divorce, a loss of a parent, any time you had to take care of a parent emotionally or a parent's responsibilities. Some later agency patterns are formed in response to an adoption or the birth of a sister or a brother. Possibly in fear of being sent away or being in competition with your sibling, you began to feel you must earn love by being especially good. Because you had an earlier connection with a parent who did not need you to be in agency, you are likely to feel your own core feelings and desires more clearly than someone with early agency.

This type of agency is usually in the service of being seen as "good" and, at the same time, to get what you want in a relationship. Agency then takes the form of "It's only fair" unilateral bargaining. As a child you may have made one-sided, unspoken agreements: "If I'm good enough, Mommy will love me and buy me the toy I saw yesterday. Then I won't have to ask; she'll just know and bring it to me."

Later as an adult, this same contract, still unspoken but justified as a feeling in the body translates as, "I'll do the dishes; then you'll have sex with me." If your unsuspecting partner says "goodnight" and goes to sleep, you may feel a righteous rage of indignation. This form of agency carries a tone of wishful or magical thinking that is played out in the game of, "If you really loved me, you'd know what I need and want and make it happen."

Although they often cooked together, Ellen always served the food, automatically giving her husband Tom the larger or better portion. One day, after years of this routine, Tom cut the left-over pecan pie and gave himself the larger piece. Ellen was horrified. The belief was so ingrained, she had never mentioned to Tom that she felt morally bound to the rule that the one who served had to take the least and graciously honor the other person with the best. Unaware of her unilateral contract, Tom thought that she always gave him the larger piece because he was bigger. So, when he served the pie, he merely did what she had inadvertently taught him to do.

LATER AGENCY SEX TRAPS

- Your sexual contract may be, "I'll do you, then you must do me—whenever I want." This often works at first, but before long, it becomes evident that your partner never recognized, much less agreed to, the second part of your contract. Even so, you may feel justified in your, "It's not fair" rage.
- You are probably a practiced, considerate lover, and in turn you want desperately to be thought well of. Your partner's sexual satisfaction is taken as an expression of how well you've done.
- There is often a tremendous requirement that your partner be completely, ecstatically satisfied with your performance. Asking, "Was it good for you?" begs for agency applause, but no amount of applause will ever be enough to make you feel good about yourself for long.
- You provide for others what you want for yourself. Sara says, "I love you, Tom," with the hope of hearing, "I love you, Sara." Agents rarely ask directly for what they want. So in sex, you have to have a crystal ball to know how to please them.

- A man pays for dinner and expects to have sex. A woman goes to a room with a fellow executive. They have wonderful sex, and she spends the night. She expects him to pay for the room. Both have made unilateral contracts based on their gender role idea without bothering to negotiate or even inform their partner.

ATTEMPTS TO
STOP THE HABIT

ONCE YOU REALIZE that the process of agency is eating away at your life, you may try to stop. There are may strategies you may have already tried that don't work. Some can become just as destructive and enduring as agency itself.

Super-Agency: The first strategy most good agents use is to pour on the agency one last time and fix everyone, once and for all. The hope is that everyone will stay well and love them forevermore. This agency overdrive can keep you doing the "agency dance" faster and faster for years.

Permission: "Let me go, please. See how good I have been. Please give me permission to stop," pleads the exhausted agent, hoping to preserve love and appreciation while protecting against rejection and abandonment.
Unfortunately the agency target can't break the agent's addiction, no matter how much permission he or she gives. Unless the self-agency source is reopened in the body and the decision made from within, it's still agency.

Counter-Agency: This third attempt belongs to the rebellious counter-agent who adopts an oppositional stance to his or her own agency, believing this proves that he or she is not really in agency. However, by doing the opposite of what people want, the counter-agent is actually just as stuck and controlled by others as is the agent. To be for a thing or against it is the same in that you are still not using your volition.

If you become a counter-agent and exchange your determined helping through self-sacrifice for defiance and martyrdom, your physical and emotional symptoms become even greater. Opposition not only keeps you from releasing the body holding pattern, it exaggerates it. This approach activates the six traits of the As If character style and is nonrelational. Heightened character style leads to isolation until, desperate, your attempt at revitalizing the relationship activates agency and the cycle starts again.

The secret counter-agent pretends on the surface to go along but doesn't follow through. Agency is now but a thin veil of "niceness" over character style and expressed in a destructive manner.

Another aspect of counter-agency is vigorous boundary setting. You can't reverse the agency habit by setting extensive limits on others. This only compounds your way of seeing the problem as outside of yourself. Besides, you will still have all the body deadening, closing, and shrinking that comes with agency while you sit in your circle or boundary not doing what you feel bad for not doing. As long as you think agency is about other people, you will remain stuck with it.

Somebody Must Leave or Die: Because agents believe that their pain comes from their relationship, they believe the only way out of this pain is for someone to leave. Since they don't know how else to be loved or be in a relationship—other than as an agent—there is little hope. With a chronic feeling in their body that they are bad, it's hard to feel good enough to leave or to tolerate feeling additionally bad for leaving. It is also next to impossible to muster the volition to leave. No matter how defective their target, it is hard to escape when so much of one's self is invested. For one or all of these reasons, longtime, long-suffering agents often fantasize about their own death or their partner's death as a way out.

You may have tried to get out of agency to your parents and family by leaving town. But no matter how mature you are, if your parents move closer to you and you haven't done something to change your internal process, all your old feelings of inadequacy, incompetence, and lack of volition will return as strongly as if the separation hadn't occurred.

Agency, which attempts to protect the fearful psyche, won't change if someone leaves, dies, or becomes permanently "fixed." You carry this way of being inside of you, and this is where it must be changed.

Jessica is finally alone, and a feeling of relief creeps into her body, a feeling of not having to pay attention to anyone else. Her thoughts turn to Bert and their marriage.

When Bert came home from work, she listened to his problems and talked to him so that his feelings from the day's turmoil turned to calm. She gave him the assurance and inner confidence he needed. He loved the attention she gave him. He thought she was so special and often said, "Jessica is perfect; there is no one like her." Jessica, in turn, felt loved, wanted, needed, and secure. It was a perfect marriage to all who viewed it.

"Our life was 'nice.' Why did I feel increasingly distant, isolated, and alone? Sometimes I felt like I was his mother or caretaker, responsible for him emotionally," Jessica says.

There were a few problems others couldn't see. Sex, for instance, didn't work. The more Jessica tried to be just right and do all the right things, the less sexual she felt. The more she tried to please her husband, the less real her tenderness and loving became.

Bert loved and needed her. He wanted more than anything to please her. But the more he wanted to please, the more pressure he felt, and the less sexual desire he had. As his desire dwindled and began to slip away, Jessica assumed it was her fault, so she increased her efforts to please him, in bed and out. The excitement quietly withered. They both felt impotent.

"Bert is gone now, and there isn't anyone else. So why do I still have this horrible shrinking feeling in my body? The divorce is final and I am alone." Jessica liked the pleasant feeling of being alone and responsible to no one but herself. Even so, in her mind she replayed old scenes, trying to figure out what went wrong, what she could have done differently to change the course of their marriage. She felt she was still responding almost hypnotically to something other than herself, some external force, some voice, some need she kept straining to hear.

"Enough of this! Enough!" she shouted internally. "Bert's gone! I can do my own life now. The first part of my life I did for my parents. The second part I did for Bert and the kids. This time is just for me! Now is my time! I don't have to do anything to please anyone but myself."

The thought was thrilling and it sent a tingle up her spine. The excitement lasted only a moment; then the void came and the despair began.

"My God!" she panicked. "I don't know how. I don't know what I want or like, or what I can do. I only know about other people."

When the alarm clock rang to end her meditation, Jessica crawled out from the closet thinking, "Now who was I supposed to call? What is it I have to do?" She could feel the tension return. She straightened the clothing, rearranged the shoes on the floor. "So, it's come to this! The only way I can feel myself and get away from taking care of others is to hide in the closet and meditate."

When you are successful and your agency begins to subside, you may feel the emotional fears, "I, or someone will die," or, "No one will ever love me and I'll be alone forever." These are just the fears that, as a child, caused you to become an agent, and throughout life they are liable to scare you away from self-agency experiences. Every time we try to change any long-held body-mind patterns, our protective cover yells danger as loudly as it can. It takes courage and willpower not to let these ghost feelings scare you. The exercises in chapter 7 and the agency mantras in chapter 2 will help you move through the impasse.

RELATIONSHIPS
CAN BE HEALING

ALTHOUGH WE CAN and must say the good parent messages and the agency mantras to ourselves and deal with all of the secret themes we harbor in our bodies, we also need support and validation from those we love and respect. Though you can't truly take these affirmations in from others until you are able to give them to yourself and believe them, when this interior work is accomplished, an affirming response from another can help reopen the wounded heart and calm the desperate cry to be loved and valued.

Only the one who carries the wound can tell another the right words and feel in his or her body whether they fit. Peter says to Lucy, "Tell me the words you need to hear right now." Lucy replies, "I need to hear that I am not bad, I haven't done anything wrong, and that you want me." Peter repeats these words exactly as she says them, not adding or changing them in any way. He respects that only she knows the combination to heal her old wound. Lucy stops to sense how these words feel in her body. If they are the ones that open her heart and touch her soul, she will know it. If not, she will need to rephrase them until they fit.

Even when they fit, she may be tempted to find a reason not to believe them and miss this healing opportunity. Lucy will have to trust Peter's words *before* he can prove them through actions.

If Peter thinks the words have something to do with him, he is liable to change them a bit or not be able to say them at all. The words are the key to her closed and injured heart. If Peter's character style won't let him say them at all or won't let him say them exactly the way she said them, *the new wound can be devastating*. It can crystallize the suspicion that the relationship is bereft of compassionate consideration. This is not a time to joke, be stingy or rebellious; such behavior will be felt as terribly abusive.

Between partners, there are several classic messages that address agency injuries to the heart. They are powerful, positive, adult affirmations. For example: "You're a good man (woman). You haven't done anything wrong. I love you, and we are going to work this out." You can begin with these and then add the ones that come from your body and speak to your soul.

When looking for these opening words, keep the sentences short, simple, and to the point. If they are too long or complicated your partner will not be able to remember them exactly. If they are not to the point, they will not fit.

CHAPTER FOURTEEN

Arena 4: Existential-Transpersonal

THERE'S A LARGE FIELD of knowledge that deals with changes of consciousness, the mystery, the wonder of life and death. This area explores the spiritual aspects of life. It is the thread of inquiry and insight that has wound through most religious pursuits since we began to try to understand our passionate body urgings and answer the questions, "Who am I?" "What's it all about?" "What is the source of joy?" "What is love?" and more.

On this journey, there are differences in comfort between a native and a tourist. Some people have an inner familiarity and understanding that comes with awakening. For them the transpersonal journey is like returning home to a long lost memory in their body. Others do not have this comfort of the native; their openings are more like exploring uncharted territory. For them understanding awakens a new interior source of self-validation. Many of these explorers never really develop a deep interest in understanding or acquainting themselves with this new territory, and they always remain visitors.

For natives to have a deep core-to-core experience of awakening with their partners through heightened sexuality and intimacy it can feel like a wonderful amplification of an old familiar territory of heightened consciousness. They are simply natives returning home again along another path, that of erotic sexuality.

Regardless of where you fit in, native or tourist, what you learn in *The Intimate Couple* will give you the opportunity to enter and inhabit these rarefied altitudes consistently.

Don't be upset if it takes awhile before you feel like a native. There are many stages of change to go through, and this takes time and courage. It is not easy to be so vulnerable, open, loving, sexual, and passionate—at one with the spiritual aspects of life, yourself, and your partner.

For some, sex with a heightened charge will be just a loving, wonderful sexual experience. Perhaps their lives will be a little better and they will feel more hopeful. Others may find a profound personal awakening that amplifies the spiritual aspects of their entire being.

Some people seek out the spiritual with a vengeance and try to take it by force. They may look for a short cut to God through sexuality. But what seems to work best is to be grounded in the core sense of self and the witness "I am" experience (chapter 7). The secret is in the opening of your heart and having compassion for yourself and others, as well as in your sexuality. You must relish your authentic Self and bring it to life.

There are a number of paradoxes that you must accept as the body-mind exercise opens you to a deeper interior consciousness. One of them is living with impermanence. Nothing, not the hair on your head or the rock you sit upon, remains the same; it is all changing. At the very same time there is something about us that always was and always will be. We are mortal, and we will some day die. This is inevitable. The challenge lies in how fully you participate in your life, how fully you live it. To do this you must become comfortable with change and transformation.

Impermanence

We are transforming every moment of our lives. We can see that our bodies change. At the same time, we experience changes in our assumptions. We look at our being and our whole world view in a different way. As you experience this exercise it will be clear that something remains the same. Something is dying, and something is changing and coming to life as we grow.

Begin: Sit up straight, take about five full breaths. As you do, relax any tensions that you become aware of in your body. Try each step before you read the next one.

Step 1: Closing your eyes for a moment, remember when you were a very small child and imagine that you are riding on a tricycle. Reach your hands out as if you are this child placing your hands on the handlebars.

Open your eyes and look at the back of your hands as they rest on the imaginary tricycle handlebars. Are these the same hands that were on the tricycle when you were a child? In fact, they are not even the same molecules or the same skin or the same bone, but they are the same hands, so something remains the same.

exercise one

Step 2: Again, close your eyes and this time imagine you are a little older, reach your hands out as if they are on the handlebars of your bicycle. Open your eyes and look at these hands. Are these the same hands that were on your tricycle? No, again they are not the same hands, but something is the same, isn't it?

Step 3: This time, close your eyes and imagine that you are driving your first car. Place your hands on the imaginary steering wheel, and as you turn the wheel, open your eyes and look at the back of your hands. Ask yourself, "Are these the same hands that were on the tricycle, the bicycle?" No, they aren't, but something remains the same.

We do not see the world the same way as we saw it from our tricycle, our bicycle, or our first car. With time we change and, as we change, as we live longer, we no longer have the same desires or needs that we had at earlier times of our lives. We may no longer wish to climb as high; we may no longer be as excited about jumping out of airplanes or moving from relationship to relationship. But something remains the same, and has continuity over time, an interior body experience of witnessing your life's journey.

The witness, this steady, immutable part of yourself is self-sustaining. It provides you with a vantage point from which to view the process of your life. To do this you must be able to identify your being with something separate from that which is consumed by life. For instance if you look at a log being consumed in a fireplace and you identify with it, you will feel very uncomfortable. If you identify or think of yourself as the fire, you will have a different experience. Fire is not consumed and is a basic element and will always exist.

If then you can find something in your being that is outside of time, constant, something that is not consumed by age or change, then you can begin to explore new territories with comfort.

As a witness, with the "I am" core body experience (chapter 7), you can more easily learn from and live with change. Otherwise, all you can do is hold on and, in your grasping, shrink your aliveness, your body, and your hope. But in shrinking you lose the feeling in your body of a continuity of being that transcends.

THINGS THAT CAN HAPPEN ALONG THE WAY

ANYTHING THAT APPRECIABLY alters your body or mind changes your way of being. Passionate erotic sex, intimacy, and love alter both. Erotic sexuality and, most importantly, the opening of your heart can and do lead to a deep change of consciousness. This will, in turn, change your world view. If you think you see the world differently from the time you were riding on your tricycle to driving your first car, that is child's play compared to what this shift in consciousness can bring. No wonder cultures for millenniums have used practices such as body opening, breathing, movement, chanting, dance, disidentification with psychological struggles, and sexuality as a catapult for spiritual transcendence. In *The Intimate Couple* you will find all of these aspects.

With a transpersonal experience, you may awaken to a heightened awareness: knowing, seeing, hearing, and sensing things far beyond what you are accustomed to. This may scare you. You may feel that the illusive answers to the mysteries of life are now being revealed to you. These answers may shake the foundation of the assumptions that you base your life upon, leaving you feeling that you don't know anything for sure any more.

"What we see and call reality is only a tiny portion of reality—a fraction of the infinite made manifest through our perception. The more extended our perception, the more the infinite is made manifest. If it is your wish to go beyond the narrow pathway that most travel, to walk amongst the stars; you must first walk toward your fears, cast off your close armor of lies and then risk the terrifying dazzle of truth."
REVEREND DANIEL PANGER,
FELLOWSHIP CHURCH
PUBLICATION,
SAN FRANCISCO, CALIFORNIA

Your perceptions of time and space may be altered. Your senses, such as vision and hearing, may become intensified. You may see lights, colors, and energy around people. Taste, smell, and touch may also become intensified. You may become hypersensitive and find yourself emotionally touched by everything you see at the movies and no longer able to tolerate those that are violent.

You may become more aware of universal human experiences. For instance, while you are making love you might have a body experience that you are, at that very moment, doing what human beings have been doing throughout time. Although you may have already known this intellectually, the new body experience may cause it to feel profound.

If you are not accustomed to these experiences, you may worry that something is wrong with you. Don't worry. These experiences are extremely common even though they are not generally discussed. In fact, more often than not, they are kept secret.

Another transpersonal experience is heightened intuition. For example, you may follow a gut feeling to telephone someone and have them say, "How did you know I needed you right now?" You may know more about what people close to you are thinking and needing, more than is comfortable.

You may come to feel deeply that you are an expression of God, that the "God" you seek is within you. People have very personal, very different experiences that they call God. Some see God as a particular being or person, others as an energy, a life force that is in all things. This experience is a personal, nonverbal certainty.

If you did nothing more than body exercises such as yoga, you would be walking a path very parallel to what people have done for thousands of years. Just using the body-opening exercises in *The Intimate Couple* can produce very deep psychological and physiological changes. You may have a reawakening of early psychological patterns and the possibility of moving into transpersonal states. When you add the breathing to the body work, you greatly intensify and deepen your experience. Some people have very profound psychological insights; others have no psychological impact whatsoever. But they have the same openness and understanding of life's processes, and a softening of heart. If you work on yourself using the psychological chapters as well as on a body and spiritual level, you can achieve deep transformations.

When you do the combination we present of body-opening exercises, psychological work, and high-charge breathing, the energy in your body will amplify. This heightened energy released to circulate through the body is called Kundalini energy by yogis. This charge of energy in the body is often felt as heat, tingling, or vibrations. This hyper-energy was once thought to be released sequentially, segment by segment of the body starting at the base of the spine and moving up the body to higher centers of consciousness. We now know that the energy need not follow this ascending pathway.

Building this energy is extremely pleasurable to most people. They feel more alive and at the same time more calm, creative, and interested in life. And yet, there are those who feel frightened by the heightened experience of aliveness in their body. They are likely to hold back with their body to slow down the experience of aliveness—what yogis visualize as the Kundalini energy being stuck. This is the same as the energetic holding patterns in chapters 7 and 10.

Knowing that these experiences have been familiar to so many others may relieve any anxieties or uncertain feelings. These are healthy signs, not strange, dangerous, and obscure things happening to you. You can perfectly well deal with them with the information provided in the exercise chapters for calming and grounding your body. If your charge feels too much at any time, you can do the exercises for lowering your charge. If you feel uncomfortable at any time you can just hold your breath for a few moments or push against a wall (see chapter 7).

The openness that one achieves through erotic sexual lovemaking can sometimes create a vehicle for transcending or going beyond self-imposed limitations to transpersonal experience. For those who have not yet established a stable core body experience of self in which to turn, the openness may feel like a loss of self-identity, and may therefore feel uncomfortable. Without knowledge of this process and a familiarity with core experiences, there can be a temporary loss of the familiar experience of self. People can misunderstand the experience and fleetingly have thoughts that *they*, rather than defensive body-mind patterns, are dying.

When the initiation to transpersonal experience happens in a sexual context, the marvelous awakening may feel so overwhelmingly powerful and revealing it may never be approached again. Years later, in a very different situation, perhaps with the death of someone close, falling in love, or the birth of a child, another opening, another initiation to the transpersonal may occur. Then it may be recognized for what it was: a gift rather than something to fear. Sometimes, it takes years before a second opening occurs. Unfortunately, if it comes towards the end of life's journey, then one is apt to mourn the time lost for living in this open state of grace.

Many people are more afraid of transcendence when it is opened through sexuality because they fear they will get hooked on sexuality or on their partner rather than remain on their spiritual path. In modern cultures, it is often difficult to understand the experience of using erotic sexuality to awaken different levels of consciousness.

Just as we invest a place, a person, or an object with spiritual meaning, so must we raise the nature of our relationship. Although each of us must realize that we are alone on this journey, when we bring spirituality to our relationship we are not alone.

"What is a mystic? One who knows no answer, one who has asked every possible question and found no question is answerable. Finding this, he has dropped questioning. Not that he has found the answer—he has simply found one thing, that there is no answer to be solved, not a question to be answered, but a mystery to be lived, a mystery to be loved, a mystery to be danced."

RAJNEESH, *MORE GOLDEN NUGGETS*, 1989

LOVE ON THE TRANSPERSONAL JOURNEY

WHEN THE FEELING of impermanence takes up residence in the bedroom, most people believe this indicates that the relationship is in trouble or that someone is going to leave or die. They are not aware that this is more a transpersonal issue felt in their body than a relationship, health, or sexual problem.

The challenge of impermanence is in knowing how to cherish your lover when everything else is changing. How do you treat your lover if he or she is experiencing a transformation of consciousness? How do you treat a lover who is not experiencing the opening to consciousness that you are? The answer is the same for both. The answer is in staying with the immediacy of the moment. You can feel this immediacy with an infant or with a dying friend, because you have no way of controlling the inevitability of their fate. In both situations every moment is precious, and you must emotionally show up or miss the experience.

Opening your heart with love, compassion, and understanding is all you really need to do. This is not a time for competition or lies, just absolute authenticity. You must speak without agency, without wanting something from your partner or trying to explain or fix them. Love is a willingness to live with acceptance, a knowing that you can't change your partner or provide his or her interior journey. You can help your partner by taking care of your own fragmentations and being honest, present, equal, and relational. These brief moments of understanding, union, profound acceptance, and transcendence are ecstatic glimpses of eternity, the world of the mystic.

If you understand how to be with a person compassionately and fully without attachment, then you can live as a conscious lover.

How often we see people who regret and mourn the wasted chances for deep love and sexuality when they were not able or not willing to let go and follow their heart's inner voice, to move toward their partner with love and passion. Being ecstatically in love and joining with your partner creates the experience of the deepest wonder and joy and, at the same time, confronts you with the essential aloneness of life. And it challenges you to sustain your interior sense of self and be willing to join with another.

Sexual participation can range from just satisfying yourself or your partner on a reflexive level, to ecstatic participation that moves past ordinary reality. "The crossover between sexuality and religious ecstasy is a well-known phenomenon, whatever the religious context it occurs in. No matter

"How often attachment is mistaken for love! Even when the relationship is a good one. Love is spoiled by attachment, by its insecurity and pride; and then, when love is gone, all you are left to show for it are the 'souvenirs' of love. Scars of attachment."

RINPOCHE,
THE TIBETAN BOOK OF LIVING AND DYING, 1992

The Kundalini Chakra System

body-mind awakening

The awakening of consciousness that comes with the opening of the body is an integral part of *The Intimate Couple.* The experiences you will discover in mind and body are not new. To those who have practiced mind-body traditions, the experiences are a format for the transformational process.

All traditions concerned with opening to consciousness—the Sufis, Cabalist or Hebrews, Hopis, Taoists, Christians, Japanese mystics, and others—discovered and noted energy emanating from and circulating through major centers of the body. The segmental system of energetic holding patterns, first laid out by Wilhelm Reich, corresponds to these traditions and our segmental approach.

The oldest and still the most universally understood system comes from the yogis of India, dating back five to seven thousand years. In the yogi Kundalini system, the body is the central component. For an understanding of

the body mind approach, it is most useful to review this system. (See *Total Orgasm* and *Body, Self and Soul,* Rosenberg, for further information.)

The yoga system is based on the Yoga sutra, or writings, of Pana Mangali. The word yoga comes from the Sanskrit word "to yoke," to link two things together. Yoga provides a link between our everyday awareness and the source of consciousness, the spiritual or God. This link allows us live in tune with this consciousness in our everyday lives. There are many yogic disciplines, but the one most similar to what we present is the Kundalini chakra system. The energetic holding patterns in different segments of your body correspond to this chakra system. Other cultures have used this common information for many years, and it can provide you with a clue to possible psychological or physiological components associated with energetic holding patterns.

how 'spiritual' the cosmological urge may seem, it is, I want to emphasize, thoroughly grounded in the tissues of the body; meaning it is part of the bodily self." (Berman, *Coming to Our Senses*, 1989)

KEEPING A CLEAR PERSPECTIVE

THE PROCESS OF CONSCIOUSNESS is a lifelong journey whether you are in a relationship or alone. Yet for some people, the onset can be quite rapid and accompanied by immediate and overwhelming clarity of universal knowledge. As the body-mind opens, many insights emerge faster than they can be integrated. These insights often feel like a direct communion with a deity; some are right on and do represent a shift in consciousness. Others are infused with distortions and are laden with unresolved issues of the nursery, and an acting out of the character style and agency arenas. The Spanish poet Antonio Machado (Berman, *Coming to Our Senses*, 1989) said it this way:

> In my solitude
> I have seen things very clearly
> that were not true.

The dilemma is what to believe and follow. This can be a struggle if you lose your humor. For humility you must have humor. Only humor can cut through the blind assurance of revealed experience. As Umberto Eco states in *The Name of the Rose,* "[Humor] throws us back on ourselves, gives some psychic distance from the things we are so certain of."

There are too many odd and bizarre things in life, too much irony, too many misperceptions and faulty mirrors to believe anything at first appearance with absolute certainty. Perhaps the best way to judge the importance of things is to see the humor in them. Anything that requires a devotion to seriousness must be viewed carefully for, if you can't have humor for perspective, then you won't see things very clearly.

The same is true for the psychological arenas: primary scenario, character style, and agency. When they are seen as insurmountable struggles and used to justify our behavior in the present, we lose our compassion for ourselves and others. When we take ourselves too seriously, we lose our objectivity. Humor and detachment must accompany our soul to help us witness our personal process and see ourselves clearly on our journey. Humor provides the laughter and the joy to lighten our step along the spiritual path.

"The real goal of spiritual growth should not be ascent (going up to God) but openness and vulnerability (compassion and love) and this does not require (ecstatic) great experience but, on the contrary, very ordinary ones. Charisma is easy; presence, self-remembering, is terribly difficult and where the real work lies." (Berman, *Coming to Our Senses*, 1989)

Remember the old Tibetan saying: "The highest art is the art of living an ordinary life in an extraordinary manner."

CHAPTER FIFTEEN
Fragmentation, or Intermittent Insanity

IF YOU ARE IN an intimate relationship and don't clear up your own fragmentation, your negativity and distorted feelings can cause your partner and your relationship to fragment. Fragmentation can strain even the best of relationships to the breaking point.

Couples in therapy often insist on arguing about what happened *after* a fragmentation occurred rather than uncovering the source of the upset. They complain about the irrational, cutting words thrown back and forth. A reiteration of "He said… She said…" can only deepen their own fragmentation and push both people farther apart.

A common but often tragic misconception is that the things people say or do in this state of "intermittent insanity" are the *real* truth. *This is not correct.* When a person is fragmented, his or her utterances and actions are clouded, warped, and exaggerated. The symptoms of fragmentation are an expression of childhood injuries repeated in a current situation. You may be fragmented in more than one arena: primary scenario, agency, character style, existential-transpersonal. The underlying source of each fragmentation, not its glaring symptoms, must be acknowledged before any current issue can be resolved.

Most fighting is caused by unacknowledged fragmentation. Fighting does not work, no matter how "fair." It only inflicts more wounds, leaving its own scars. An argument that is not easily resolved means that a deeper problem is not being recognized and dealt with. Fighting is what couples do instead of sorting out and resolving their problems.

STEPS OUT OF FRAGMENTATION

It is possible to be fragmented in more than one arena at the same time. The way out of multiple fragmentations is to follow the sequence: primary scenario, agency, character style, then existential-transpersonal.

WHEN YOU ARE FRAGMENTED is not the time to try to work out existing problems with your partner. Take time out to write in your journal and bring yourself back to a state of well-being by doing the steps out of fragmentation that follow (and the sustaining integration series in chapter 7). Have the courage to stop an argument as soon as you realize that you or your partner, or both, are fragmented. Agree that you will work on the problem in your personal journals, each finding his or her own part. Then set a specified time when you will return to discuss the problem anew.

You need a place to take your rage and let off at least a little steam. In your journal, exaggerate your hurt and anger. Write as fast as you can, letting all your feelings emerge and spill onto the pages. Don't spill them onto your partner. Put your upset into perspective by following the steps out of fragmentation and shift yourself energetically out of this body experience.

Steps out of Primary Scenario Fragmentation

Scenario fragmentations, by definition, are reenactments of childhood themes of emotional injury. In the primary scenario chapter, you learned to identify the themes most likely to fragment you. Using your journal, follow these six steps to find your well-being. Each step is necessary to insure the results you are looking for.

Step 1: Acknowledge that you are fragmented. Identify your symptoms: emotional, physical, mental, and behavioral. In particular, pay attention to loss of sensory awareness and feelings of negativity and hopelessness. Identify where you feel these symptoms in your body:

"I'm holding my breath; my shoulders are tense; my stomach aches; I can't see clearly; etc."

Step 2: Acknowledge the temporary nature of fragmentation by writing: "I have been fragmented before; I will be fragmented again; I have gotten out of it before, and I will get out of it again." Notice if you feel any difference after writing this.

Step 3: Get present by doing a sensory-awareness exercise. You have fallen into the past and out of your body. Bring yourself back by doing a body exercise, such as the sustaining integration series. This will further bring you back to your senses and a somatic sense of self, the "I am" body experience. *If you are split off,* use your eyes to become energetically present. Aloud, quickly list the colors and objects you see. *If you are cut off,* do a body awareness exercise. Say, "I can feel my back touching the chair, my feet on the floor. My jaw and belly are tight, but I can relax the tension with my breath." Start slowly with your head, neck, chest, arms, etc., one segment at a time.

Step 4: Find when and how you became fragmented. To do this, think back to the last time you felt good. You may have to go back several days or weeks or even

longer. When you think you have identified the time, look back two more days to see if that was far enough. Now, start checking: Was I okay in the morning? at noon? at night? Come forward in time, looking for the trigger for your fragmentation. You will find many upsets and clouded perceptions *after* the point you fragmented, but these are not the trigger. You must find the first one.

Step 5: Search your memory for the childhood injury that parallels the current upset. The temptation is to identify an injury that occurred later in your childhood rather than in its earliest origins. Always try to go as far back as you can to the inception of the theme. Once you have discovered the childhood injury, figure out which good parent message would have made a difference in your life had it not been missing.

Step 6: Identify which good parent message was missing in the current fragmenting situation. Is this the same message missed in childhood? Can you give this message (or messages) to yourself and take it in from others when it is given? Do you disqualify the person bearing the message? How is this message, or lack of it, a theme in your current life?

If you couldn't find the triggering event in step 4, write the good parent messages from memory. If you memorized these messages when you read them in chapter 2, you can use them now to help yourself out of fragmentation. Finding the missing message (or messages) will help you identify the triggering event and the childhood injury. The ones you don't remember are the ones that are most apt to have caused your fragmentation. Then proceed with steps 5 and 6.

Note: After you follow these steps, if you are not fully out of your fragmentation, you may be fragmented by more than one arena. Try the agency steps next.

Steps Out of Agency Fragmentation

Agency fragmentation occurs when:

(1) The body feeling of "I'm bad, and I've done something wrong" is activated.

(2) Your omnipotence causes you to blame yourself because you can't fix your agency target.

(3) Your target doesn't stay fixed.

(4) You feel emotionally split in deciding whether or not to help someone else at your expense.

(5) You have done something in your own behalf and broken the old family rule of agency. The earlier in childhood you learned this benevolent goodness, the more entrenched the habit, the more intractable your fragmentation, the less available is your sense of core self, and the less interested you will be in sex for yourself.

From the scenario fragmentation exercise you have already realized that you are fragmented, acknowledged that this state is temporary, gotten back to your body and the present, found the triggering event, found the childhood parallel, and found the missing good parent message. And though you might feel better, you are still fragmented.

In your journal, proceed by doing these five steps out of agency fragmentation.

Step 1: Identify the emotional, physical, mental, and behavioral symptoms that tell you that you are in agency fragmentation. Don't skip this step. You will need this information later when you are not fragmented, to differentiate for yourself between loving and agency.

Step 2: Locate the trigger for your agency fragmentation:

(a) You fear that you have done something wrong.

(b) Your target didn't get fixed or stay fixed.

(c) You have set your body in a ready mode for agency.

(d) You tried to get your sense of well-being from the outside.

(e) Someone didn't live up to your unilateral contract.

(f) You've gotten into a "nonentity" panic because you have abandoned yourself.

(g) All of the above.

Step 3: Read the agency mantras (chapter 2). They are healthy statements that most people feel all the time. If you can't feel their truth in your body as well as in your mind, you are not living honestly with yourself. This dishonesty will surely keep you fragmented.

Work with these mantras until you feel in your body which one (or ones) you have not remembered in your own behalf. Figure out what is keeping you from believing the truth and you will discover the way out of your fragmentation. Remember, you have a right to believe and act on these mantras and not feel badly about yourself.

Step 4: If you haven't already done so, do a body practice such as the sustaining integration series to enliven your core body self. In particular, do an exercise that both opens your chest and builds a charge, such as the fish position with high-charge breathing, ending with the witness "I am" experience in your upper chest.

Step 5: Use your self-agency to complete an action in your own behalf, one you can feel in your body as emanating from your own volition. It won't do any good to do something in reaction to someone else. If you have made any unilateral contracts, clear them up. Find out what your side of the bargain is and what you want in return. Try the Character Style steps next if you are still fragmented.

Steps Out of Character Style Fragmentation

It is *your* character style that can cause you to fragment, not someone else's. As you learn to recognize and accept the aspects of who you are, character style will be greatly reduced (chapter 12). Character style fragmentation occurs when your abandonment, inundation, or the abandonment-inundation As If profile is aroused, and you respond by acting out the traits of your style in a way that works against you.

To work with character style fragmentation, begin with the scenario and agency fragmentation steps above. Then write these steps in your journal.

Step 1: Identify the symptoms—emotional, physical, mental, and behavioral—that let you know you are fragmented by your character style.

Step 2: Write the five or six primary traits of your style (see below). As you write each one, identify which one (or ones) has become so exaggerated and rigid that it has caused you to fragment. You may have to write the traits of all three styles to figure out which is causing your fragmentation.

Step 3: Identify the childhood situation that caused you to adopt this trait. What belief did you form due to this identified experience? Does this belief perpetuate your attachment to this trait? What feelings and fears did you experience back then? Using these traits is likely to evoke your childhood feelings and fears. The feeling in your body is the voice of the injury that happened to you as a child. It is not who you are today. You are in charge and do not have to protect yourself like a child.

Step 4: Some situations will only require you to rectify the problem within yourself, as in step 3. Others will require that you make restitution for a problem you caused while acting out your style in fragmentation. Using your journal, follow the inside/outside exercise on the next page.

Abandonment Character Style Profile
- I Will Do Anything, Just Don't Leave Me
- No Matter What, It's Never Enough
- There's No Such Thing as Too Close
- Constellate Around Someone or Something
- Hyper–Body Awareness, Sensuality, and Vulnerability
- I'm Hyper-Vulnerable and Aware of My Body

Inundation Character Style Profile
- Separate and Removed: I Am What I Am
- Cut Off from Feelings and Emotions
- Defined, Rigid Boundaries and Assumptions
- Literal, Right or Wrong, Black and White Assumptions
- Physically Cut Off and Emotionally Armored

Abandonment-Inundation Character Style Profile
- Automatic No: Nobody Can Tell Me What to Do
- Have an Idea of How Things Should Be and Cling to It
- Treat Myself and Others as Objects
- Authenticity Gap: Tend to Lie Up or Lie Down
- Intimate Relationships: Not Too Close, Not Too Far Away
- Feel Split Off from Self, Body, Emotions, and Aliveness

Inside/Outside Exercise: Authenticity Reality Check

When any of the four arenas cause fragmentation, your perspective can become distorted, causing your character style and agency patterns to heighten and take over. When this happens, it is hard to know the difference between what is coming at you from other people (outside), especially your lover, and what comes from you (inside). With this confusion the problem is more likely to escalate than become resolved.

Work first on your part of the problem (inside). If you can let your guard down and admit your own underlying issues, your partner may feel safe enough to do the same. *Refrain from using your partner's admissions to prove your point.* If either of you does this, it is no longer safe to explore together.

Determine, on a scale of one to ten, how much of your fragmentation is caused by your own inside assumptions. This assessment will help you evaluate what and how much is coming at you from the outside.

Inside

Check Your Assumptions: What do you think happened? How does this fit with your primary scenario, agency, or character style traits? Ask yourself, for example: Am I fragmented because I have an idea of how it is or ought to be? because I think someone just told me what to do? because of my lack of or rigid boundaries? Have I lately reality-tested the assumptions I hold so dear? Has my grandiosity been punctured, my unilateral contract been broken? Is this the same as what happened in my family of childhood?

Check Your Balancing Act: Ask yourself: Is the bond of my relationship really threatened or broken? Do I have to be angry, indignant, hurt, or withdrawn to get enough breathing room or get even? Is the lack of attunement just a sign that my character style is acting up? Am I fragmented because someone just acted as if they were separate from me, or because they got too close?

Check Your Crisis Meter: See if you have gone back to an old habit of making a crisis where there isn't one. Say, "This is just my character style (agency or primary scenario) acting up. I don't have to make a crisis out of it. I'm not helpless. I can accept my character style (agency or primary scenario) with humor. How have I made a crisis this time?" For good sex, you particularly need C-H-C: Know this is not a **C**risis. Keep a sense of **H**umor. Have personal **C**ourage.

Check Your Intention: What is your intention toward your partner? Are you hurt and trying to get even, control, or change your partner? Do you believe your partner's intention is positive toward you and the bond, the breathing room, and the attunement between you? If you assume your partner has a negative intention toward you and you don't check it out, it will fragment you.

Outside

Take Action: Your fragmentation won't go away if there is something on the outside that is undermining you, especially if it's triggering your agency or character style. Example: If your partner constantly keeps you waiting, won't be on time, won't make commitments, and you feel abandoned, you must set limits or you will find yourself in a perpetual state of fragmentation. Your partner can neither stop your feelings of abandonment nor be perfect all the time, but if he or she can't make and keep a reasonable commitment, you may not belong with this person. With agency, if you are ignoring or otherwise not doing something in your own behalf because you fear it will interfere with your partner's well-being or he or she will be upset with you—you are likely to remain fragmented. You must act in your own behalf or you will remain fragmented. If you have caused a problem or injury due to your character style, you will have to make restitution: Apologize and make up for what you have done.

Bracket Off: How can you take care of yourself if you can't act immediately? You may find temporary relief from fragmentation by making a decision to set the problem aside, promising to readdress it at a specified later time. But to avoid a deeper fragmentation, be sure to keep your promise.

EXISTENTIAL-TRANSPERSONAL FRAGMENTATIONS pull on our soul and cause physical and psychological pain and crises, forcing us to confront the human dilemma of how we are to exist in a world that is in constant flux and the inevitable moments of despair. These larger, more spiritual issues are often brought to our awareness by a threat to our own survival or that of our loved ones—surgery, illness, serious accident, death, or a deepening realization of the aging process.

The crisis may be a perceived threat to our existence—a reversal of finances, loss of a job, home, or other possessions; and powerful events such as earthquakes, floods, fire, and hurricanes, which can shake the false security upon which our beliefs of permanence are based. Another type of crisis is one of awakening, which may occur when you become a parent, fall in love, join in marriage, engage in erotic sexuality, or do body-mind practices that push the barriers aside. Few of us are prepared for anything like full aliveness and the seeing and knowing that come with this degree of consciousness. Many fragment when they get exactly what they have been wanting and working for.

Some people raise every mundane glitch in their life to the level of a life-or-death crisis, which elevates the ensuing fragmentation to the existential level. When this happens, simple fragmentations become impervious to the less complex psychological solutions of the primary scenario, character style, and agency arenas. Therefore, it is important to know the difference between a psychological fragmentation and an existential one.

Although the feeling in your body may cause you to feel that way, primary scenario, character style, and agency issues are not life-or-death crises. You will not die if your partner leaves, if you are inundated, or if someone does not agree with your idea, love you, or think well of you. Changing the level of fragmentation from a psychological basis to an existential crisis is not necessary and is destructive.

For instance, those who have a high abandonment anxiety may constantly fear that they or their loved ones will die. They may act as if their very existence is threatened if someone doesn't come home on time, that is, if they can't get proof from their partner of unconditional love from every interaction. The excess drama of treating a fragmentation as an existential crisis will take you deeper into the abyss rather than taking you out of fragmentation.

People who faced death at a very early age may carry the body memory of their existential crisis close to the surface. They can interpret every obstacle as an existential crisis, and fragment. Others who elevate everything to a crisis may not have been wanted at conception or may have struggled for existence in utero, during childbirth, infancy, or an accident or illness in their youth. They might have been raised by a parent who lived in danger, fear, or anguish due to the death of a loved one, the ravages of war, economic poverty, or spousal abuse. When this is true, some of the same feelings are incorporated into the child's body voice, making life more difficult than necessary.

Existential-transpersonal issues need to be addressed and separated from every little disappointment of life. These fragmentations must be worked with in the psychological arenas so life can be lived more easily. Here are some underlying issues likely to emerge and engulf you in existential fragmentation.

Existential aloneness is an experience that tests the fabric of relationship. Even as you embrace your lover and join with the deepest affection, you know in your heart that this blissful union cannot negate the knowledge that you are alone in life no matter how close you are to another. You alone are in charge of living your life as a separate being.

For some, profound aloneness doesn't surface to consciousness until the last moments of life. For others, there is a constant nagging. In a relationship it may sound like, "If you really are the right one, why do I feel so alone? Why don't you save me from my isolation?" Subtle variations on this theme often leave insurmountable doubts in the best of relationships and can lead to recurrent fragmentation.

One of the major ways one is awakened to the spiritual is through tragedy or loss, an event that feels so shattering that we cannot cope. Then it is only with the shift of consciousness to the witness—a body sense of deeper knowing—that we can survive with our sense of self intact. This internal support is also necessary for a relationship truly to become a spiritual union, a joining of a core-to-core experience.

The shattering of the hope or promise of a relationship can cause a profound existential fragmentation. If the hope invested in a relationship is a substitute for living your own life, and this relationship or the hope in the relationship is lost, life itself feels lost.

Unfortunately, sometimes in agency we make a unilateral contract with God, or whatever we see as a higher power. We promise to be as good, honest, forthright, and authentic as we possibly can and not ask for much of anything for ourselves. In return, we expect to be protected and favored by God or the powers that be.

If we then suffer any reversal of fortune, such as loss of a loved one or a legal or social injustice, we may feel betrayed and possibly forsaken by God. Fragmented, we may then lose not only our hope in life but our sense of spiritual comfort. Then, considering ourselves fallen angels, we may turn our backs on God and abandon ourselves as well.

We must have faith in the moments of our worst travails. Our hope can return if we can find our personal meaning from even the greatest tragedy, for all of life is our teacher. Life does not have to be a journey of despair or pain.

Death is something we can't think about for very long without fragmenting. Yet avoiding it keeps us distant from the realities of our lives. This is why a serious illness can become an existential as well as a psychological and physiological crisis. To a weakened physical condition, we may add the fear of death. For some it does not take much more than a minor cold. But somewhere during the course of the illness, we realize that perhaps we are only ill and this is not our final passing. Then, as the feeling of hope arises, we summon our life energy and begin to heal ourselves. In this way we bring ourselves out of the "existence crisis."

Most of us accept the fact that we are going to die "some day." But when it no longer remains a thought but is felt in the body, the deeper awareness can shift to fragmentation. We can only hope to survive physically for a limited time. Even if major advances take place in medical treatment, we can't be assured of any prolonged longevity. If we compare our allotted time to the thousands of years humanity has inhabited the earth, we realize the paltry few we really have.

If, by chance, we do catch a glimpse of death, we may be totally unprepared and terrified. Once fragmented, we may try to stabilize our well-being by rushing back into our busy life pattern and reestablishing our defensive cloak of denial—until we catch the next glimpse of death.

A life lived in denial of death offers little comfort for living. It is spent holding on, fighting ineffective little skirmishes, and running away. But, like dealing with any bully, you eventually have to stand and face death.

It is said in the Buddhist tradition that a truly conscious person will look forward to death with joy. A person who has done the work and preparation through meditation can expect to move toward death without fear. Those of us not in the Buddhist tradition can at least live our lives *without regrets*.

Impermanence is not just for the aged, although as we grow older, it confronts us more directly each time we look in the mirror. Impermanence is an experience right here and right now. Each look in the mirror confirms our changing body but also confirms that which remains the same. We can develop the skill and courage to deal with the inevitable.

The Witness, your interior sense of self, is the first capacity lost with fragmentation. When you are fragmented you lose your internal support system, your awareness of the witness somatic experience of self and sense of well-being. The most important thing to do is get back to your body. Start with the sustaining integration series (chapter 7). This will bring you back to presence and intensify the "I am" experience. Once this is established, sit up and meditate by focusing on the "I am" feeling in your chest.

Feel the well-being and the silence. Any time the same thought comes up

"There is no chance of getting to know death if it only happened once. But fortunately life is nothing but a continuum dance of birth and death, a dance of changes. Every time I hear the rush of a mountain stream or the waves crashing on the shore or my own heartbeat, I hear the sound of impermanence."
RINPOCHE, *THE TIBETAN BOOK OF LIVING AND DYING*, 1992

again and again, write it down in your journal. Then return to a silent meditation. Each time you return to meditation from writing in your journal, you may have to take 10 to 20 breaths to renew the "I am" feeling. Other meditations, prayers, and contemplation are all extremely helpful, too.

There are no exact steps out when you are fragmented by issues of this existential arena. The process is one of using your volition and living life fully. There is no solution to your existential dilemma other than to find meaning in your life and to live as consciously as you can.

When you are fragmented, be sure to do the steps out of the other psychological arena fragmentations first. You may be surprised to find your well-being return. When you are not fragmented by these arenas, you will face existential-transpersonal issues more easily.

FRAGMENTATION PREVENTION

BECOMING FRAGMENTED at times is inevitable; however, you can avoid its constant intrusion in your life by consciously using the tools for body-mind well-being that have been laid out. You have learned how to regain your well-being once you are fragmented, but it is best to stop a fragmentation before it happens.

The use of a journal is the best tool for sustaining your well-being. Take just a little time every evening to record an entry. With the following exercise, you can watch for your upsets before they cause you to fragment.

Emptying-Out Exercise:

Review your day, hour by hour. Is there an encounter that triggered feelings or remains unfinished or that has fragmented you? Use your body to sense when something just doesn't feel right, is upsetting, or unfinished. When you reach a moment that feels uncomfortable, explore it to find the reason for your discomfort, then find what you have to do or say to resolve the discomfort. Sometimes creating a dialogue in your journal with someone will help. The good parent messages, agency mantras, and character style traits can help you find your key for resolution. In your journal, complete what is unfinished. You may or may not have to say something to someone else at a later time. Usually the journal is enough. This exercise will create a major shift in lowering the level of unconscious abandonments and inundations that you carry in your body.

EXAMPLE: As I sit with my journal, I begin to write, "All was well…except at lunch. Why was that upsetting? What do I feel in my body? I feel something in my chest. I feel unfinished. What is unfinished?" I review back through my lunch hour. I remember a conversation, a brief moment, when Joe asked me about Bob. He then told me how angry he was with Bob. I felt put in the middle, like I had to take sides. I changed the conversation. I thought it was all over, but I still have the sick feeling in my body. *How is that like something in my past,* in my family? It is *the same feeling I had when* Mom wanted me to take sides with her about Dad. I never could win in that triangle, and I can't win in this one. *My fear is* that I will lose one of them as a friend if they argue. Then I will be abandoned. I don't have to say anything to Joe. I just have to remind myself that I'm not bad because I couldn't fix my mother and I can't fix Joe. Oh, its just my *agency.* I can stay out of their problem."

Questions to ask yourself about an unfinished or upsetting incident: 1) What is the feeling in my body? 2) How is this feeling like something in my past? 3) Which arena am I struggling in? If you write about your feelings you might find out how you are acting your arena themes without knowing it.

Collecting small upsets results in larger ones. People are more apt to place blame on the final upset that seemed to tip the scale. But to get out of fragmentation you must work with the first, triggering upset, not the last, symptomatic one.

Fragmentation can be triggered by small slights: the bank teller closes the window just before your turn; a colleague shifts his eyes away during a conversation; a friend describes someone else favorably; your husband takes out a stick of gum and doesn't offer you one; your wife didn't get the hint that you wanted to put the kids to bed early because you wanted time with her alone.

Although they seem slight and unimportant, these everyday emotional injuries accumulate, permeating your body and your emotions. They affect your moods, distort your attitudes and assumptions, creep into your relationship, and reduce your availability for intimacy and erotic sexuality. Working in your journal can release the tension from unfinished situations, which can otherwise build up to an explosive fragmentation.

Falling in love is easy. Keeping it alive takes commitment. If you want a change, you have to do something different. Start by examining your relationship; then clear out the damaging hurts. All relationships, even the healthiest, need cleaning out from time to time. Injuries are unavoidable, but healing them is always possible.

SEXUAL ECSTASY
for the
INTIMATE COUPLE

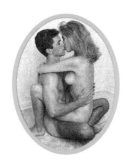

C H A P T E R   S I X T E E N

The Ambiance of Sexual Lovemaking

HEIGHTENED ORGASTIC RELEASE can offer brief universal changes of consciousness, intense feelings of love, and luminous moments of spiritual awakening, actualizing the deepest expansion of being. These powerful psychic insights and profound body releases of energy are well known to travelers in the state of ecstatic sex. But to become a permanent resident in Nirvana is not the intention. It is equally as important to bring these profound openings back to earth and ground them in the everyday existence and aliveness in your body and relationship. Without this grounding, ecstatic experiences serve no greater role than a psychedelic drug experience. More love, sexual pleasure, and satisfaction are the ultimate rewards for building a heightened charge.

Altered states of consciousness can be remarkable, but they can also distract you from your own body sense of self, mutuality, and spirituality.

Once you start making love, throw the book out; or at least lock it outside the room. Prepare your body; bring little body remembrances, thoughts, insights, movements, and plenty of breathing, a little at a time. You need not make a project out of this. Trust what you have learned through your body and mind—feel it and practice through the exercises and masturbation. Don't memorize the information as a how-to list. When you make love sexually

"Sex is one of the most sacred acts because it is through sex that life arrives and it is through sex that you can penetrate to the very source of existence."

GUNTHER,
NEO TANTRA, 1980

with your partner, savor each sensation. Allow your movement, breath, and sound to express your passions.

Following are further opportunities for exploration and insight written to help you through the unknown, the untried, the unexplored. Sex is fun and exciting, especially when you know how energetic excitement works in the body. Use this knowledge in your own unique way to bring greater understanding to your relationship and to enhance your lovemaking.

In a committed relationship, it is mutuality that allows people to feel like soul mates. We all long to be seen, heard, and valued for who we are, not for whom others wish or expect us to be. We want to be loved, known, and understood as we truly are—at our core—beyond the words and actions we present to the world. We long for reciprocity and parity with our lovers— the rhythmic give and take. We long to assume that our chosen partner has the consistent positive intention toward us that is so necessary in a loving relationship. We all want to be with someone with whom we can share our deepest thoughts, hopes, and desires. Mutuality is heightened when you have a worldview, hopes, values, and dreams in common.

And when sex matures into ecstasy, these feelings of mutuality are manifested at a body-energetic level, a core-to-core coupling with another being. This in turn fuels mutuality and helps support what is now an undeniable total body experience. Once you experience this ecstasy on a body level, you will know without a doubt that you don't want to live without it.

ROMANCE

ROMANCE IS PRIMARILY BUILT on idealization. Everybody wants to have the feeling of romance in their relationship—to feel that something about their partner is special. Most often people build romance on the positive virtues their lover actually embodies—honesty, wisdom, beauty, etc.—but these virtues are usually idealized qualities that make one feel hopeful and romantic.

Idealizations are projections of hopes and longings that originate from within one's self. Sometimes we search in others for something we feel is missing in ourselves; instead of trying to develop this virtue we try to gain it by merging with another. Other times we value a virtue we admire in ourselves and wish to find the same in another. Either way, chances are that our romantic idealizations say more about ourselves than our partners.

When we try to satisfy our primary-scenario longings through romance, our dearest of secret themes, particularly gender prejudice, show up on parade. Finally character style—that outdated, protective, psychic guardian of our shallow, fragile persona—joins them. They all appear costumed in idealizations as if at a Hollywood premiere.

In this way, romance fogs our perceptions. We project our romantic hopes on our unsuspecting partner. The hope is that this time it will all be different. Unfortunately, projection does not allow us to see who our lover really is. As we dance with our own shadow, our partner feels left out, unseen and unknown.

Being aware of your emotional issues is critical to sexuality because if you are not intimately familiar with them, you will not recognize when you are unconsciously projecting your expectations and uncomfortable parts of yourself onto your partner. What you don't accept in yourself can be mistaken as being part of your lover. Conscious sexuality requires conscious lovers—those who can see their partners clearly, with all their faults, and still allow and support an ample portion of romantic idealization. Romance is like spice added to food: Too much overpowers the individual flavors, and too little means blandness.

What people usually call romance are the extra special enhancements that soften the heart: a candle-lit dinner, a canoe ride in the moonlight, a shared glass of wine, a bouquet of flowers, dancing on the terrace, walking hand in hand barefoot on the beach—all the wonderful, crazy, spontaneous things that light the spark of hope and love. With romance we transcend everyday existence for a little magic.

So don't be stingy; take a chance on romance. Experiment with the unexplainable, the wonder, the mystery of mutual attraction. Do or say something to let your partner feel good about himself or herself in a romantic way. When people say, "I want more romance," they mean, "I want you to idealize me." They want to hear, "You look beautiful (or handsome). I like your body. I like to touch you. I like your smell. You are a wonderful cook. You are so brilliant, clever, sexy." So if you feel it at all, say it. Even if you can't say, "I love you," try saying, "I'm loving you right now."

Everyone has a right to feel idealized and special at times. This is nothing to worry about. You won't get trapped. Only your character style prevents you from giving what you and your partner so desperately need. Not being able to accept the compliments involved in the idealizations of romance can also be due to character style. A major consequence of character style is that it inevitably ruins both romance and mutuality.

Many fairy tales with characters such as Sleeping Beauty, Cinderella, and Prince Charming are based on the wish to fulfill universal romantic longings. A fantasy based on longings has a dreamlike quality. When you make love to a fantasy you take the risk of waking up a few years into your relationship and finding that the fantasy has worn thin and the person you are with is a stranger. This is painfully disappointing and can cause you to feel foolish about yourself and betrayed by your partner. Fantasies based on a great night of sex, without the foundation of a relationship and love, can fade even faster. When you have an ecstatic core-to-core erotic body experience with your partner, you no longer have to weave a fantasy because you have an authentic body experience of reality far richer than you can imagine.

Romance can be a ticket, the gift, that allows two hearts to make a mysterious journey to new depths of being together. Sex will be a part of this journey, but the final destination is far beyond sexuality.

Anima/Animas Projection

We are each made up of both masculine and feminine characteristics. As Robert Johnson wrote in *She*, "C. G. Jung, in one of his most profound insights, showed that, just as genetically every man has recessive female chromosomes and hormones....so too every man has a group of feminine psychological characteristics that make up a minority element within him. A woman, likewise, has a psychological masculine minority component within her." Jung called the man's feminine side *anima*; the woman's masculine side he called the *animus*.

Awakening the anima/animus principle in each of us is an integral part of the inner journey of emotional growth. At some point in adulthood, a man accepts his softer and gentler yin side and a woman accepts her more aggressive and powerful yang side. Gender prejudice and other arena themes can interfere with this inward self-acceptance journey. To feel whole we must each accept our "other" side. But when we deny ourselves this completion, the search turns outward.

People can go on a fruitless search to find a part of themselves in someone else. Then, when they are looking for a mate, what is sought is actually a romanticized, disowned part of self. Another attraction is to one's own mirror image and what we would be like if we were the opposite sex. The lure can be so enticing that many peo-

ple leave marriages, have affairs, or are on an eternal search for their beloved knight on a white horse or princess in a tower.

Sometimes when we find an anima/animus, because it is a part of ourselves, we feel complete and believe that we have found our true love. This experience brings on a feeling of relief that we've found our "better half." The feeling is wonderful, horrible, scary, and exciting, and it often comes with the body feeling of wanting to become one, wanting to merge, crawl inside of, or gobble up the loved one.

As this match-made-in-heaven proceeds, the illusion fades and we see that the object of our affection is not all we thought. We awaken one morning wondering how this person we loved so much could have changed so drastically. Feeling severely betrayed and devastated, we say, "Who is this person in bed next to me?"

This theme can ruin families and relationships and project itself on future generations. It is far better that you take on the task of finding your own interior counterpart. Then, instead of projecting it onto someone in the outer world and falling in love with it, you can honor it within yourself. In this way you can be in your relationship as a whole being, with no need to make unreasonable demands of your partner to fulfill longings that are best fulfilled on your own.

SEXUAL AFFAIRS — MONOGAMY'S BETRAYAL, the secret affair, is a symptom of something not working in a relationship. The act of infidelity is often a cry for help, an attempt to break the cycle of old patterns that are impossible to live with. There are many reasons for affairs as well as different types. Besides the desire for excitement, fun, revenge, or experimentation, there can be an urge to spark a mate's interest through jealousy, to cause hurt, to punish, or to gain breathing room by creating distance between oneself and one's partner. Alcohol and drugs can also create distance or blur a person's sense of boundaries, which may lead to affairs.

There is also the affirmative affair. In an emotionally destructive marriage, the affirmative affair is an attempt to regain confidence in one's self and one's sexuality, to affirm one's femininity or masculinity, to re-own one's body and sense of self. It is driven by the need to find a new source of reflection and, in this way, find value as a person. The affirmative affair often achieves this goal but damages the primary relationship more than either party can handle.

When there is a sexual affair, one's partner always knows. They do not always know the actual facts of the affair, of course, but they can feel in their body that something is wrong. A break in any part of the bond of the relationship can be felt. This is also true when there is an infidelity of the heart—when love, without sex, is given to another. This can be to another adult or in the form of excessive attention to one's own children.

Long-term infidelities can keep a couple together by providing excitement or a way to escape from the relationship struggle. This, of course, doesn't confront, much less resolve, the injuries and dissatisfactions within. When energy, body, interest, and emotions are split between a primary and a secondary relationship, a person is forever vacillating, waiting for a crisis to change the situation, yet praying that it never happens. When one relationship balances or off-sets the other, you never get a true feeling of what is or could be. Eventually you have to face your core issues before either relationship will work.

Some people do love each other and yet still have sex outside their relationship. But, when a person opens up his or her body as through *The Intimate Couple* exercises, sex with anyone other than the one he or she loves becomes more and more uncomfortable. In this case, something comes to an end, either the affair or the marriage.

Agency, that penchant for either not being aware of one's own needs or blatantly giving them up to attend to another, kills the aliveness of sexuality in a relationship. It can drive one or both of the partners to find sexual excitement outside the relationship, even when they love each other. Agency extinguishes the erotic spark. This works two ways. For the agent, it is easier to feel sexually alive with someone he or she doesn't care about, particularly a stranger they will never see again, because the act itself doesn't trigger an agency response. For the partner of an inveterate agent, sex outside of the relationship may be the only way to feel the genuine spark of erotic sexuality again rather than just a partner's compliance, duty, or eagerness to please.

Character style can cause affairs in ways too numerous to mention. With the As If abandonment-inundation character style, for instance, if one partner says wistfully, "I could forgive you almost anything but your sleeping with someone else," the other feels controlled. The body experience of this is like a virtual command and provokes the automatic "no" response and a compulsion to have the forbidden affair. Each aspect of the As If character style, when it is acted out of a high level, can drive a partner to seek relief in a safer bed.

Intimacy, sexuality, and eroticism are problems for those with a high fear of both abandonment and inundation. They are often the first to break the pledge of fidelity because they are disassociated from their inner source of aliveness and continually seeking an experience of aliveness from others.

The person with a high fear of abandonment will never leave, but in order to protect against ever having to face abandonment, he or she may keep several relationships going. There never-enough longings can drive their partner away and into the arms of another who doesn't need such constant reassurance and can be satisfied more easily.

The person with a high fear of inundation will often seek meaningless affairs so she or he doesn't have to make emotional contact but can still have sexual gratification. The partner left behind may then seek an affair of the heart (sex is usually not their problem) to keep from dying of emotional starvation and loneliness.

People who are uncomfortable with intimacy use intermittent affairs as an ongoing means to create distance in their relationships. This works only for a while; eventually they are bound to gain more distance than they bargained for. For some people, affairs can be a habitual but futile attempt to attenuate old longings and psychic wounds.

Bringing in a third partner, having a threesome, can be an attempt to revive waning feelings of aliveness, love, sexuality, or eroticism. This type of external stimulation can be exciting, but it never lasts long. It is like giving artificial respiration to the ambulance driver while the patient quietly goes under. The attention is aimed in the wrong direction. It is the relationship between the two people and the internal aliveness of each that needs attention. A succession of new and different sex partners will not accomplish this. Excitement, once aroused and originating from within, can last as long as there is a breath left in your body. It is not dependent on age or the length of the relationship.

Usually the problem that leads to an affair isn't solved through having other relationships. An affair can be exciting and fun but, in the long run, someone will get hurt and the bond of the primary relationship will be broken. The price is often greater than the excitement merits.

Some people, you may have noticed, can forgive infidelity, while others remain forever isolated and tortured by the betrayal. The greatest, most enduring pain is felt not necessarily because of the affair but because it triggers feelings of betrayal in the psyche. Too close to the core, too closely parallel to an abandonment in childhood, the two wounds merge into one and become too painful to bear. The injury can be so great that it ruptures the trust and hope necessary for the growth of a deeper, more intimate relationship. Unless the old and the new wounds can be dealt with as separate experiences, and unless the infidelity can be seen as a symptom of a relationship that wasn't working, forgiving may not be possible and the relationship may inevitably end.

And then the question of whether to reveal infidelity to a partner may arise. No one else can solve this dilemma for you. Many counselors are adamant in one direction or another. Avoid the advisor who knows what's best for your life. To us, the first question is not, "Should I tell?" but, "Why do I want to tell?"

Although there are many reasons for disclosure, they almost always fall into these four categories:

1. *To get honest* in the relationship, to clear up the fog of lies that has been creating emotional walls of distance. With honesty comes the hope of beginning to build an *authentic* intimate relationship.

2. *To get even,* to hurt the other person. Sometimes you feel better, but usually it just backfires.

3. *To relieve guilt.* But beware, this is usually a ploy for, "I want permission (or forgiveness) from you so I don't have to take responsibility for my actions." When you do this you are treating your partner as a parent and unfairly asking him or her to take responsibility for your actions and for creating the solution. Some try to relieve their guilt by getting their partners to carry some or all of the guilt and pain.

4. *To end the relationship.* If this is your plan, there are kinder ways.

The next question to ask yourself is, "Will telling about the infidelity create a betrayal so great as to sever the bond of the relationship?" Consider that the bond is most likely already in trouble and that's why the affair came about. Remember that telling can cause a scenario, agency, character style, or existential-transpersonal fragmentation and activate gender prejudice—often all at once. Therefore, despite the best of intentions, a disclosure may sever the already frayed bond.

Once you figure out why you want to tell, you need to answer, "Is the affair over?" and, "Am I ready to be fully committed in my relationship?" Find these answers before you decide whether to tell. Not telling however, is like sitting on a keg of dynamite. It leaves you with a lie in your relationship, and if your spouse finds out years later, even though you may think the affair is ancient history, it will seem like a current event to your partner. If your decision about any of these questions is not clear, working with a competent therapist can be helpful. But remember that you are the one who must live with the results of your actions. Don't pass the responsibility on to anyone else.

Remember, also, that when there is a problem in the relationship, someone will act out the symptom. An affair is only a symptom, just as a fever or cough is. Stop blaming one another. The only hope is that *both* people can see their part in creating the problem and work together to resolve it.

Our view of infidelity as a poor way to solve relationship problems is not a moralistic view but a pragmatic one. It's just too likely that the partner's scenario has made them so vulnerable to betrayal that telling will permanently interrupt the process of monogamy, trust, and hope.

COMMITMENT AND MONOGAMY

THERE COMES A TIME when two people make a commitment to one another. That commitment is actually to one's self, a decision that a relationship is the best place to be to fulfill one's own needs.

John Loves Amy:

Sometimes in the morning, before she awakens, I find myself basking in the sunlight of my togetherness with Amy. Lightly I touch her forehead, and any shadows of doubt that I feel fade from my heart. My body trembles with excitement as I think of the depth of my commitment. Saying that I am in love doesn't seem to capture the depth and complexity of my emotions.

For the first time in my life I am immersed in so many positive feelings and sharing so much of my innermost affections. I can't remember a time before in my life when I wanted to have a child, to create a new life, a new being. My devotion and my loving are expressed in so many ways; but in our sensual, sexual joining, lovemaking becomes an unexplainable erotic core experience in which my being touches hers. And yet, I do not need her. I am with her from my momentum of positive loving, not from my need to fill some vast emptiness and longing in my soul, nor from a need to fix or complete her life. I accept her as she is and cherish her inner expression of being.

To say that I am in love is like comparing a full symphonic crescendo to an amateurish piano drill. I am in love and loved and loving simultaneously. I am the act of loving embodied. Amy is the moment of loving, and she is my cherished love. I will not live without this feeling in my life. I will not do anything to jeopardize this feeling for myself. Monogamy is not the question, the sentence, or the answer, but simply the expression of my commitment to myself and to the fulfillment of my life. Even the thought of another's touch feels like an inner betrayal.

To have a feeling such as John has for Amy, you have to stop evaluating every issue as a test of whether or not you are going to stay in your relationship. Lack of commitment is often played out by a person with strong fears of both abandonment and inundation. This is torture when it's played against a partner with a high fear of abandonment. Yet commitment can help establish a body experience of constancy and stability in your relationship, then you can then pursue a deeper and better quality in lovemaking.

- Part of the commitment you make to be in a relationship is to accept the shadow aspects of your partner, the characteristics that are less admirable, right along with those that you adore. When you add the quality of love, a little humor, and compassion, you may even see these less admirable traits as quirks or endearing qualities. No one is perfect.
- No matter how right your partner is for you, no matter how much you love him or her, if your fears drive your style you can always find something to be upset about. Most upsets start from within; then you look for evidence on the outside to substantiate your feeling.
- Many people feel that being stingy with love or sex puts them in charge of a relationship. But the one who holds back, usually for self-protection, is the one who loses the most because he or she never gets to feel love.
- Loving implies an essence of consciousness and intimacy, and an ability to make this feeling known. It is not about making love to another person so much as it is about opening yourself to a state of being.

One of the most effective ways to shift your body feeling to love is to use the word *cherish*. This implies *value* and importance, a treasuring but not ownership. When you say "cherish," you communicate a generosity of spirit through your affection, excitement, sexuality, and acceptance.

THE OPPOSITE OF
LOVE IS NOT HATE,
IT IS INDIFFERENCE

AS YOU WORKED with opening and enlivening your body in previous chapters, you probably noticed that you could feel good in one part of your body and bad in another. And you could feel happy, sad, and angry all at the same time. One emotion did not invalidate the other feelings. In an intimate relationship you can also feel many feelings at the same time. It all depends on where you want to place your focus. It is your choice; you can decide.

Many people believe that if love is not unconditional, then it is not really love. Actually, in healthy adult relationships, there is no such thing as unconditional love. Everyone does and should have limits. Unconditional love is for infants, and if we were lucky we had our share. But love does not survive consistent poor treatment, abuse, or neglect. Sometimes, people who believe in unconditional love expect to receive the good mother messages from their partner no matter how poorly they behave. They say, in effect, "Take that. Now will you love me?…Okay, then try this one. Now do you still love me?…You're angry? I knew you didn't really love me."

In a long-term relationship one must keep a larger picture in mind. You must be able to remember in your body that you love someone, even when you are not feeling it. Constancy is the feeling that your sense of self, the bond of your relationship, the love between you and your partner, is consistent over time, even when you can't feel it. Constancy is a body experience that can't be felt if you are fragmented, split off, or cut off. Therefore, it is important to develop a part of yourself, the "witness," that can remember that the bond is stable, your partner is a good person, and these upsetting feelings are just temporary. You must also be able to differentiate between not liking a person's behavior and not liking them as a person. In a long-term relationship, you will surely be angry at some of the things your partner does, and at times you may dislike or even hate her or him. This does not make you bad. You can hate and love at the same time.

Yet, emotionally beating your partner up with your anger is abusive and destructive to both of you. Anger is a bandage we put over hurt so as not to feel pain. When you are angry, write in your journal whenever possible before you discuss it with your partner, and definitely before you engage in sex. Most fragmentations, even small upsets, have little or nothing to do with your partner anyway—even though, in anger, it is easy to point out exactly what he or she did wrong. Sometimes just beating on a pillow can dislodge your anger or frustration so that you don't project it onto your partner. But eventually you have to get to the source of the upset. This you can do through the steps out of fragmentation (chapter 15). It is extremely important that you recognize and take care of your own fragmentations.

Some people use anger to generate excitement for sex. Sometimes saying angry words to oneself can arouse sexual passion. But this can be very abusive to your partner, not just physically but emotionally, especially if you are making love and thinking, "I hate you. I hate the way you touch me. I wish you would go away and leave me alone," or, "Fuck you. I'll show you who is in charge." There is a difference between loving and hostile energy, and that difference can be felt.

Sometimes joining physically, as in skin time (chapter 1) can help you move past a temporary upset. If the bond between you is solid and you have established a positive intention toward your partner and your relationship, physical closeness can usually let you see your upset in a new light. Your part in the upset is likely to become apparent and help you out of fragmentation. You may feel the humor of the upset and even feel a closer physical bond.

| MARRIAGE | WHY SHOULD WE get married? We have been living together for years, so what is the point? The answer is usually based more upon your feelings about yourself, marriage, and family than on your commitment to your partner. There are a number of reasons that people give themselves for wanting or not wanting to marry: |

- Some see marriage as the death of individuality, a loss of freedom, a constraint.
- Some see it as a promise of security and constancy, a promise of forever and ever, "Till death do us part."
- A desire to become a family is an incentive to marry. This may or may not include having and raising children. But sometimes a person who does not

want children is surprised to find the longing for family develops after marriage.

- Sometimes a person is hesitant to marry because their partner does not feel like family. But, paradoxically, this feeling of family is often not aroused until the couple marry.
- Some see marriage as a financial partnership and a form of security.
- For others marriage means a commitment to agency, an agreement to abandon oneself and take care of another.
- Some think of marriage as making the relationship legal, or official, in the eyes of their community and family.

There are many legal, moral, religious, personal, and psychological reasons for getting married or not. But a marriage ceremony is also a ritual, in which the commitment between two people is witnessed by their community. Our western modern culture has left us with a severe poverty of meaningful rituals, rituals that can touch the core, the archetypal sensibility in our being. As we have become more modern, rituals have become less and less understood as essential to meaningful living. In earlier times, we would have never dreamed of embarking on a journey without first receiving the blessing of a holy chief, witch doctor, priest, goddess or god, sovereign, or tribe elder. Ritual has been used in every culture to evoke spiritual support and a depth of meaning for transitions in life.

True marriage is more than mere practicality, it is a soul-to-soul joining and inner commitment. For many people it is necessary to share this joy, to let the world know and witness the union.

PREVIOUSLY MARRIED

FOR PEOPLE WHO have been married before, there is more to consider than the issue of commitment. If the past experience was positive, there are often fantasies and comparisons that get in the way. If the experience was painful, the fear of repetition or the hope of being saved and reestablishing a new sense of self-esteem can add obstacles or even adversity. Children from previous marriages also can bring more complications.

"I am not sure that I can love so fully, so innocently, again," is probably the most common feeling. "I can't give everything this time; therefore, I am not sure I can get married," is someone who was married in agency and does not wish to again make a commitment to agency. After a marriage has ended, and a person is single, one's sense of self may seem more readily available, and he or she doesn't want to lose this. Both marriage and agency are a choice. *And the choice for one doesn't necessitate the other.*

Marriage between two adults who have lost their innocence through life experience, and who are no longer considering children, will always feel different from marriage the first time around. One is not better or worse; the new commitment is a reflection of who they are today.

AT WHAT AGE is your apex of sexuality? This revealing exercise will help you find your truth. Have a pen and paper handy, then close your eyes and take a few full deep breaths. Now, answer this question for yourself, "At what age will I or did I reach the peak of my sexual excitement and ability?"

When you have the answer, open your eyes and draw a little mountain like an upside down "U." At the peak place the age you chose as the apex of your sexuality.

What you believe is what you get is as clearly demonstrated in the aging process as in sexuality. If you believe that twenty years of age, or even forty, is the apex of your sexual desires or potency, then your interest, body, and behavior will follow your belief. Yet if you change the age at the apex of your trajectory to seventy or eighty, then forty is only a minor step along the way, and your life will continue to be exciting for a longer period of time. The question is, "When do you believe you are over the hill?"

If you believe your interest in sexuality will peak at fifty, then be assured your interest in sexuality will begin to diminish the minute you've blown out your fiftieth birthday candle. Sexual interest and level of participation is really more a function of belief than anything else.

If you have difficulty finding the passions of love, sexuality, hope, and joy, look more to a holding pattern in your body than your age or your relationship. In our youth, floundering under the pressure of awakening hormones, what did we know of love, of transcendence, of inner beauty? Maturing brings wisdom, life experience, and the openness to explore deeper into the core self and not be so willing to give up one's true self. There is a new ability, without reserve, to join with a lover in erotic loving passion—no longer in a rush to experience sexual release. In fact, people tend to become less defensive and more sensual as they age and, as a result, often start having the best sex of their lives.

As you age there are many changes, both physical and psychological that do occur. One is hormonal. With age, for a great many people, blood levels of a large variety of hormones lower. Some of these hormones are a key factor in sexuality for both men and women. With the advent of hormone replacement therapy couples do not have to remain subject to the effects of low hormonal levels. As hormones lower it often produces a chemically induced emotional impact and in addition can trigger an existential crisis since this signals one is moving closer to the inevitable conclusion of life.

With these changes, some men and women say, "Well, at our age sex is just not important." Yet, if they divorce or their partner dies, and after a mourning period they meet someone else, surprisingly, sex springs to life—better than it ever was in youth. Erotic expression reawakens secreted pleasures and vitality.

Passages of life can affect sex tremendously. What you enjoyed at fifteen may not be satisfying at twenty-five, and what was exciting at twenty-five may not do at forty, fifty, or eighty. But that does not mean that our ability, interest, pleasure, or frequency have to diminish with age.

Many men fear they will lose their ability to maintain an erection as they age. When a man maintains his general health, this apprehension is based more on the fear than on reality. A far greater danger in aging is not losing genital rigidity but gaining a rigidity of attitude. Fixed beliefs lead to psychological and physical atrophy.

Any part of the body that is immobilized or not used for any length of time will decrease in function. The sexual organs are no exception. The idea of "use it or lose it" is very applicable. Regular orgastic and ejaculatory release is an important part of maintaining physical as well as mental health for both men and women.

Not having a participating partner is no reason for not having a healthy sexual release for yourself. For many people masturbation is a primary source of sexual satisfaction. Masturbation can also help couples with different levels of sexual desire and different needs for frequency. Finding a balance, particularly at times of physical or emotional distance, or when one person is in poor health, is very important. Sex is an important source of aliveness and vitality in life. Don't let it slip away through neglect.

HEALTH PROBLEMS

ANYONE CAN LOSE INTEREST in sex if plagued by general health problems, particularly fatigue, low blood sugar, and inadequate nutrition. Of course, pain or stress of any sort causes the body to shrink and not feel sexual or alive.

Lack of exercise or other activities, such as sex, contributes to lack of desire more than age does. Many a simple yoga or exercise class has revived a waning sexual interest by waking the body and psyche. Exercises in *The Intimate Couple* are specifically geared to do just this.

It is our prejudice, our fear of aging, and our lack of comfort with the erotic that make us treat older people as though they were not sexual beings. To neglect mature needs for skin time and sexual satisfaction is inhumane. One of the most repressive and cruel facets of geriatric care is the unavailability of privacy for physical, sensual, and erotic companionship. Sexuality and erotic feelings are not reserved exclusively for the young.

MEDICATIONS

AS WE AGE, we become much more sensitive to substances than we were when we were younger. Standard drug dosages, necessary food intake, even alcohol tolerance, changes. Our normal pattern at thirty can't be continued at forty or sixty or beyond because we are more sensitive to everything and because we are emotionally more vulnerable.

Many common over-the-counter drugs can increase muscular fatigue and decrease alertness and body moisture, for example, saliva and vaginal secretions. Younger people may also find that these drugs affect them physically, their sexuality included. Some common prescription medications also have dramatic side effects on sexual potency, arousal, and desire, as well as general aliveness.

These symptoms can often be avoided if the side effect is brought to the physician's attention, but older patients are often reluctant or embarrassed to talk to their doctors, particularly about sex, so they fail to ask important questions or give relevant information. They assume their symptoms are just part of the aging process, which they have to accept. This is not so. Many elderly people have iatrogenic, or medically induced, symptoms that end up being treated with additional medications. This often occurs when a person is being treated by several different doctors and no one is monitoring the overall picture and the interactive effect of the medications.

Major offenders are antidepressants, blood-pressure drugs, ulcer drugs, appetite suppressants, diuretics, antipsychotic drugs, and sedatives or sleeping tablets. Combine a few of these drugs, add a lack of exercise, and you'll find it hard to find your glasses, your memory, or your aliveness, let alone a sexual feeling.

Different drugs affect people differently so, *before you give up on sex, determine when you started losing interest or function and see what drug you began taking around that time*. There often is a connection.

With the increased sensitivity brought on by aging, you may find the exercises in *The Intimate Couple* affecting you more easily. The opening to aliveness that the breathing and movement bring may occur more quickly. Therefore you may not have to do as much to get a positive sexual effect. In addition, as you do the exercises you may find that you become more sensitive to the amount of drugs you use and need less. Be sure to check your physical reactions to medicines with your physician once you start exercising. More aliveness may mean less need for medication.

CHAPTER SEVENTEEN

Engagement in Sexual Lovemaking

MANY PEOPLE NEVER ENVISION the possibility of making love for hours and hours, of going on an ecstatic excursion and riding on wave after wave of passion that alters perception of time and place and also sensation. Sexuality and sensuality over time blend into a slow, undulating dance of love. Long acts of love build and build and your body releases into one orgasm after the other. You kiss and hug, touch, smell, and taste over and over, and make love again and again. You have a little bite to eat, make love again, drift into sleep in each other's arms, then make love again. The longer and more often you make love and have orgasms, the more your body softens and your inhibitions melt, and the more excitement you'll feel and the deeper

A Guide for the Considerate Lover

Erotic sexual lovemaking is an expression of your whole being. Now is the time to participate fully. Be considerate. Bring your love and your positive intentions to your love-making.

- Keep your heart and body energized so that you can express your love to your partner. But don't give your-self away or there will be no one left to be a lover.
- Each time you touch or look at your partner, shuttle to the emotions and sensations in your body. From there, with love, express in actions and words how you cherish your partner as a human being (as in the "I-Thou" exercise).
- When you touch your partner, move slowly and with exquisite awareness of his or her energy. Never move in too fast or go past his or her energetic boundaries, or yours. Remember, the edge of the boundary is where excitement builds.
- Let your face, breathing pattern, and sounds express the joy and excitement you are feeling. Think of how cats purr when they are being stroked.
- Listen for your next move with your heart, not your pelvis.

body-mind awakening

- Find your own energetic excitement and emotional warmth. Then, using your own volition, meet each of your partner's requests with enthusiasm.
- Stay excitedly present and let your excitement grow with each interchange.
- Enliven and revel in all your senses: sight, taste, smell, touch, and sound—each can be its own turn-on.
- Don't form a preconceived idea of what your partner's response should be; you are bound to be disappointed and invasive.
- *Don't expect from your partner what you are not willing to give.*

In the beginning of an intimate relationship, when making love is new, energy, fantasy, planning, anticipation, and excitement are free-flowing and abundant. Lovers focus on one another, on the relationship and the sexuality they so excitedly anticipate. But as time passes and familiarity sets in, their attention inevitably shifts and changes.

From who you are today, right now, in the moment, turn toward your lover. Focus lovingly, with positive intention, on the one who once captivated your heart. Prepare for erotic sexual lovemaking with the same considerations you once enjoyed. Embrace the changes that have occurred in you, your mate, and in the life you share.

your ecstasy will be. The slower you make love, the more you are able to feel the emotions and sensations.

Unfortunately many people believe that ecstatic sex is magic and is *only* good if it happens spontaneously and mysteriously. Superstitiously they believe that talking or thinking about it very much destroys the magic. They may occasionally have really good sex, but it remains sporadic and has little chance to deepen—and they live in fear of upsetting a fragile sexuality.

For a banquet of pleasure you really have to create the setting, inside and out. Sex is like lunch: If you don't set time aside for it, you may miss it. Sex can be more like a feast than a snack, but this takes time and planning and has more to do with pleasure than just physical need. You can't really make love when you are exhausted, when your mind is on something else, when the kids are going to bang on the door at any moment, or when you have an appointment you have to dash to. Anything that has to do with intimacy takes time to build.

It is not necessary to make love at the banquet level all the time. Quickies can be wonderful fun, too, especially once a new level of sexual potential has been established. An inability to set aside a time for sex is usually a character-style problem, an inability to make commitments without feeling told what to do. There always seems to be some excuse, and sex just ends up not happening at all.

THE LANGUAGE OF SEXUAL LOVEMAKING

MANY PEOPLE HAVE never known a safe atmosphere where they could talk about their emotional feelings and desires, much less their erotic or sexual ones. To do this, lovers need a shared language of sexuality to express what they feel and want.

Many people say, "I don't have to use words, I just *do* something physical and she or he knows." Approaching the body directly can feel very crude or invasive; it can also be misunderstood. But language is part of the respect, honesty, and romance of sexuality. In previous chapters, we emphasized communicating through energy, touch and other senses, movement, and breathing, but here we are specifically focusing on verbal language. Some words can be erotic but not romantic; others can be loving but not sexual. All can add to your sexual lovemaking.

Language can be used to talk about sexual activities and sensual parts of the body. It can also be used to heighten romance, as in poetry, which speaks to our hearts and soul. Language is an important means of expressing feelings of love and desire. Yet language must be more than just sexual words. It must also be used to express the feelings of love and erotic excitement.

The language of sex without love is offensive. Without a softening of the heart, without the erotic spark, there is no sensual excitement. One must not be stingy with words. You must be able to say, "I'm sorry," or, "I love you," with a generosity of spirit.

Some people are able to be sexual but not talk about it. Others can talk a good game but are short on action and skill. Some can't have the feelings of sexuality without the words. They often like the most erotically-charged sexual words, saying, "I love it when you talk dirty to me." Others are highly offended by such language. But most of the time this is not eroticism, it is a depersonalization, a splitting or cutting off from the body, which enables one to speak to another in distant, objectifying terms.

Words having to do with sex are particularly loaded with emotional and psychological meaning. This means that you have to be sensitive and pay attention to the words you choose *and their effect on your partner*. Some people, due to their character style, have a persistent "foot in mouth" disorder. They force their partner to say no to sex or closeness by using the one word he or she cannot handle. This is neither an issue of prudishness nor one of language. This is hostile, distancing humor very common to character style.

Many people are relatively inhibited or uncomfortable talking about anything to do with sex, much less talking about it in specific terms that refer to their own body parts or sexual behavior. They aren't able to describe what they want, and yet they become angry and hurt when "down there" and "not like that" doesn't get them what they want. You must be able to communicate to be understood.

SEX WORDS

IN TURNS, say each word listed below out loud. Then discuss what the word means to you, any negative connotations you attach to it, and any emotional feeling the word engenders in you. For each word, also discuss the words or phrases you use between the two of you in place of that word. Then discuss what word or phrase you would *like* to be spoken in your sexual relationship.

Word list: penis (testicles, scrotum), vagina (clitoris, labia, majora and minora), cunnilingus, fellatio, sexual intercourse.

Any discomfort felt in saying a particular word is usually due to the connotation that you give to it. Rather than avoid these words because of your discomfort, write in your journal to see if you are harboring negative emotional associations about sexuality. Some people try to avoid the uncomfortable associations by substituting words of another culture. Penis and vagina are sometimes named with the Sanskrit words "lingam" and "yani." Another avoidance is giving pet names to genitals, such as "George" or "Mr. Wiggly" for a penis. Other words are avoided because of their lusty quality. For some, the acknowledgment of sexuality is bypassed through use of euphemisms, "Let's sleep together." Any bypass raises a problem when it avoids rather than deals with negative connotations. Remember, genitals of both men and women have many parts. For accurate, clear communication, you will need to become specific. Try this experiment.

Step 1: Close your eyes. Imagine that you are feeling a desire to engage in oral sex, that you feel comfortable approaching your partner and asking for what you want. At this moment in time, do you desire to *give* (participate in oral sex with your mouth on your partner's genitals) or to *receive* (your partner's mouth on your genitals)?

Step 2: What choice did you make? Would you feel comfortable asking for what you want with your partner? Do you consistently ask for the same thing? How did you make your decision? Did it have to do with how you felt in your body, or what you thought your partner might like?

Some people can only ask to receive, and others to give. People high in agency usually ask to give. Others make silent, unilateral contracts, giving with the hope they will receive, becoming angry when their message isn't understood and their secret contract isn't honored.

BUILDING CHARGE DURING INTERCOURSE

YOU HAVE ALREADY PRACTICED most ways to build a charge in your body. Below is a summary of these approaches and new information for how they affect lovemaking. And, of the following, only the last involves the genitals.

Presence and Contact

Have you ever had sex with someone who is "not there"? What did it feel like? Terrible? Like making love to a corpse? Have you ever had sex when *you* weren't present. Could your partner do anything to change how you felt?

Don't try to force your partner to be emotionally or energetically present during sex. It's impossible and can feel so invasive that she or he can't help but become more split off or cut off. Don't make presence a battleground. Each person has to choose through their own volition to be present and "show up" for sex.

If you think your partner is not present, it may actually be *you* who is vacant or gone. Do a presence exercise for yourself rather than saying anything to your partner. He or she may suddenly appear, fully present, as you focus on your own presence and not on your partner's.

When uncomfortable feelings arise, allow them to be felt. They are just feelings and are not dangerous. If you indulge feelings of abandonment, an opening emotion, you are likely to open yourself to a mood of painful feelings. Inundation, a closing emotion, is likely to cut off your ability to build and feel energy and other emotions in your body. By staying present, the sharing of the charge will more than double the excitement. Practice the sensory awareness exercise presented in chapter 3, page 56, naming colors and objects you see around you. While making love, it is more exciting to do the following variation.

Look at the color changes in your partner's body—at skin color, texture, moisture. See: how his or her lips change color and how genitals and nipples change size, color, and shape; if your partner is flushed or has turned pale in any particular segment; if your partner is holding or tightening any part of his or her body; if he or she is trembling, vibrating, or in any way releasing in any part of the body. Look at your body in the same way. Bring your awareness to the colors, tastes, aromas, and sounds of erotic sexual lovemaking. Enjoy them.

Clues that your are split off are: feeling detached emotionally, as if you are watching yourself making love instead of participating; fantasizing too much about another person, another time, or another way; lack of feeling or numbness in your body; being lost in thought, making tomorrow's grocery list, solving a problem at the office, looking for something to be critical about, especially if it concerns your partner.

The best and fastest way to come back from being split off is to use sexual positions that allow you to make eye contact with your partner. This helps focus your attention, shifts you into your body, tunes you into your partner. There is nothing that will inhibit presence and sexuality more than not activating your own volition. Even when you are approached for sex, you still have to make your own decision to be there.

Remember:
- If you don't wish to be present with your heart and sexuality, you will be split off.
- If you are performing, you are not authentically yourself or true to what you feel, and therefore not present.
- When your heart is not open, you are not loving; part of you is not present and you limit your total orgasm.
- You can't enhance your energy unless you are present, and you can't share it unless you and your partner are in contact.
- Your vulnerability and the closing of your heart can cause your partner to split off.

Containment and Boundaries

If you consent to sex reluctantly, you'll feel pushed, invaded, and used. Making love when you don't want to violates your integrity. The only boundaries you can maintain in this circumstance are through the physical tightening of your body or splitting off. You are apt to fragment, lose your sense of self and identity for a while. Maybe for quite a while. Is it worth it? "Doing it anyway"—for someone else even though you don't want to—is an act of agency.

Many people fear that they will lose their identity during sexual contact, lose their boundaries, give themselves away, surrender everything. One way to avoid this feeling is to imagine your boundaries like this:

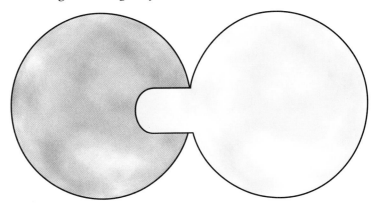

Is the boundary of the circle on the left consuming or joining the one on the right? Is the circle on the right joining or invading the one on the left? During intercourse women may feel joined or invaded; men may feel joined or entrapped. It's all in how you look at it. Imagining the boundary diagram can help you reorient your perspective and reestablish your boundaries and sense of self-containment. You have a choice. The diagram actually shows that neither gives up anything to join. If the loss of boundaries during sex is not a fear of yours this will have little meaning for you.

In order to avoid loss of self-identity, some people raise boundaries like walls. This allows them to show up, feel in charge, and not feel invaded, but it is not relational and does not allow for any real contact. This rigidity squelches the possibility of a high charge. The best boundaries are those that are established through finding your sense of self and setting your own pace and limits rather than pushing against someone else.

You can maintain your self "I am" experience and boundaries and also have the feeling of surrender during lovemaking. You don't give up yourself, your heart, or your body to your partner. You *join* with him or her, and this mutuality can change the level of consciousness for both people. When people feel a sense of self in their bodies, they don't have to set boundaries, they just have them. We are, as long as we are alive, separate beings and separate souls. Our feeling of joining in mutuality is a momentary and delightful change of consciousness.

A lack of limits is not what makes sex great. You don't have to like to try everything. In fact, if you do not have limits, you are not paying attention to your body and are using sex for other purposes, such as performance, avoiding intimacy, or satisfying longings.

Volitional Choice

Volition, defined in Merriam-Webster as, "the act or power of making a choice or decision," carries its own charge. It is an act of showing up, of acting on your own free will. When you are not acting on what you wish for yourself, it is a performance and is the kiss of death to sexual aliveness.

Using volition that emanates from your core experience is not the same as the reactive, "Don't tell me what to do." The automatic no is a rebellious, oppositional stance; it is nonrelational and lacks the vitality of a core experience. Just because someone else has an idea doesn't mean you are being told what to do or who you are. Volition includes *the choice to be receptive* to your partner's choices and your own. It is character style rather than volition when you reject your partner's desires simply because the wishes did not originate as your own. If you do not use your volition to make decisions and choices that involve not only yourself but your partner, you will have less excitement to fuel your charge.

Thinking and Fantasy

Your fantasy life is another important way to build excitement.

Close your eyes and think in detail about the last time you had a passionate, satisfying sexual experience. Remember the sights, sounds, smells, and how you felt in your body. Do this for about ten seconds. Now pay attention to your body and notice that you are probably more excited than you were before the fantasy. Such a fantasy about times past or future can heighten the excitement you feel with your partner.

Fantasy is not a betrayal or a thought crime. Actually, many people form an image of their partner that came from a remembered special moment or previously used position that was particularly exciting to them.

Memories

Let your mind carry you back to the time when you felt the first rush of sexual desire with your partner, when you first met, when you first touched, or when you were alone for the first time. Remember the excitement of anticipation, of touch, smells, and tastes. Arouse these memories until your body fills with the delight of the remembered sensations. Recall when sex was your idea, generated from your own deep desires and longings, when you knew it was what you wanted more than anything. When the erotic desire

body-mind awakening

reaches your heart, approach your partner the way you want, at the time you want, and ask for what you want. Pleasure yourself in all the ways that feed your ecstasy. Delight in all the sensations of love and sexual pleasure you can generate from inside your body through the memories of what it was truly like before other patterns of duty covered these feelings. From the core of your sexual being, indulge yourself in delicious satisfaction.

Fantasy is a problem if it is the only way you get your excitement. If you constantly make love to a fantasy or a former partner instead of your mate, it may indicate a problem with your relationship. It may only be your character style acting up to create distance so you can feel safe in intimacy.

Fantasy is misused when you try to control your excitement by thinking of unpleasant or negative images. A man worried about premature ejaculation, for instance, might make himself think about rotten garbage or being at work, etc. This image may keep him from ejaculating, but he isn't in charge of his excitement; he just splits off from it. Lowering his overall charge and disengaging from his body awareness are both major factors in causing premature ejaculation. Besides, it feels terrible to the partner. How would you like to have sex with someone you know is fantasizing about something disgusting while being with you? The exercises in chapter 10 that help you spread out a charge are much more effective.

Breathing and Movement

A key factor in heightening your charge during sexual lovemaking is to apply the orgastic pattern you learned in the exercise chapters for building a charge through breath and movement. The sustaining integration series will also help you in building and spreading your charge.

Sensuality and Eroticism

Sensual, erotic movements of the body are contagious and can turn you and your partner on. *Bringing sexual energy to the senses and fully enjoying this pleasure is what we call eroticism.* We usually think of people enjoying their eroticism by touching someone else's skin, smelling, tasting, or looking at them. In addition, using the orgastic pattern exercises, you can move your sensuality into the erotic energy of your body: open to it, feel it, and move so it flows through your body. All you have to do then is tune in, feel, and enjoy it.

Arousing Eroticism Experiments

- Once you have a feel of the whole-body orgastic pattern, *upper and lower body,* try to move this way while standing up watching yourself in the mirror. Add slow, erotic music and move very slowly, undulating with the orgastic pattern in mind. Really move your pelvis and your energy with it. Let your abdominal muscles be free.
- Learn how to go inside and free the flow of erotic energy and then shuttle to your partner and enjoy the feel of your partner's body, his or her tastes, smells, sounds, how your partner looks in all her or his nuances.
- Take a cold mango, papaya, or nectarine and rub it on your and your partner's nipples and genitals. If you prefer, whipped cream or chocolate will do, but make sure to apply only a thin layer or you might get caught up in the flavors and miss the body beneath. If you let yourself become erotically aroused by these tastes while you are licking or sucking genitals and nipples, it will increase your sensory experience.

Genital Stimulation

Stimulating the genitals is natural and very pleasurable but is a limited source for building a charge. If you are depending solely on this stimulation to heighten sexual charge, remember that when you focus on the trigger, you move toward orgasm or release before you have had a chance to build a larger charge. Focusing only on the genitals severely limits the possibilities for heightened sexual lovemaking.

Since the genitals are a delightful source of pleasure in sexual lovemaking, there are a few things you need to know.

- Stimulation of the genitals or nipples is best kept to the level of charge in the body. In other words, if you stimulate the nipples, vaginal area, or penis hard and fast when a person's charge is low, it will probably feel uncomfortable. In addition, the discomfort will cause the recipient's body to tighten and close down in an attempt to tolerate the excessive intensity. (See page 54, chapter 3.)

- The genitals of women, like lips, are lined with mucous membrane tissue that doesn't form calluses, so rubbing can chafe. Be gentle, stroke lightly, and don't stay on one spot too long. Extra lubrication is helpful. These tissues can become sore and tender very easily and, when this happens, it is likely to affect the desire phase the next time you want to have sex. Men, try this little experiment: With the fingers of one hand, pull your lower lip down. With one finger of your other hand, rub back and forth across the mucus membrane inside your lip. Do this for about one minute. How does this feel? Imagine doing this without let up for about fifteen minutes.

- Approach your partner's genitals with reverence and love. They can create life. Don't treat your partner's genitals as if they are mechanical gadgets used to start a fire.

- Genitals are supposed to have a light smell and taste.

- You can't possibly know what feels best to another person. Only your partner knows how much and where, and of course this is continually changing: Even though you may know one moment, you may be wrong the next. Communication is imperative. Respect what you are told; ask for what you want. Yet don't give directions like a traffic cop. Don't just emphasize what is wrong. An, "Oh, I like that," will get you a lot further than a, "No, not like that."

- Don't use your hand or fingers to touch your partner when your tongue will do the job. Oral sex is so pleasurable for both participants that the distinction between who is receiving and who is giving melts away.

- With vaginal intercourse, the penis should enter slowly at first, as too abrupt an entrance can cause pain. The vagina adapts rather quickly if given a chance. Sometimes when a penis enters a woman it hurts her. Most often it is because there is a tightness inside, near, or around the PC muscles, uterus, and cervix, and the penis touches these sensitive, tight spots. If a woman moves slowly she can use the man's penis as a tool for internal massage.

The entering of the penis brings about many psychological feelings for both lovers. Hurrying is often an attempt, by one or both partners, to avoid these emotions and usually creates more problems than it resolves. For the man it may be an attempt to avoid the possibility of losing his erection; for the woman, it may be a fear that she will miss her orgasm if he has one first.

A man's penis, although he is often hesitant to say so, can be very sensitive. Rough handling, sharp teeth, or sucking very hard can all be painful. Never blow into or place anything into the urethral opening at the tip of the penis. If a man is not circumcised and his foreskin is tight, manual stimulation can be very uncomfortable. In addition, this can cause the covered head of the penis to be as tender and sensitive as the vagina mucus membrane. Bending an erect penis can also cause pain.

MUTUALITY IN BUILDING, SPREADING, AND RELEASING A CHARGE

SEXUAL LOVEMAKING is mutuality in the fullest sense. It takes the decision of both partners to want to be there at the same time, to open to deep feelings of caring. It takes the desire, means, time, and experience to create a rhythm between lovers that attunes to both, that becomes a creation of their joining in body and spirit.

Erotic sexual lovemaking is going in to find the lover within and bringing this fullness to the joining. It is a willingness to honor and appreciate the aliveness and vulnerability that sexuality enhances in your partner and in yourself. It is a willingness to be both a leader and a follower with courage, even when feeling timid or wanting to be in control, to allow your sexual lovemaking to express appreciation for the privilege of intense shared experience, for being so close to the experience of life, of being alive.

What you have learned in your body from doing the exercises for mutuality (chapter 9), you can now bring to sexual lovemaking. Remember that you learned how to build and send energy within yourself and between you with the moving heightened energy practice. You learned what it feels like when either partner isn't present and how to come back into contact with the presence eye-alogue and how to deepen the relationship with the "I-Thou" experience. The silent conversation practice showed that you can speak through your touch and that it is also important to use your words to touch, explore, and clarify.

The experience of dancing with energy brings mutuality to full bloom and is the rhythm that makes for the most memorable, extraordinary sexual lovemaking. The position for sensing each other can be used for emotionally and energetically joining with your partner as you begin to make love and as a completion during the satisfaction and intimacy phases. You can continue this emotional, energetic feeling with slow lovemaking, especially when you first join genitals in intercourse. As you join, try being rather still and slow, both of you using the contractions of your PC muscles only (chapter 8) to awaken the body and stimulate lubrication. Always remember to breathe fully and use the movements that you have been repatterning in your body.

PRESSURE POINTS

PRESSURE POINTS can be used in conjunction with techniques you have already learned for releasing segmental holding patterns. The results can at times be instantaneous. Some holding patterns will not release unless you work with the segmental exercises; others will not release unless you work with the psychological component. Yet, once worked with and released by other methods, if the holding pattern returns, the use of pressure points can be magical.

Pressure points are like openings to one's inner excitement, pathways by which you can make a deeper connection to your partner. As you touch, caress, kiss, and connect during sexual lovemaking, try bringing your attention to the points. (See chart below.) Think not just about touching them but about passing your energy through them to your partner. Touch them with your fingers, lips, tongue, nipples, penis, clitoris, vulva. You can use them to build and spread a charge. You can usually tell when you are right on the pressure point as it will be a little sensitive to the touch.

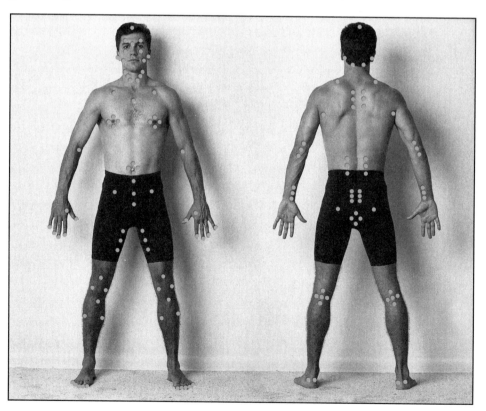

Pressure Points of the Body.

It is easier to build a charge in the extremities of your body and move the energy toward the genitals or the heart than the other way around. Excitement will spread out and build as you move toward these centers of the body. The closer you get to the genital area, the more the excitement moves exclusively toward release. So the points at the heel, bottom of the foot, and in between the toes are more sensual when kissed, touched, massaged, sucked, etc., than the points on the pubic bone, which tend to be more sexually exciting.

You can also start at the top of the head to build excitement. You can rub, scratch, kiss the top of the head and also the ears and ear lobes, back of the neck, under the chin, mouth, eyes, eyebrows—all are very sensitive points. Do not ignore the shoulders or the area *around* the nipples of both men and women. Most people are not aware of how sensitive men's nipples can be.

The points above the pubic bone and below the navel are also extremely sensitive. Stimulating them in a woman moves the charge deeper into the vaginal canal, even to the uterus and ovaries. Stimulating them in a man will move the excitement to the base of the penis, scrotum, and testicles. The points at the hip bone and on the buttocks and the sacral area are very important because they move the energy from the front to the back of the body. Many holding patterns are in the back as well as the front. There are four points around the anus that can be stimulated without touching the anus itself. All can increase pleasure, but especially the ones on either side. Stimulating the anal area is probably the most effective way to release the holding pattern in the back of the pelvis during intercourse. When people "hold back," the body interprets it as a message to tighten the anus and pelvic floor.

There are three points along the inner thigh that are very sensuous and move the excitement from the genitals to the legs for grounding and back to the genitals. And don't forget the spot behind the knees that is the back side of the holding pattern in the leg. Stroking, kissing, and fondling these points not only feels good but moves the charge rapidly to the pelvis. No matter whether you start at the bottom or the top, by the time you reach the genitals you will have built much more of a charge than if you had started with the genitals.

MASTURBATING TOGETHER

MASTURBATING TOGETHER can be fun, erotically stimulating, and often full of surprises. It is also the best way to teach your partner what you like, and learn how to touch your partner the way he or she prefers. Some people can bring themselves to orgasm when alone but find it difficult or impossible to have an orgasm in their partner's presence. This is usually character style. Many women can't have an orgasm with intercourse alone and need manual stimulation. If her clitoris is more than about an inch and a half from her vaginal orifice, it will not be stimulated automatically by the motions of intercourse. Of course, if her charge is high enough this will not much matter as her whole clitoral-vaginal area will trigger her release.

If, man or woman, you can only achieve orgasm in one position, it can become quite limiting to you and to your partner. While alone, build to a high charge in your favorite position, the one in which you can stimulate yourself to orgastic release most easily. Lying on your back, side, stomach, etc., make sure that you are comfortable in knowing that you can bring yourself to orgasm. Then next time, shift your position to one that is less familiar, one that is conducive to sexual intercourse with your partner, such as lying on your back or sitting up. Don't expect your partner to be able to do for you what you can't do for yourself. Then try the following experiments.

FEMALE PELVIC
HOLDING PATTERN

THE FEMALE UTERUS and cervix in the pelvic area are very vulnerable to emotional distress. When this happens, the uterus and cervix tend to tighten and form a holding pattern. This can deaden a woman's ability to feel sexual desire. She may wonder why she doesn't feel sexual even though nothing seems wrong in the relationship. As she searches for a reason, she may criticize herself or place the blame on her partner. Either is an easy pattern to fall victim to. This holding pattern can also cause intercourse to feel painful.

Working on the physical block is the most direct way to release the holding pattern and an ideal opportunity for assistance from a partner. But, since all physical holding patterns have a psychological correlate, the block will return if the stressful situation continues. She must discover what triggers her tightening, withdrawing response and do something about it.

Cervical Release

Begin with the woman building a charge. The higher her charge, the easier she will achieve release. The best way to do this is by using the sustaining integration series (chapter 7). Moving to a knee-chest position (see *Total Orgasm* or *Body, Self and Soul*) uses gravity to align her uterus. In this position, she can use her hands to massage her uterine area from the outside (lower belly, below her navel) while she continues to breathe fully. Remain in this position for approximately two to three minutes while breathing fully.

During vaginal intercourse, if a woman feels discomfort as if her partner's penis is bumping against tender areas, she can first ask her partner to stop and pull out until her tension subsides. They can consider using other forms of sexual lovemaking for a time.

If she would like him to help her release her tight holding pattern, they can raise her pelvis by placing a pillow under her buttocks. In this new raised position she may no longer feel the discomfort.

If the discomfort remains, she can ask her partner to again enter her vagina

Masturbation Practices

The four guides below provide variation to sexuality and solutions to common sexual difficulties. Take your time and choose the pace most comfortable for both of you. These steps are not meant to be done during one sexual lovemaking period. During these exercises, don't forget to breathe and rock your pelvis to build and maintain your charge, as you learned in the orgastic pattern exercises. Make sure to use a lubricant for the following exercises.

Exercise 1: *Show and tell.* While together, at the same time or in turns, masturbate, showing your partner what you do to pleasure yourself. Show your partner how you bring yourself to release by masturbating to orgasm.

Exercise 2: *Show and teach.* Each partner in turn, teach your partner what you do to bring yourself pleasure and orgastic release through masturbation. Sit with your back to your partner, between his or her legs, in front of a mirror with the lights on. (If there is enough difference in body size that it is uncomfortable to reach around to the genitals, sit side by side.)

As the partner sitting in front, the teaching partner, place your hands on

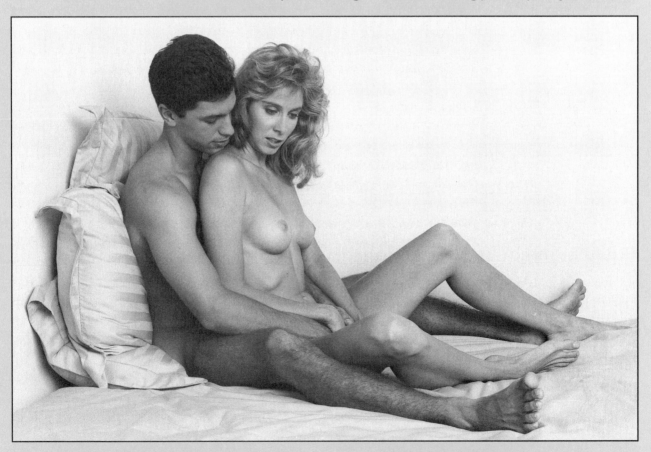

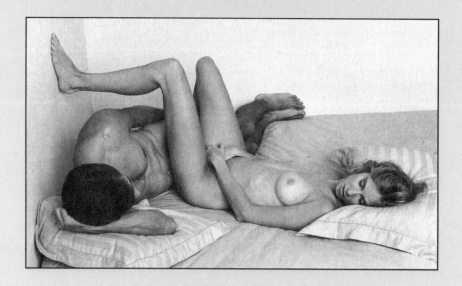

your own genitals just as if you were masturbating yourself—while your partner's hands are placed on yours. As you move your hands and fingers to pleasure yourself, your partners hands will automatically follow yours. Show your partner the pressure to use, the speed and direction of motion that you enjoy, anything you can think of that you would like done. After it feels to you that your partner understands your touch and rhythm and where and how you like being touched, reverse the hand positions so that your partner's hands are on your genitals and your hands are on top. Now in this hand position as your partner touches you, provide a little guidance. Breathe fully with your partner as he or she masturbates you to release.

Exercise 3: *Transition to intercourse for women.* In addition to an enjoyable variation, this works very well for women who have difficulty having an orgasm during intercourse. Both partners breathe to build a charge. The man lies on his side across the bed (if you're using a bed), facing the headboard or wall. It's best if you find a corner so both people can put their feet against the wall for grounding. The woman lies with her knees raised and her legs draped over man's hips, feet against the wall. Their bodies will form a cross. They are aligned so the man can insert his penis into her vagina and she has room to provide her own manual stimulation.

In this position, the man inserts his penis into her vagina. The woman masturbates herself to orgasm while the man's penis is inside of her. After she has had an orgasm, in the same position, the man can then thrust or move inside her vagina until he releases to orgasm.

Variation. The woman lies in any position in which she can masturbate to orgasm. Together, with a little ingenuity, find a way for the man to insert his penis into her vagina. She then masturbates to orgasm. Once the woman can bring herself to release with the man inside her, the transition from masturbation to intercourse is usually very easy.

Exercise 4: *Transition to intercourse for men.* In addition to being a variation for pleasure, this works well for men who have difficulty relaxing and ejaculating in a woman's vagina. The woman is on top, sitting facing the man. She can sit behind his penis so they can both watch; she can sit in front of his penis which is more private for him; or she can move forward to his mouth for oral sex while he masturbates himself. He masturbates until he feels he is ready to release, then he inserts his penis partially into her vagina. She can accommodate for this by raising slightly to her knees. He continues to masturbate with his hand, rocking his pelvis, moving in and out of her vagina until orgasm. If she has not already had an orgasm, she can then have one through manual or oral stimulation or through intercourse if his erection is again aroused.

with his penis. While he remains still, the woman can now be in charge of moving in a way that his penis massages her interior areas of discomfort. Breathing deeply, she can rock her pelvis with her breath in the orgastic pattern. It is difficult for a woman to feel interior holding patterns in this segment, but if his penis touches a tender area she can identify and bring her awareness to the held area. As she identifies the tender areas in this way she can at the same time, use her own hand to externally massage them from the outside.

When his penis touches a sore point, it is best if both partners stop moving so that his penis remains gently touching her tender area. This will help her focus attention on the specific area. As each tight, tender area is identified, without moving she can practice softening and relaxing the pelvic tension completely with a full, letting-go breath. You do not have to try to change the tender holding pattern. The woman just needs to relax and accept it. Tightening against the pain keeps the holding pattern intact. The acceptance of the pain can allow the body to relax and release the holding pattern.

If the tenderness or holding pattern does not easily go away be sure to check with your physician.

The woman will probably feel the released energy from the holding pattern stream to other parts of her body. Don't be surprised if there is also a release of emotions such as anger, sorrow, or sadness before sexual desire returns. Emotions held in the uterus cause the holding pattern; if they emerge during the massage, they do not have to be solved by either partner at that time. They only have to be witnessed. If there is anything to be resolved, it can be done later in the journal.

ORAL SEX

THE MOUTH IS A SEXUAL ORGAN as much as any other part of the body, and a primary source of erotic expression and reception. It is a wonderful source of sexual gratification. If sexuality is seen as a total body experience, then sucking becomes as important as genital stimulation. In its own way, oral gratification can be as great a turn-on as genital stimulation. Oral sex is very common and natural.

As long ago as the 1920s, marriage manuals recommended oral sex to married couples, with one manual describing it as the "genital kiss." (T. H. Van Velde, *Ideal Marriage,* 1926, as quoted in Michael et al., *Sex in America,* 1994) It was presented as something you might do for a partner if you wanted to express physically how intimate and emotionally close you felt. It was seen as a special gesture, not as something that would normally be part of your sexual practices.

This view of oral sex as special to particular moments began to soften in the 1950s with the reports from the Kinsey studies revealing that oral sex was fairly common. The resulting change in sexual advice books was that it was recommended as a technique especially satisfying to women. By the 1970s, the sex experts began saying that oral sex could be part of the sex act for every couple, whether or not they were married. It became less of a special gesture and more of a routine, expected sexual practice. Now college textbooks discuss oral sex as a "technique for arousing your partner, a marked transformation from the old view of it as a deeply significant emotional act by married or well-established couples." (Michael et al., *Sex in America*, 1994)

Sucking is our first primitive source of pleasure and the first way we learn to comfort ourselves and soothe our longings. The pleasure, erotic excitement, and satisfaction gained by sucking is not exclusively felt in your mouth. Your lips, tongue, throat, face, nose, and brow, too, are integral parts of the giving and receiving. They are used often in the expression of love in the form of kissing and nuzzling. Besides, the oral and pelvic segments are very reciprocal, so kissing, sucking, and using your tongue or nose (as with the Eskimos) turn on the pelvis.

When it comes to oral sex, who is giving and who is receiving is difficult to answer. Oral sex and sucking opens the mouth, throat, and chest segments of the body. Sucking is an effective way to connect the split between sex and love—that is, sucking can open both the pelvis and heart and join the two. Being made love to by your partner's mouth is not only stimulating and exciting but is an expression of full sensual, erotic acceptance. An act of oral sex embodies giving and receiving at the same time.

Oral gratification is indeed pleasurable, but the pleasure is greatest when you are enjoying adult sexuality, not attempting to satisfy childhood longings. Because the mouth is a source of pleasure and offers a way to explore and learn about anything and everything, young children put everything they can into their mouths. Later, in adulthood, kissing is enjoyed, then necking, and then oral-genital stimulation, all of which can harken back to childhood oral satisfaction, or injury if it's associated with rejection or neglect. You can't change the past, but you can come to terms with old longings. Then sucking can allow for a deeper excitement throughout the body.

Biting and sucking are closely related. Because sucking can arouse associated longings, people often bite rather than suck. But, in avoiding the longings, the biting can bring out feelings of anger and aggression. If you are angry, work out the problem. Don't bite, or try biting a towel or another nonliving object. No wonder that sucking and biting become associated. When sucking is frustrated or punished, the child begins to bite: fingernails, cuticles, ends of pencils and pens, pipes, toothpicks, etc.

When sexual pleasure is at its height, some people feel the urge to bite, but this tends to lower the charge for both people. They may be able to release into orgasm, but the orgasm will be diminished. Also, biting your partner can be quite hostile. Next time you feel the urge to bite, try sucking instead and see how it opens your heart and helps to release other holding patterns.

Food often satisfies oral longings, so is it any wonder that eating is often associated with sex? Food is an excellent foreplay to sexuality. It can set the mood for erotic sensuality. Part of the ancient Tantra ritual, in which sexuality is a path toward enlightenment, is a specific eating ritual to heighten the charge. An interesting note is how the French are known for their cuisine and for their oral sex.

We have a desire for sucking that is separate from nutrition or feeding and childhood longings. It is interesting to note that thumb sucking has been prohibited almost as much and as strongly as has masturbation. Perhaps this stems from the innate understanding that it has something to do with erotic gratification and expression of sexuality.

ANAL STIMULATION

MANY MEN AND WOMEN find anal stimulation or anal intercourse to be very satisfying. Anal sex can facilitate a release of a posterior holding pattern in the pelvis. For men, anal intercourse can stimulate the prostate gland, analogous to the G spot in women, and with genital stimulation bring about an orgastic release. But remember, if a charge is high enough, it stimulates all areas in the body and stimulating triggers can become less important.

Early toilet training, punishment for enuresis (bed-wetting), and enemas are often the beginnings of a posterior pelvic block. The nerves from the brain that control the anal sphincter do not function adequately until about 18 months of age. Therefore, if forced to retain feces before the anal sphincter is functional, the child must pull up on the muscular floor of the pelvis instead. This is very painful, as anyone knows who has tried to make it to a toilet when they have a stomach virus or diarrhea. When children learn to turn off this pain in the pelvic floor, they can develop a block or a numbing holding pattern. When the anal sphincter finally does come under their control, the block is already in place along with psychological associations and a host of other symptoms.

If you wish to engage in anal penetration, here are some cautions to observe. The rectum is very vascular and sensitive, and it takes time to adjust to being penetrated. This means that you must enter slowly and gently. The use of a good lubricant is imperative to prevent the tearing of tissue.

Foreign objects placed in the anus can tear or damage the delicate tissues, so be very careful of sharp objects, fingernails, etc. Once inside the rectum, anything that isn't tethered can very easily get lost. Many people have spent hours in the emergency room to have removed an unbelievable array of objects—gadgets, vibrators, balls, carrots, cucumbers, scarves with knots, etc.—all meant for stimulation and fun.

A most important caution to remember is that anything that touches the anus should be washed thoroughly before touching other parts of the body, particularly the vagina. Vaginal infection can easily occur if you are not careful. Because there is a vast blood supply in the anus and the tissues are fragile, there is potential danger from diseases that are passed on through contact with blood, such as hepatitis and AIDS-related disorders.

<table>
<tr><td>

DRUGS

</td><td>

ALTHOUGH SOME DRUGS may heighten sexual experience, when sex is a drug-influenced experience, the good feelings become associated with the drug rather than the partner. If the drug is eliminated, the desire and even the very ability for satisfying sex can go with it. In fact, drugs—both "uppers" and "downers"— depress the body's actual ability to build a charge. Drugs separate you from the "I am" sense of self-experience in your body. Whether they stimulate, depress, or otherwise alter one's sense of self, in the long run drugs create a disassociation from the body and core self. They also cause distortions in the fabric of the relationship, which can alienate lovers.

</td></tr>
</table>

Some drugs seem to release sexual inhibitions, but they actually do this by causing a splitting off. In this way you may numb your sensations and, certainly, your ability to build a high charge. When people use drugs in an attempt to solve psychological problems around sex it generally backfires. Instead of solving their problems, they are more likely to create new and more difficult ones. Splitting off with drugs limits contact between partners during sex. And, as we keep saying, contact with your partner in love and intimacy is one of the most important factors in really good sex. The one who is taking the drugs always says, "It doesn't affect me." The partner not doing drugs always feels isolated and lonely.

Pain and Sex

The fascination with inflicting pain during sex is not rare. It's easy to identify abuse and pain when whips and chains are used and even more obvious when there is physical fighting, brutality, or physical restraint, as in bondage or sexual slavery. But this process is not limited to the kinky rubber-clad set.

For many, inflicting pain is more subtle and not even recognized as such. Many couples inflict pain emotionally by having a fight. To either build or release a charge, they emotionally abuse each other, causing the stress of fragmentation. Sometimes, they do this by threatening abandonment or inundation; then they make up, feel closer, and have sex. This kind of foreplay is hard on the two people and on the bond of the relationship.

Stress or pain inflicted from the outside is an attempt to break through holding patterns in the body. Sheer exhaus-

body-mind awakening

tion or over-stressing can indeed cause the muscles to release, making way for a charge. But because pain causes a constriction and a constricted container is small, the release will be small. Pain is used primarily by people who, because of their holding patterns, have difficulty feeling more subtle emotions and sensations, have problems with intimacy, and have trouble letting go into release. So, pain is used to open the body from the outside like puncturing a balloon. It replaces inner excitement, charge, release, and surrender.

Most of these behaviors are a substitute for a body core sense of self and an interior aliveness. They are a substitute for an ability to share love, tenderness, and caring with a partner and enjoy sensuality and the thrill of a truly erotic experience.

CHAPTER EIGHTEEN

Sexual Positions, Releases, and Satisfaction

IF YOU CHECK OUT ANY SEX BOOK with 101 positions, you will see that most of the positions limit the building and containing of sexual energy for one or both partners and often inhibit the release into full orgasm. Some actually inflict outright physical discomfort and can be injurious to your back or neck when you're in the throes of orgasm. It is important that the positions you use to engage in sex are mutually caring and supportive. We will teach you new ways of evaluating and choosing positions for yourself and your partner. If you don't like a position or it is uncomfortable, don't do it. On the other hand, if you never try anything new, it's hard to keep the aliveness going.

Besides just being physically uncomfortable, many positions carry psychological associations that can provoke couples to fight out character style, agency, and scenario themes. Sex is not a battleground. It is important not to make it one. No position should be painful, demeaning, permanent, or imperative. Keep your sense of humor and dispense with the character-style rigidity of, "No, I can't keep it up in that position," or, "I can't have an orgasm unless I can be in that position and therefore I won't have sex." Be willing to experiment. You never know till you try it—you might like it.

SEXUAL POSITIONS AND RELEASES

IF YOU ARE IN A POSITION while having sex that doesn't allow for full, free movement of your orgastic pattern, your ability to build a charge will severely be hampered on the physiological energetic level. Movements that replicate the orgastic pattern build and spread your charge throughout your body and let you feel the streaming of energy. If you know what can and can't heighten a charge, you won't think something is wrong if a particular position is pleasurable but doesn't send you into orgasm. But change the position slightly, and the new position can boost your ability to build and contain your charge.

Understanding the principles of the five freedoms (see box, page 258), you can use them to evaluate all positions for yourself. The following guide addresses positions for penis-vagina intercourse.

THE "MISSIONARY" POSITION EXPERIMENT

IF YOU TAKE THE TIME to physically try this experiment, you will feel what the five freedoms are all about. You will need your sense of humor to learn from this experiment.

Step 1: Women: pretend you are a man having sex with a woman. Move to the floor and assume the male missionary on-top position. Notice what you feel

The Five Freedoms

There are several criteria necessary for sexual positions to permit your orgastic pattern to function fully. What we call the "five freedoms" are necessary to enable your body to build, contain, spread, and release energy for sexual orgasm.

1. The freedom to see and make eye contact. To maintain intimacy and exchange energy you must be able to have eye contact. Making love in the dark won't work. Positions like rear entry don't allow for eye contact, but you can solve this by using a mirror.

2. The freedom to move your pelvis. To build a heightened charge you must be able to rock your pelvis in the orgastic pattern. If you tighten your abdominal muscles you will cut off the charge, diminishing or even halting your orgasm.

3. The freedom to move your neck and head. Because it is closely correlated to the movement of your pelvis, your cervical segment must be able to move freely for a full orgasm.

4. The freedom to move your chest and breathe fully. Your chest is the site of breathing to build a high charge. It must also be free for loving emotions and a body feeling of self. Without this ability to open your heart and soften, sex is devoid of lovemaking.

5. The freedom to keep your feet or knees grounded. You cannot rock your pelvis without using your stomach muscles unless you can stabilize yourself by pushing with your feet or knees. Grounding is strongly correlated to your eyes, so it is also difficult to remain present when you are ungrounded and is difficult to tolerate higher levels of intensity, sexual or intimate.

and where you feel it in your body as you act out the man's role. Notice how you have to support yourself with your arms or elbows so you don't crush your partner. Notice how hard it is for you to breathe, how tight your back, chest, and arms are because you're holding yourself up. Notice how supporting your body with your arms affects your breathing. Now lower yourself and pretend to insert your penis into your partner. Keep your pelvis close enough that your imaginary penis could be inside a woman. Now, rock your pelvis in an orgastic pattern as if you were a man, and breathe deeply to build your own charge. No, don't pump your pelvis up and down, rock it. Enough said.

Step 2: Men: Lie on your back and pretend to be a woman. Spread your legs open very wide to accommodate an imaginary male partner. Try to rock your pelvis in an orgastic pattern. Remember, you have to keep your neck relaxed and stomach muscles loose and look into your partner's eyes. Now pretend that your partner is on top of you. Breathe deeply and smile like you are having a good time. Stay present. Don't laugh. This is the most common position many women experience. Now you know why women are always asking to be on top.

Notice that the position is relatively impossible for both partners. The missionary position is a very common position in which people have sex, yet it has little potential movement for either partner so is not the best for building higher levels of charge or containment, and it makes release difficult. Read on to see what you can do to make this and other favorite positions better for each partner.

Man-on-Top or Missionary Position

Inherent Problems in This Position

This is a very popular position, but if you tried the exercise above you are aware that there are several difficulties.

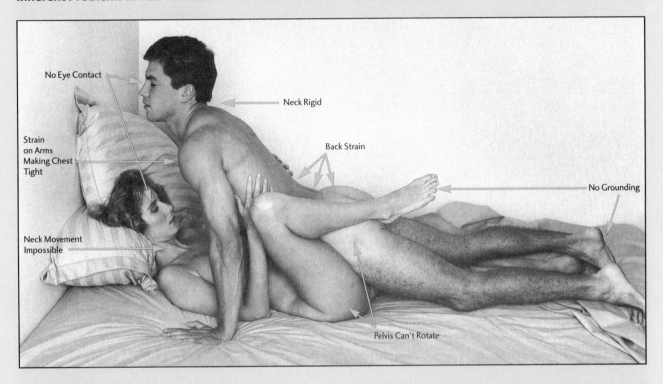

No Eye Contact

Neck Rigid

Strain on Arms Making Chest Tight

Back Strain

No Grounding

Neck Movement Impossible

Pelvis Can't Rotate

Evaluation

Start your evaluation by using the five freedoms to assess this first position.

(1) You *can* both make eye contact, but the cervical segment is often compromised in doing so. **(2)** The man can easily move his head, but because of the stress on his shoulders and arms, his cervical segment is fairly immobilized. **(3)** His breathing is also somewhat restrained from the tension on his arms that he must maintain for support, even if he is on his elbows. This tightens his chest and back. **(4)** In this position it is difficult for him to move his pelvis. He will probably have to stiffen his whole body and then raise and lower it in a pumping motion rather than isolate and rock his pelvis. This can limit his charge, and the stress of the position pushes him toward an earlier orgasm. Unless he already has a high charge, he may ejaculate prematurely, i.e., before his charge is high enough for a full orgasm.

(5) Neither his knees nor his feet are fully grounded. But he can remedy this by moving his feet to the head or foot of the bed and bracing them. Then he can push and rock his pelvis. The strain of this position can cause severe back pain for many men. Chiropractors love the Monday morning business it brings them.

Now, let's evaluate the woman's sexual potential in this position. **(2)** She probably can't move her head and neck, particularly if her head is on a pillow. **(3)** With a man on top of her, it is not likely that she can breathe fully with her chest. **(4)** The man's weight usually precludes her ability to rock her pelvis. **(5)** If her legs are in the air, she can't ground herself to rock her pelvis. With her legs in the air she is, in effect, in a stress position. If she already has a high charge this can force the energy to spread through her body, creating a deep streaming feeling. She can exaggerate this by straightening her legs and pressing out with her heels.

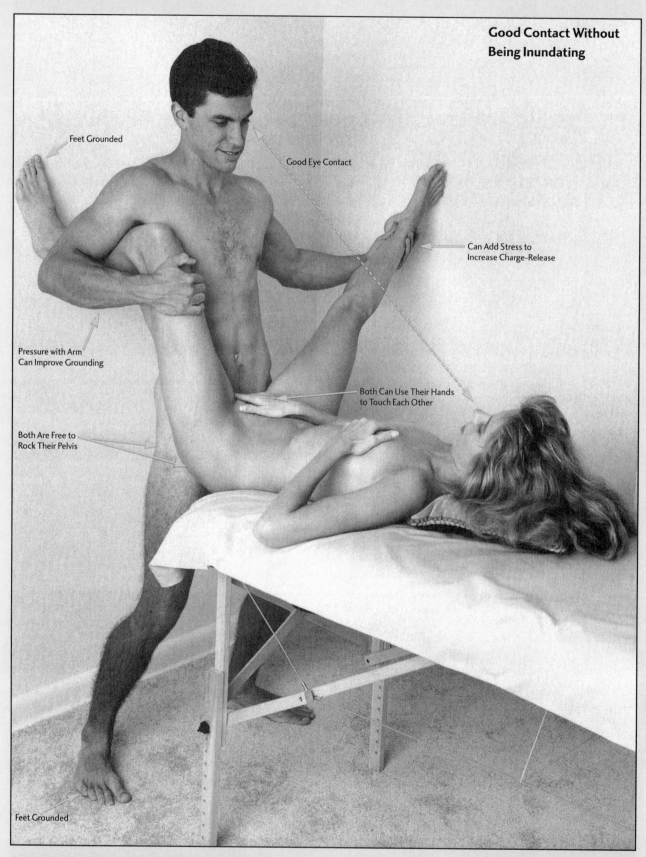

Good Contact Without
Being Inundating

Feet Grounded

Good Eye Contact

Can Add Stress to
Increase Charge-Release

Pressure with Arm
Can Improve Grounding

Both Can Use Their Hands
to Touch Each Other

Both Are Free to
Rock Their Pelvis

Feet Grounded

But this still does not help the woman become fully grounded.

If her legs are wide apart, in the air or not, it will be difficult for her to contain a charge. If her feet are firmly grounded, she can then squeeze with her knees as in the ball squeezing exercise in awakening your body. This can release her pelvis and assist her partner in rocking his.

Since this is an emotionally as well as physically satisfying position for many couples, what can be done to make it better? The primary change you can make is to get the man off of the woman and onto his knees or feet. If the woman were to lie on a massage table (or any high counter) with her feet on a wall or counter top, she would be in a very free position. If the man were to stand between her legs, his pelvis as well as the rest of his body would be free to breathe and move. They still maintain good eye contact, their hands are free to caress each other, and they are both grounded.

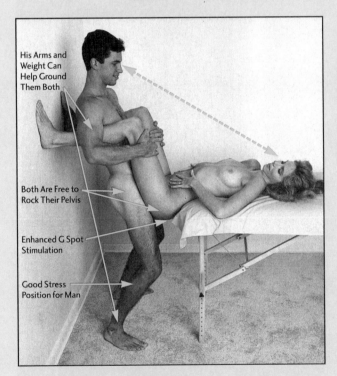

His Arms and Weight Can Help Ground Them Both

Both Are Free to Rock Their Pelvis

Enhanced G Spot Stimulation

Good Stress Position for Man

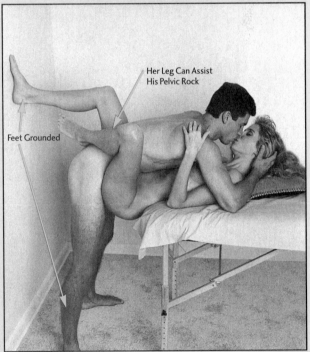

Her Leg Can Assist His Pelvic Rock

Feet Grounded

If the woman can let her buttocks hang slightly over the edge of the table, the man's penis is in a position to rub her G spot, just behind her pubic bone. As you will see later in the positions that enhance release, he can now stress his leg muscles (quadriceps), bending his knees slightly. This can both spread the charge and trigger a release.

A variation of this position is for the woman to lie on a bed (or counter) with her feet on the floor, wall, or counter, and the man to kneel between her legs. In either of these positions, the woman can move forward into more of a sitting position and/or the man can lean forward. This can bring them into closer body-to-body, skin-to-skin contact.

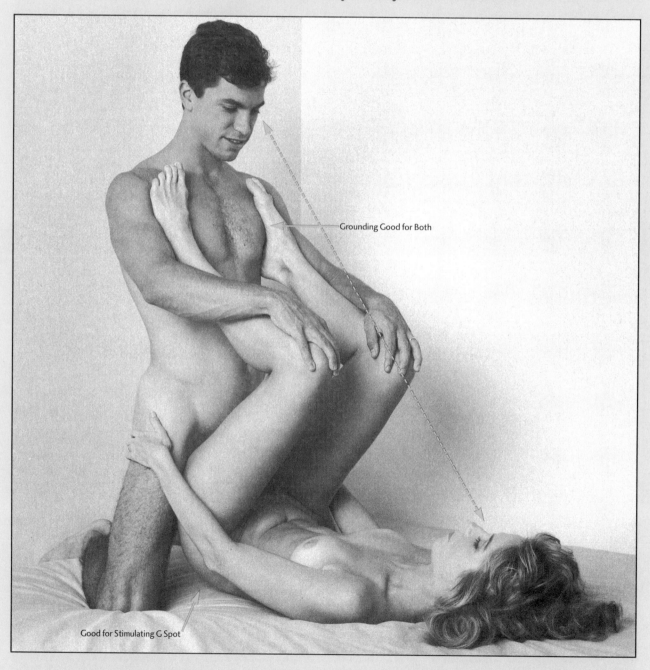

Grounding Good for Both

Good for Stimulating G Spot

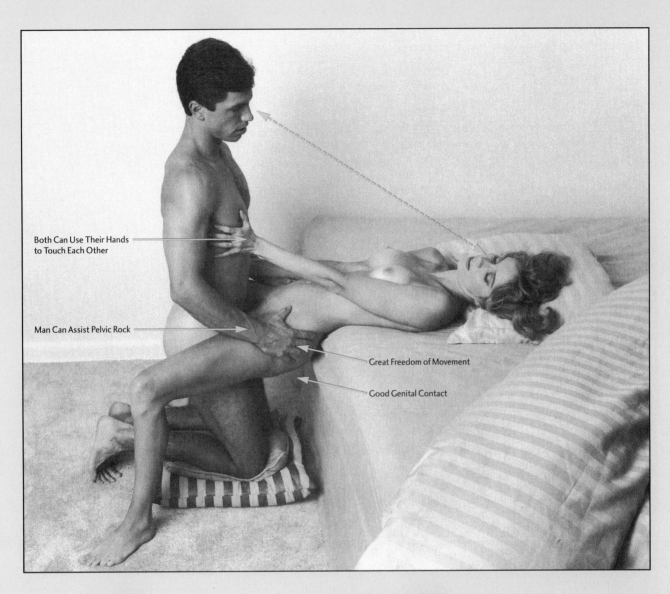

Both Can Use Their Hands
to Touch Each Other

Man Can Assist Pelvic Rock

Great Freedom of Movement

Good Genital Contact

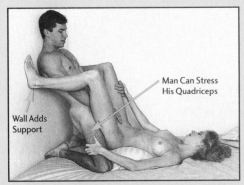

Man Can Stress
His Quadriceps

Wall Adds
Support

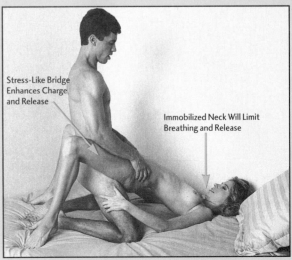

Stress-Like Bridge
Enhances Charge
and Release

Immobilized Neck Will Limit
Breathing and Release

Woman-on-Top Positions

Inherent Problems in This Position

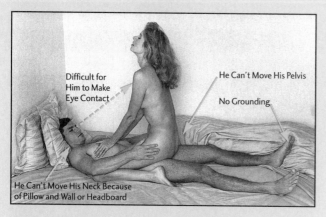

Difficult for Him to Make Eye Contact

He Can't Move His Pelvis

No Grounding

He Can't Move His Neck Because of Pillow and Wall or Headboard

Many women say this is the only position in which they are assured of an orgasm because it allows them to move in a way most stimulating to them. There are many variations, including the woman facing away from the man. The most popular version is the woman facing toward the man.

Evaluation

Use the five freedoms list to assess this position. **(1)** The possibility for eye contact is good for both partners. **(2)** If the woman can allow herself to move freely in this more exposed position, her head and neck can balance the movements of her pelvis in the orgastic

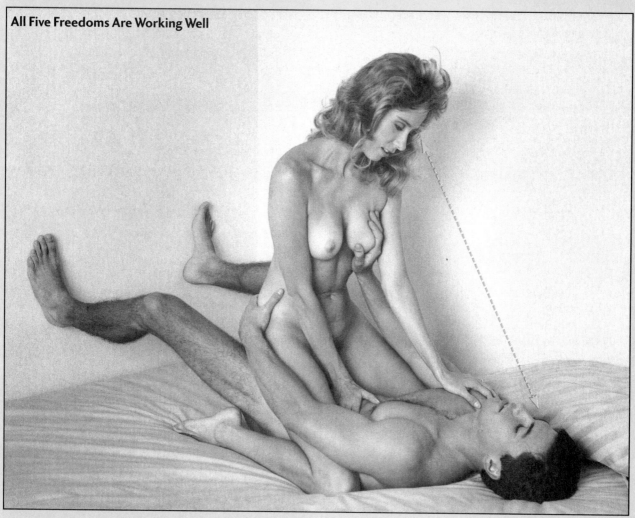

All Five Freedoms Are Working Well

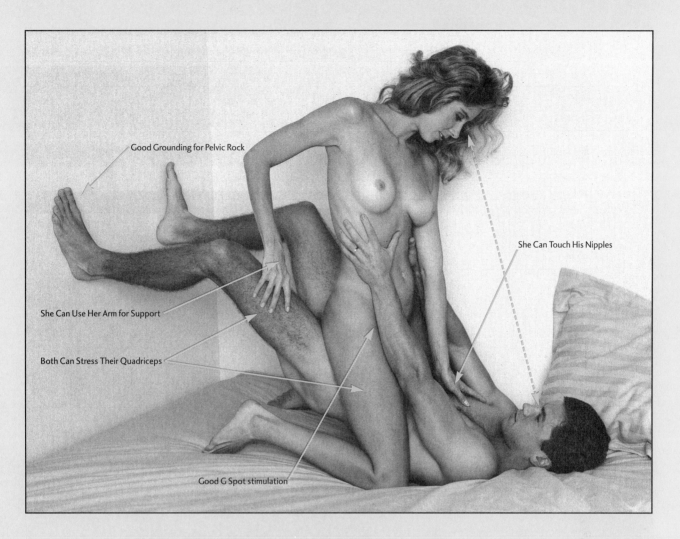

Good Grounding for Pelvic Rock

She Can Touch His Nipples

She Can Use Her Arm for Support

Both Can Stress Their Quadriceps

Good G Spot stimulation

pattern, helping her build and release more easily. **(3)** As she doesn't have to support her weight with her arms or his weight with her chest, she can breathe fully. She can easily lean forward for kissing, rubbing her upper body skin against his, and caressing herself or her lover with her hands. **(4)** On her knees, she can easily rock her pelvis. She can also rotate her pelvis in a more circular motion, stimulating her whole vaginal area and spreading her pelvic charge. If she is too concerned with how she looks in this upright position, though, she may stiffen her body and tighten her stomach muscles. This, of course, will cut off or diminish her charge and orgasm. **(5)** She is grounded by her knees and can stress her quadriceps to spread her charge and trigger orgasm.

The man, on the other hand, **(2)** usually has his head on a pillow and therefore can't move his head and neck freely, which creates an artificial cervical, as well as reciprocal pelvic block of energy. **(3)** If she lies flat on his body with all her weight he will have some difficulty breathing. **(4)** As his legs are flat or relatively so, he will have difficulty rocking his pelvis. **(5)** His feet, without something solid to push against, remain ungrounded and unable to help him retain presence, push without tightening his abdominal muscles, or build a charge.

The primary change needed is for the man to become more grounded. He can accomplish this by putting his feet against the wall or headboard. If he places his feet even higher, as in the "feet against the wall" position in chapter 7, he can move his pelvis more effectively. His penis will enter the woman in the direction of the rear-entry position which, again, is more able to stimulate the G spot. And, if he wishes, he can stress his legs to trigger an orgasm. To be able to move his head and neck, he simply has to get rid of the pillow, though if his feet are raised high against a wall, the movement of his neck and head still may be limited.

If the woman wishes, and she has a high enough charge, she can lean back, stress her quadriceps, and trigger an orgasm. She can also create stress for spreading and releasing a charge by placing her feet on the ground or bed and squatting while she is sitting on his penis. It is somewhat difficult to rock her pelvis in this position, but this variation for athletic women can open the pelvis easily, and the energy that's released can cause her to burst into orgasm.

In another variation, the woman can straddle the man facing away from him. This is interesting as a divergence but, in all likelihood, her clitoris will not be in a position to be stimulated by his body or penis. Self-stimulation and charged breathing will help enjoyment. As eye contact is lost, use a mirror to maintain intimacy.

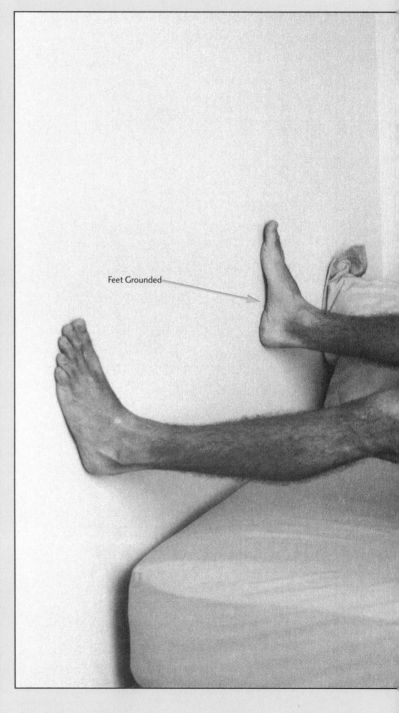

Feet Grounded

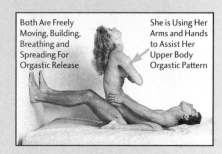

Both Are Freely Moving, Building, Breathing and Spreading For Orgastic Release

She is Using Her Arms and Hands to Assist Her Upper Body Orgastic Pattern

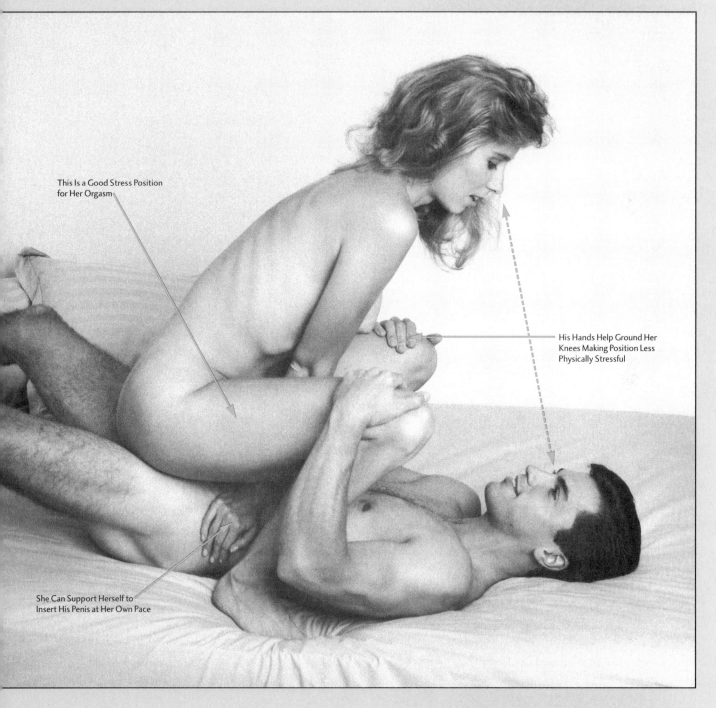

This Is a Good Stress Position for Her Orgasm

His Hands Help Ground Her Knees Making Position Less Physically Stressful

She Can Support Herself to Insert His Penis at Her Own Pace

Rear-Entry Positions

This is a good position for deep penetration, and for stimulating the G spot, for the man to stress his legs, to trigger an orgasm. It is also a position often used to avoid intimacy. If the woman lowers her chest to the bed, the position can help realign a tilted uterus, which can be a source of discomfort for her (see chapter 17).

Evaluation

(1) In this position eye contact is most difficult. This can be remedied by using a mirror. If the mirror is somewhat to the side it will restrict movement less. For rear entry, both partners can be on their knees at the same level on a bed, floor, counter, massage table, etc. Or, while the woman is kneeling on a higher surface, the man can stand behind her with his feet on the floor. **(2)** The man can easily move his head and neck. **(3)** There are no limitations to full-charged breathing. **(4)** He can rock his pelvis freely. **(5)** Either his feet or knees are grounded. His hands are free for caressing or are placed on her hips for balance, and he can lean way back and stress his quadriceps as an orgastic trigger. Because of the possibility of deeper penetration, he must take care, when first entering her, to be slow and gentle.

The woman can be on her knees with her upper body in an upright position or leaning on her hands or elbows. **(2)** Her head and neck are able to move freely, depending only on the placement of the mirror. **(3)** Breathing may be difficult if her chest is pressed too close to the bed or floor. **(4)** She can move her pelvis quite freely. The internal stimulation can be intense, particularly if she continues to build her charge. But she is not in a position for her clitoris to be stimulated by intercourse alone so, if she is moving toward orgasm and has difficulty in building or releasing, she may need additional manual stimulation by him or by her own hand. This same position can be done while standing (see standing positions on pages 272 and 273).

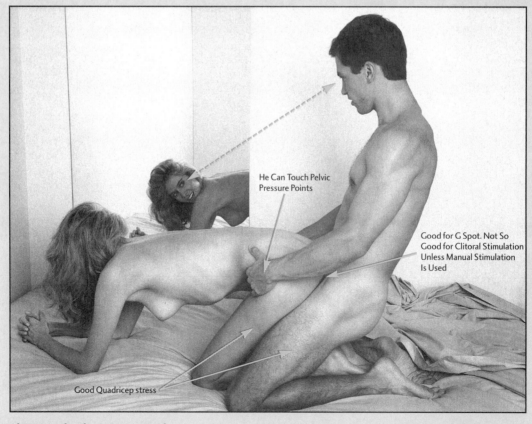

He Can Touch Pelvic Pressure Points

Good for G Spot. Not So Good for Clitoral Stimulation Unless Manual Stimulation Is Used

Good Quadricep stress

Scissors Positions

Scissors positions are the favorites of some couples, possibly because they are positions of relative equality and because neither partner is greatly exposed. Moreover, both partner's hands are free for caressing one another.

Evaluation

(1) Eye contact is relatively easy. **(2)** Head and neck movement may be stifled by pillows, by lack of grounding, by lying on one side and trying to balance, or by trying to see each other. **(3)** Both partners are able to take full-charging breaths. **(4)** The problem with this position comes about when either tries to rock his or her pelvis. Instead of rocking, the pelvis is more apt to twist. This does not allow a wave of movement and energy to travel up the spine, neck, and head, nor does it place the body in the orgastic pattern. Furthermore, with a charge, this rotation has the potential to cause painful back strain. **(5)** The knees and the feet are usually ungrounded.

Scissors positions work best if both partners can place their feet, or at least one foot, on a wall, counter, or piece of furniture. This allows each person to be grounded and to rock his or her pelvis in an orgastic pattern. This works best in a corner so that there is a wall for each person to push against.

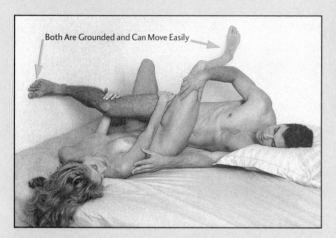

Both Are Grounded and Can Move Easily

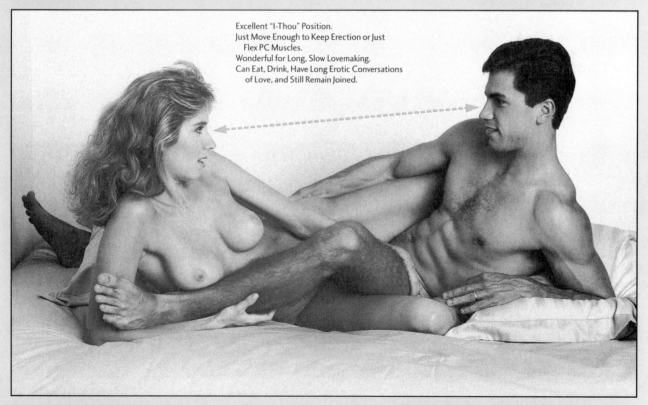

Excellent "I-Thou" Position.
Just Move Enough to Keep Erection or Just
   Flex PC Muscles.
Wonderful for Long, Slow Lovemaking.
Can Eat, Drink, Have Long Erotic Conversations
   of Love, and Still Remain Joined.

Spooning Position (Side-by-Side)

Spooning is mainly a cuddling position. It allows wonderful body-to-body contact. Penetration is not as deep and intimate contact is not as intense, but this position sometimes feels safer as the woman's back is to the man. If the woman moves too much his penis will slip out. If she moves too little, she is apt to feel passive and "done to." Although she can somewhat touch her partner with one hand and, certainly, herself, his hands are more in a position to caress and stimulate her.

Evaluation

(1) Eye contact is not possible unless there is a mirror available. **(2)** The head and neck, probably supported by pillows, arms, etc., are only partially free for movement. **(3)** Breathing pattern is not limited. **(4)** For the pelvis, the motion is more of a pumping than a rocking one and therefore limits the full body movement of the pelvic rock and orgastic reflex. This rotation movement can cause back injuries. **(5)** If each person has a wall, head- or foot-board, or other stable object to push against, they will be more able to move in an orgastic reflex.

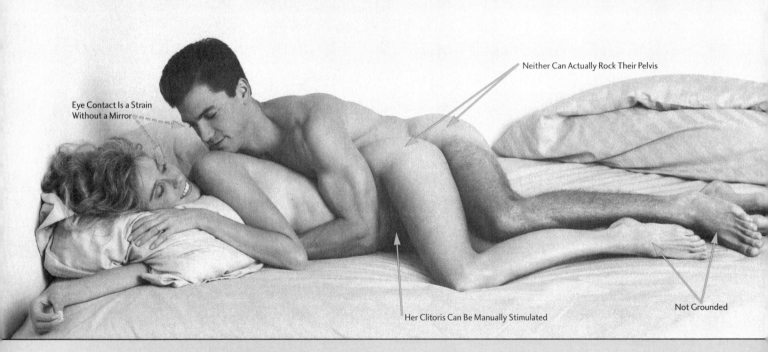

Eye Contact Is a Strain Without a Mirror

Neither Can Actually Rock Their Pelvis

Her Clitoris Can Be Manually Stimulated

Not Grounded

Sitting Positions (Woman-on-Top)

In this position, the woman is on top. Women like this position because, if their feet are touching the ground, they can move their pelvises very easily and, at the same time, stress their legs. Men in this position have an opportunity to take a more passive position. The opportunity for intimacy is great.

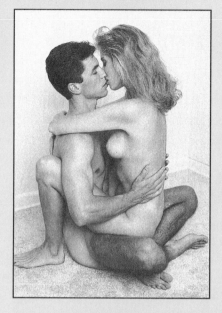

Good for Kissing and Sensuous Contact

Use PC Muscles as Part of Long Slow Lovemaking

Good for High Charge Breathing, but Does Not Allow for Much Movement for Either

Not Good for Orgastic Release as Orgastic Pattern Is Inhibited

Evaluation

(1) Since both partners are facing each other, eye contact is good. **(2)** Neck and head are also free for movement. **(3)** Chest and breathing are also free for both. **(4)** The man on the bottom can't move his pelvis freely while the woman on top can, particularly if the knees or feet are grounded. **(5)** Both people have the possibility for grounding their feet.

For sensuous contact, the man can sit on the floor with his legs crossed in front of him yoga style. The woman can then sit on his lap with her feet on the floor behind him. While she can rock her pelvis more easily than he can, this is a better position for the containment phase than for orgastic release.

If you have an armless rocking chair, the man can use his feet to rock his pelvis in an orgastic pattern. The woman can hold the back of the chair for balance.

On the bed, a woman can sit on the edge while the man kneels on the floor. In this position both can rock their pelvises.

In a variation of this position, the man can sit on his knees on the bed with his back to the headboard or wall. With his back against the wall for support he can tuck his feet in at head of the bed. The woman can sit on his lap, straddling him, holding onto the headboard or anything solid for support. If they move away from the wall when he has a high charge and is ready for orgasm, and if he then leans back, he is in an extremely good position for total body orgasm. If she is flexible and has a high charge, she can lean back and also use this position to spread her charge through her body and release into a total body orgasm.

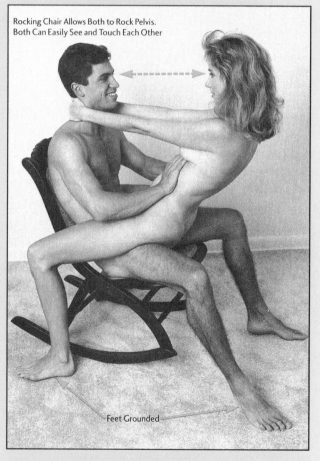

Rocking Chair Allows Both to Rock Pelvis. Both Can Easily See and Touch Each Other

Feet Grounded

Standing Positions

In this position, both partners are able to move freely. The primary difficulties are finding ways to maintain balance and to make up for any height differences. If there is something sturdy overhead to hold onto, such as you might find in a shower or doorway, either partner can hold on and stress the upper body. This can release blocked energy in the chest. If the lower body is also charged, these centers of charge—the chest and pelvis—join, which can be quite powerful and feel like a total body orgasm. Balance can be compensated for if one person leans against something solid.

To compensate for a difference in height, the shorter person can stand on a step or stool. Be sure to add enough room so that both can bend their legs slightly to stress the quadriceps.

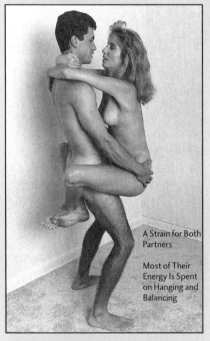

A Strain for Both Partners

Most of Their Energy Is Spent on Hanging and Balancing

Inherent Problems in This Position

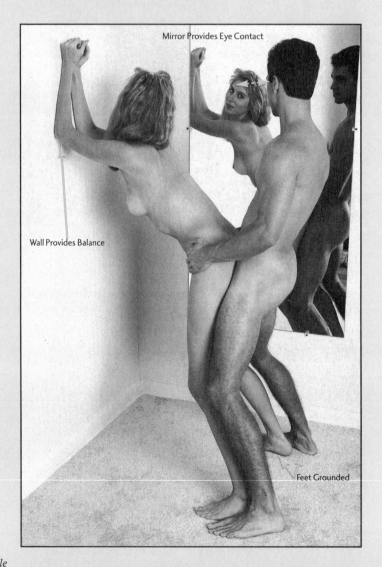

Mirror Provides Eye Contact

Wall Provides Balance

Feet Grounded

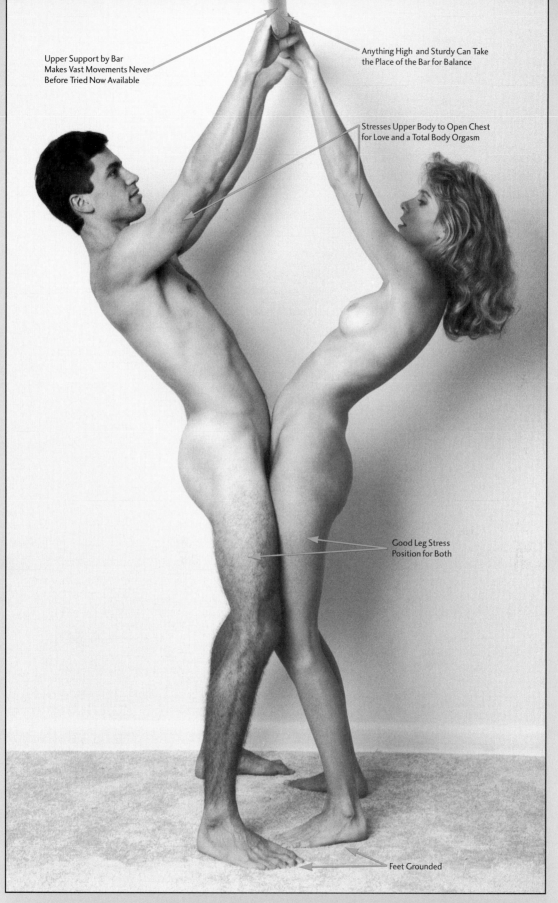

Upper Support by Bar
Makes Vast Movements Never
Before Tried Now Available

Anything High and Sturdy Can Take
the Place of the Bar for Balance

Stresses Upper Body to Open Chest
for Love and a Total Body Orgasm

Good Leg Stress
Position for Both

Feet Grounded

Remember, an orgasm is like a reflex: set it up and it will happen. With a high charge almost anything can trigger your orgasm: a touch to your genitals or nipples, a thought, a stress position. Just paying attention to the waves of sexual energy in your body can escalate your charge, letting your contained energy overflow into orgasm.

MOVE TOWARD RELEASE by heightening your charge, not by pushing or straining but by relaxing and softening your body. The higher your charge when you release, the greater your pleasure. Even while you're having an orgasm, you can increase your charge more and more through movement and breath.

When your partner is moving toward orgasm, don't withdraw your excitement or presence. Don't become distracted just before your lover's orgasm. Sometimes your partner's heightened excitement just before orgasm can scare you into turning way. This is apt to be interpreted by your partner as a devastating rejection, a negative statement about his or her erotic sexual excitement, openness, and vulnerability. Such an abandonment can cause a severe emotional injury. Instead, show your pleasure, encouragement, and your excitement. This adds to the mutual charge and helps your lover flow into bigger and better orgasms.

If either of you is getting sore from the friction of intercourse, switch to using a lubricated hand, your tongue, or mouth, but try not to interrupt your partner's building toward orgasm. If you continue in pain, though, you'll avoid sex the next time around.

Heightened orgastic release can offer brief changes of consciousness, intense feelings of love, luminous moments of spiritual awakening, and an expansive sense of self.

Approaching Orgasm

Many of the ways you enhance your lovemaking are mind-to-body, such as fantasy or instructing your body to move in a particular way. But as you approach orgasm, it becomes more and more important to allow your body and its sensations to supersede your mind. Give up thinking for a while. See what your body feels and wants, how it naturally moves. Let your body, not your mind, move with your lover. Look at your partner. Use your heart to feel your love. Bring these energies to orgasm. As you approach orgastic release here are a few reminders.

- Move so it feels particularly good to you.
- Don't tighten or push. Focus on the charge rather than the release.
- Move toward orgasm with anticipation and courage.
- Move your pelvis easily in a steady rhythm, keeping stomach muscles soft, moving in the orgastic pattern. Find your own rhythm from inside your own body.
- Don't be afraid to stop and reconnect with your body rhythm if you need to.
- Allow your upper body to move freely. Ground your feet or knees.
- Suck, lick, or kiss to greatly facilitate orgasm in you and your partner.
- If you have difficulty releasing, stress your quadriceps.

If your sexual arousal and charge are high enough, a release may occur spontaneously. Yet, additional stimulation is both pleasurable and helpful. An orgastic surge can be triggered by stimulation of erotically sensitive areas of the body, erotic thoughts, fantasies, by a lover's erotic energy, or through any excitement of the senses.

The most common triggers for orgasm are, of course, the genitals—clitoris, G spot, penis, and prostate. Other erotically sensitive areas are the mouth, throat, nipples, anus, neck, ears, skin, pressure points, and parts of the body not usually touched (such as back of the knees), inner thighs, buttocks, bottoms of feet, between fingers and toes, etc.

Some people have certain rituals, visualizations, or thoughts that they use to trigger orgasm: sights, pictures, smells, music, or other sounds or textures. Some triggers are conditioned through association with masturbation or other first sexual experiences. These body-stored memories are retained as powerful, conditioned aphrodisiacs. Sensory experiences are usually easily mobilized through body memory.

- **Simultaneous Orgasms.** Simultaneous orgasms are not only unnecessary, they often cause you to miss half the fun. When you are fully engulfed in your own orgasm, it's hard to stay present and fully enjoy your partner's orgasm. It's not necessary to try to have orgasms at the same time. More often than not, striving for togetherness will just heighten your character style or agency response and interfere with at least one person's release. The whole idea of simultaneous orgasms came from a time when loss of boundaries, surrendering to each other, was the goal of intercourse. It was thought, "If you don't have an orgasm at the same time I do, you don't love me." Losing one's sense of self to a partner does not support the deeper experiences of sexual intimacy.

- **Intensified Orgasms.** As you approach the point of orgasm, try changing your breathing to very rapid, deep charge breaths. Take 25–50 of them. This will delay your orgastic release but, after taking the breaths, keep moving your pelvis and you will approach the point of release very quickly again, but with a higher charge. Rest a while; let your charge spread. Do this two or three times, increasing your charge each time. Finally let yourself release into orgasm.

If you have trouble releasing, it may be because you are overcharged. If so, change your position to one where you can either stand or be on your knees. Stress your quadriceps for a few minutes, continuing to move your pelvis while having intercourse. Stay present as much as you can and you will have a full and intense orgasm.

Women, if you wish, after your orgasm, take another 50 or so breaths, and your charge will be right back up and you can have another orgasm. Men, keep breathing, enjoy the satisfaction of your orgasm and ejaculation, rest for a few moments and you can begin making love all over again. (See chapters 4 and 8 for multiple orgasms and orgasms without ejaculation.)

If you still find orgasm difficult with a partner, pay attention to your character style and gender prejudice themes, loss of boundaries, splitting off, and agency—all major contributors to this struggle. A person with a rather high inundation response might need to establish a little breathing room to have an orgasm: they may try a position that limits contact, such as rear entry. It may help trick your character style by telling yourself, "I don't really want to have an orgasm."

SATISFACTION AFTER
SEXUAL LOVEMAKING

SATISFACTION IS THE MOST NEGLECTED aspect of the orgastic cycle. Many people never really let the feeling of satisfaction permeate their sensory awareness anywhere else in their lives—not in their work, play, relationships, spirituality, or sexuality.

Satisfaction is a feeling of closure, of completeness, felt in the body. In our busy, competitive world, a great many people seem to avoid experiencing their own satisfaction, as if they are afraid that the acknowledgment would permanently immobilize them. Some fear that if they really let themselves feel satisfaction, they would never feel motivated again. Sometimes people fear that if they were satisfied with themselves, they would not need others; if they were satisfied with others, they would need them too much. They fear that they would no longer care about goals and accomplishment in their life. For some people, the habit of not allowing satisfaction is the primary source of their unhappiness, instability, searching, and lack of well-being. Nothing seems to work, and they are constantly on edge.

People tend to withhold the little satisfactions on the way toward their goals, like the unattainable carrot that dangles in front of a donkey, keeping it moving but never satisfied. It's also like the parent who never encourages a child, never acknowledges small successes along the way, always promising that if the child does just one more thing, then he or she will be praised or rewarded. For far too many people, satisfaction, sexual or otherwise, is never reached because there is always one more thing to accomplish.

Satisfactions felt in the body not only motivate us, they are also affirmative, telling us if we are on the right track. People who don't stop to enjoy themselves treat themselves like objects. They usually have to force themselves to reach out for goals. People who really let themselves enjoy what they do tend to be more motivated. More importantly, the body and psyche need to rest and rejuvenate, and the openness of satisfaction allows for new, expanded experiences. Lives that rush from goal to goal tend to be narrow. The same is true of sex.

After orgasm, the possibilities for lovemaking, for the most profound closeness and attunement, are at its greatest. While the body is open, there is a heightened feeling of love, affection, and sensuality. There may even be a change in consciousness. But because of the openness, paradoxically, this is also the most likely time for old wounds to surface. Therefore the impulse to create distance can also be the greatest. If you need a little breathing room, be gentle and loving. Keep in mind that your partner will be at her or his most sensitive and vulnerable. Try not to abandon yourself or your loved one; stay close.

Now is when unfinished situations from scenario, character style, and agency can opportunistically rush to the surface. Let these pass. You may remember real or imagined injustices inflicted by your lover. These thoughts will only create distance and close your body tighter. Go back to the good feelings in your body and bring these to your present interactions. Postpone any argument for later. Later, write about your feelings in your journal; then talk.

Stay present. Orgastic release is not supposed to be a sleeping tablet. Don't immediately fall asleep or you will miss what those who stick around find to be the best part of lovemaking. You may have trained yourself to split off to avoid the emotions, openness, vulnerability, or joy that comes with release. Lie together, breathe slowly and deeply. Let go gently, relaxing but staying in contact. Savor moments of tenderness.

The orgastic release is only the beginning of many releases that continue throughout your body. If you continue charge breathing, it heightens these continuing releases and the pleasurable sensations, both emotional and sensory. If you fall asleep quickly, you will miss these sensations as your body continues to release. You will also miss the opportunity to further the extent of your release. Blocks in the body can hinder or stop the release from moving through the rest of your body.

At this time, if you keep your charge breathing going, you can help each other release these blocks and any deeper muscular holding patterns. If your lover lightly strokes your body while you are enjoying the afterglow of an orgasm, it feels wonderful. A simple touch will often release holding patterns that are stubbornly resistant at other times.

Skin time is now at its best. Lie close. Cuddle up. Let any interruptions fade away. Stay present. Let yourself take in the nonverbal, energetic, core-to-core sense of satisfaction in your body. Sometimes this is all you need to feel a profound healing and shift in your relationships and life.

Very lightly, almost without touching, send love with your hands. Stroke your lover. After orgasm there is often a very magical feel to the skin. See if you can feel the energetic difference. Use the opportunity of your bodies' opening to join with your partner. Be together with a commitment toward love. With a body experience of love, nothing else is needed.

Heightening Satisfaction

Self: After orgasm, breathe about 20–60 breaths with your chest, at a leisurely pace. Breathe slowly, deeply, and fully to heighten your feelings. Let the charge of satisfaction spread throughout your body.

To encourage the releasing process. Start at your feet and systematically let go: feet, ankle, knees, thighs, etc., all the way up your body. With breathing, the wave of energetic release can go on for an extended length of time.

Partner: If you watch your partner, you will notice the orgastic release as it moves through his or her body. Because you have learned to see holding patterns, you will be able to recognize remaining holding patterns after orgasm.

At times you may want to do more for your partner than a simple caress. If your partner's orgasm is separate from yours, you can help move the release past these holding patterns, so it is felt in the rest of his or her body. For instance, if your lover has a cervical block, energy may become stuck between the neck and upper chest. You can slip your arm under your partner's neck and lift slightly on his or her exhale.

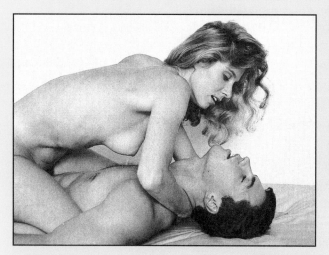

Release 1.

This is usually enough for your partner to feel the rush of orgastic energy move through her or his body, releasing and enlivening along the way. Note the changes of color and texture along your partner's body. You can use any of the release techniques you learned in chapter 10. The following are further examples of releases to facilitate the movement of the orgastic energy.

Segmental Releases, Starting with the Top Segment.
Eyes: Use the pressure point release techniques you learned, particularly those on the back of the skull that open the ocular segment.

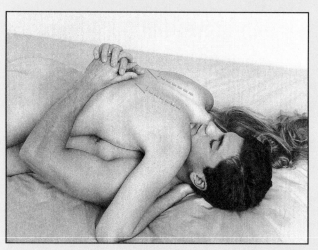

Release 2.

Neck: You can slip your arm under your partner's neck and lift as was already mentioned or you can use a towel around your partner's head and neck, lifting, then stretching and rocking as you learned earlier. Work on the holding around the upper shoulder and neck muscles.

Chest/Upper Back: This is the front and back of the same segment. You can further your partner's release by using your body weight and arms and knees.

If you are on the bottom it is easy to stroke the tight muscles of your partner's back, neck, and buttocks. If on top, turn your partner over to massage. Change who is on top and massage some more.

When you are on the bottom you can wrap your arms around your partner. If you can, reaching your arms around your partner clasp your own hands together. Press on either side of your partner's spine with the heels of your hands. Then, give your partner a "hug" squeezing your partner to your chest, slowly and gently until the air is expelled fully from the chest as he or she exhales. Release as your partner inhales. Start at the top of the spine and work all the way down the spine. Repeat this, following and assisting your partner's breathing pattern. In this way you help to soften and open holding patterns of the chest and back and encourage breathing and loving feelings.

For a man with heavy chest muscles you can use this more forceful technique. Support yourself partially with one hand and knee on the bed. Place the other knee on his upper chest and hand on his shoulder. (See release 3). As he exhales press down with your knee and pull up with your hand on his shoulder. As you help expel the air in his chest, it will relieve tight muscles. Then change your position and do the other side of his chest.

After orgasm you can release the lower back muscles using long firm strokes with your hands. With your hands massage the muscles that run parallel to the spine on your partner's back. For a big or heavily muscled man it may be necessary to add more weight. The woman can use her knees to release his back. Placing

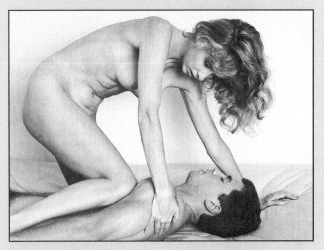

Release 3.

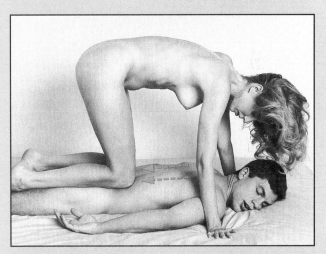

Release 4.

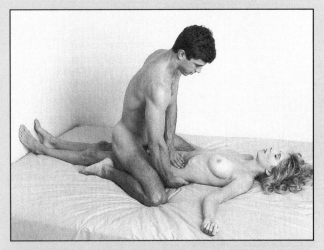

Release 5.

her knees on either side of his spine, she can move her knees down the muscles of his back and massage in the same way as if using her hands. Using her hands to support herself, she can adjust the weight applied with her knees. Be sure to stay in contact with the muscles along the spine. Check with your partner as to the placement of your knees and the amount of pressure applied.

Belly: Very gently massage in clockwise motions. Holding in the belly retards satisfaction and spread of release. Try resting a while in the knee-chest position found in chapter 17, page 250 to release the abdomen. But as this is not a body-to-body position, it can take away from the loving feelings.

Genitals: Stay away from genitals and nipples until both lovers are ready for sex again. Here is your chance to let your character style get you in trouble. Going after the nipples and genitals at this time will likely feel uncomfortably intense and invasive, and can anger your partner and create a great deal of closing and distancing.

Legs: Massage legs and feet, releasing tight muscles. The feet are particularly sensitive after orgasm. Go from head to feet and back again. This facilitates the streaming of energy.

AFTERWORD

"A soul to know itself must gaze into another soul."
HAMILL, *THE EROTIC SPIRIT,* 1996

As human beings we thrive when we have an emotional and physical connection with someone we love who loves us back.

THE PSYCHOLOGICAL, physical, and spiritual practices in this book answer most difficulties couples have wrestled with since the dawn of monogamy. The feeling that one's relationship and life are both enriching need not be elusive. We often forget to honor an interior body experience of self, the deepest and surest means of knowing ourselves and one another. This supports tolerance for intense intimacy and erotic sexuality. It is time for eroticism to be reclaimed by those within long-term monogamous relationships. Eroticism is an expression of intense aliveness and not separate from our lives or loving. We must relearn our delight in the flesh and the spirit and not deprive ourselves of this mutual joy.

The continuity of relationship can provide a safe harbor to share our experiences, travails, and soul-touching moments. Without this, for most, there is a feeling that something is missing, incomplete. In our bodies, we know without a doubt that intimate relationships are precious and worth extraordinary tending. Let this book be an opening to the rest of your life. Surpass our suggestions. Invent new ways of making love, cherishing your lover and life. Live a life without regrets. Make love forever.

Appendix

APPENDIX

The Narrative History of Your Primary Scenario

You can create a visual image of your own primary scenario, the history of the themes of your childhood, by filling out the chart that follows. Use brief descriptive words and phrases in your answers. Later this information can identify troublesome issues, themes, and fragmentation triggers. The chart creates a visual image that can provide you with many insights. You may want to draw a larger replica of this chart to provide more room for your notes.

Everyone has a unique story—a history that has become a part of her or his body and remains a significant influence throughout life. Your story, like everyone else's, is based on selective memory. Therefore, it is difficult to figure out what is really true, because many realities can exist at the same time. What you feel is true is more important than reality.

The history of your childhood is like an old familiar movie that will come to life as you remember each of the key characters in your own personal scenario. Pay attention when you have an emotional response, like warmth for a grandparent, spacey feelings when talking about your father or mother, anger or tightness when someone is mentioned. As you trace your own personal roots, picture the setting and set the scene, the year, and the place. Acknowledge what was happening in the geographical area when you were born and during the time when you were growing up. For example, 1943 in Berlin is different from 1943 in Billings or 1963 in New Orleans. Zoom in on the people of *your* past. What social and economic hardships were your parents confronted with—war, depression, emigration, death of someone close?

What you can't know or don't remember, guess about. Sometimes what you imagine your scenario to be is more important and revealing of your roots and your unconscious motivations than the facts.

Most families have an unspoken rule that no one is to notice or talk about certain truths or problems within the family. Even the healthiest families are not without limitations, injuries, problems, and secrets. Notice if you are willing to look; answer the questions directly and truthfully. It takes courage to remember, acknowledge, and reveal family secrets even to yourself. There are also many positive aspects and moments in your past that you may have been overlooking. Notice any emotionally poignant feelings in your body, those that are either uncomfortable or pleasurable. The welling up of emotion provides the most valuable information about your family.

Seek—not to blame but to understand—the true nature of your history and repetitive relationship patterns. Bring your history into the open. Blowing open your own cover is the first major step toward good mental health. Self-trust and comfort with intimacy is not built upon what is easy but upon what involves risk and authenticity.

Primary Scenario Chart (Sample)

Name _____ Date _____

Use the format of this chart to create a visual reference of your family history. Draw in siblings, add other important people and descriptions, and list important family information. Then look for themes and parallels. What you learn may surprise you. Use the questions that follow to guide you in your self-inquiry.

Grandmother Traits **GM** — Grandfather **GF** Traits — Grandmother Traits **GM** — Grandfather **GF** Traits

Mother Traits **M** — Father Traits **F**

Relationship with Mother — Relationship with Father

SELF

Scenario Themes:

Relationships:
#1
#2
#3

Re-Creating Your Story
• What was the date your parents married and where were they living at the time?

Mother
• What was your mother like at the time she married your father? How old was she? What work was she doing? What was she like emotionally? Could she show physical affection? Was she present and emotionally available, attractive, smart? What was her attitude about erotic sex and pleasure? Could you imagine her enjoying sex with your father or anyone else? Why did she choose your father? Did she get what she was looking for?

Maternal Grandparents
• What were your maternal grandparents like? Could they show physical affection? Draw in their children on the scenario map in birth order, noting how many years apart they were. Use circles for women and squares for men. What were your mother's parents' feelings about sex, marriage, men and women? What were their nationalities, cultural backgrounds, and religions? What was their relationship like? Were they present and emotionally available? What were their attitudes about erotic sex and pleasure? What was their relationship like with you? During your childhood, how did your mother's family affect her life, her relationship to your father, and her ability to parent you?

Father

- What was your father like at the time he first met your mother? How old was he? What work was he doing? What was he like emotionally? Could he show physical affection? Was he present and emotionally available, handsome, smart? What was his attitude about erotic sex and pleasure? Could you imagine him enjoying sex with your mother or anyone else? Why did he choose your mother? Did he get what he was looking for?

Paternal Grandparents

- What were your paternal grandparents like? Could they show physical affection? Draw in their children on the scenario map in birth order, noting how many years apart they were. Use circles for women and squares for men. What were your grandparents' feelings about erotic sex, marriage, about men and women? What were their nationalities, cultural backgrounds, and religions? What was their relationship like? Were they present and emotionally available? What were their attitudes about sex and pleasure? What was their relationship like with you? During your childhood, how did your father's family affect his life, his relationship with your mother, and his ability to parent you?

Other Caretakers

- Were there any relatives, neighbors, a nursemaid, or others who took care of you, that you were close to, or that were important in your life? What were they like? What was their nationality or cultural background, etc.?

Yourself

- Add yourself and any siblings to the chart by birth order, noting the years apart. What were the themes surrounding your birth? Were you a wanted child? By whom and for what reason? What was it like to be you between birth and six years old? Describe yourself. What were you like as a child emotionally, in appearance, personality, behavior? Were you a "good" girl or boy? Did you get into trouble a lot? Were you spanked or punished in some way? If so, how? What was your birth order, and what was this position like for you in your family? What was your function in the family—that is, what were you supposed to be or do for the family?

- What was your relationship with your mother, your father, siblings? To whom were you the closest? Were you and are you now able to be physically affectionate? How did it feel to be you? What were your fears or longings? What was your relationship like with your mother, your father, your brothers and sisters? What were you supposed to do to make each of your parent's lives complete? What did you do when you got hurt or angry? Who did you go to when you were hurt? Who did you talk to or share your feelings with? From whom did you get affection, your "warm fuzzies"? Did you have any pets that you were close to? How did your mother get you to obey her? How did your father get you to obey him? How did you get what you wanted? How did you make your parents crazy? What did you want when you grew up? Were

there any traumatic events or ongoing themes that have shaped your life?

- What was it like to be you between ages seven and twelve? Is your response different from what it was for birth to six? What was it like to be you between ages twelve and fifteen? Did you feel sexually attractive? Give yourself a grade from 1 through 10—1 being poor and 10 being great—as to how you felt about yourself sexually. What was it like to be you at the time you were first introduced to sex? How old were you? Was it a pleasurable, playful, life-confirming experience, or was it painful, frightening, overwhelming, or humiliating?

Significant Relationships

- Identify your significant intimate relationships, those with whom you have had an important relationship, lived with, or married. Name each significant person, one at a time, and answer these questions about them: What were their names and ages? What were they like? What was the hope of that relationship? Who ended the relationship and why? Did you have any children? (If so, write in their names.) Have you ever had a miscarriage, stillbirth, or abortion? (This question is for both men and women.) Make sure you have entered each answer on your primary scenario chart.

- When you get to your current intimate partner, ask yourself, "What was the hope and promise that motivated me to choose this particular man or woman?" What was different about this person that gave you hope? What do you feel about him or her now? Have you gotten what you hoped for? If not, what is your part in creating this outcome? What do you believe your partner's attitude is about erotic sex and loving? Were you erotically sexually attracted to your partner from the beginning? Are you at this time erotically sexually attracted to your partner? Do you feel love, trust, and affection toward your partner?

The hope or promise one holds for an intimate relationship is usually analogous to the wish to solve an emotional injury or dilemma from one's childhood, making the theme of the good hope or promise a sensitive, highly charged issue. And because of its childhood correlation it often leads to deep feelings of betrayal and emotional injury.

Scenario Review

Look back at the scenario that you have charted. What important information has been left out? Where are the alcoholics, drug users, pill takers, mental illnesses, deaths, or suicides? Were there people who were spiteful, victims, martyrs, or betrayal collectors? What are the hidden secrets, disasters, and crimes? Are there other skeletons in the closet—other information missing? Does this sound like a real story or a fairy tale?

All families have their own sets of problems and their own successes. It is common when looking back to remember what was unfinished, what you didn't get, and to forget how much your parents did right when raising you. Each generation has its own set of problems and themes to resolve. Most have at least some semblance of success and many are quite successful. Your set of problems and themes are yours to resolve in your own way.

Look for a repetition of themes from person to person and generation to generation. What are the insights and important issues that you become aware of as you review your scenario? How are you repeating what your parents or grandparents did? What are you doing or feeling as an adult as a result of what happened to you as a child?

This chart is just the bare bones. As you read the psychological sections and do the body-mind exercises, flesh out your scenario with more information and insights. Your personal history begins with your primary scenario and continues to be acted out by your character style and agency.

Sexual History—How it affects you today

This exercise is a variation of your primary scenario. It is a collection of body-mind memories that make up the history of your personal, psychosexual development. If you are already familiar with the pertinent issues of your childhood from the primary scenario review above, this simple exercise will help you discover and trace themes that influence your sexuality.

Both the primary scenario and the sexual scenario contain injurious and growthful themes from childhood. These appear as assumptions, beliefs, attitudes, body-mind holding patterns, fears, pleasures, and delights. Unfortunately our sexual scenarios are full of worn-out hurts, inaccurate assumptions, overrated sorrows, lingering regrets, and idealizations that we carry unnecessarily into our current sexual relationship. Tracing patterns that influence your sexuality is extremely useful for removing negative affects and enhancing pleasurable ones.

This will be a journey of body-mind memories. You will find that as you remember one story after the next, your stories will reveal physical and emotional patterns, giving you a deeper understanding of your sexuality.

Step 1: Find a quiet, comfortable place where you won't be disturbed. Take several full sighing, letting-go breaths. Imagine that you are going to watch a video of your sex life from the very first memory to the present. Let your memory reach back in time to the very first thing you can remember that has anything at all to do with sexuality. Once you identify the memory, see if you can remember anything at an earlier time. It may only be an image, a taste, sound or smell. It may be a full memory of an event.

Step 2: In your journal, note the age you were when this event actually occurred. Very briefly tell the story in the first person present: "I am walking. I am in the bathroom...." Tell your story as if you were watching a videotape of the event, memory by memory. Let yourself experience the setting, the place, the year, the time of day, any noises or smells, anything your senses and your body remember. Write a brief summary of your story.

As you relive your story, notice what you feel in your body, and where you feel it. If you are telling your story in the first person present and allowing yourself to feel the experience in your body, you are bound to have the same body feeling now as you did then.

Step 3: After you finish the story, write in your journal: *the belief* that you formed due to this experience; *the emotions*—the

fear and/or pleasure—associated with the story; the body sensations—what you feel in your body and where you are experienc- ing the feeling right now as you relive your story.

Some people can remember being aware of sexuality in infancy. Others don't remember anything until their teens. Most remember something at about age five or six. After you write your initial story, come forward in time and follow steps 1–3 for each event you can remember. Here are some important development markers to be sure to explore:

- toilet training, enemas, catheterizations.
- sex play, masturbation.
- same-sex sexual explorations.
- onset of puberty, secondary sexual characteristics, first menstruation, ejaculation, nocturnal emissions, first sexual exploration, first intercourse, gynecological exams; also, childbirths, abortions, miscarriages.
- any sexual abuse, rape, incest, or other traumatic experience that you can remember at any age.

When you are finished, divide a page into three columns, title them beliefs, emotional responses, and body sensations, then go back through your journal notes and find the threads that weave through your stories and link them together. In particular, review all the beliefs you developed and the emotional responses and body sensations you felt from story to story and write them in the new columns.

New Hints and Reminders for Sexuality
The Intimacy Phase of Sexual Lovemaking

- Character style is the major interruption to intimacy. With your partner are you playing out your abandonment or inundation anxieties or the six traits that come when both anxieties are combined? If your lover suggests something, notice if you feel an automatic "no" in your body. Can you go along without a struggle? Remember, "I'm going to do this—even if you want me to," or, "even if I want to," comes closer to getting you what *you* want than does a rebellious stance.
- Recall to mind what is special to you about your partner, even if it has been long covered by struggles or upsets. Experiment with any of the following as ways to trigger your feelings of intimacy and sexuality.
  - Think of a time when love was good and nourish the feeling in your body.
  - Be friendly. Bring your most positive intention and nurture it in your body. Assume and trust that your partner's intention is positive toward you even if you can't feel it clearly.
- Be available, not only in feelings and in body but with your time. Make a specific agreement for time to spend with your partner, then show up, stay present, and don't leave your erotic feelings behind. Try some of the following:
  - Offer to give your partner a massage and follow through without an expectation of something in return.
  - Take a shower and wash your partner's hair and body.
  - Take a bath together and give a foot massage in the tub.
  - Meditate together.
  - Do breathing exercises together.

- Lie together—have skin time not aimed at sex.
- Touch your partner while summoning the most passionate, kind, and gentlest part of yourself.

- Do something to express your love for your partner—bring flowers, cook a meal, clean the garage, finish a task you promised to do last week.
- Turn off the TV, even if it's your favorite program. Turn to your partner and ask what he or she would like to do.
- Before you talk to your partner about a struggle or hurt, write in your journal. Find your part in any conflict. See what you can do to resolve your disharmony. Do the steps out of fragmentation (chapter 15) and get your act together before you try to join with another. Don't try to get your partner to fix or soothe your feelings; it's not sexy or erotic. You may feel better and more intimate, but in the long run you will get more agency and less sexuality.
- If you can't resolve an argument or hurt, try to bracket it off until later. If you can't, you won't find intimacy. A little competent therapy often helps to resolve tenacious upsets.
- Intimacy is not constant. Don't panic if you can't feel it inside of you. If you have a solid bond between you, it will return.

The Desire Phase of Sexual Lovemaking

- Choose to have sex for your own satisfaction, not to please or get something from your partner, or to avoid making waves. Stop and consciously choose.
- Play "Remember when…" Talk about times when you first met and felt loving, when sex was new and special. Notice that when you talk about good times there is a temptation to step into old betrayals, old leftover hurts. *Don't do it*. It is a surefire destroyer of intimacy no matter how you joke, for there is always an element of hurt left in your body, waiting to be reactivated. If you open these doors, you will find yourself up to your nose in deep water. Intimacy can be quickly deadened, and it can take a long time to heal the breach.
- Feel the erotic, energetic sensations of arousal and desire in your body as you talk to your partner. Choose any topic that's pleasant and erotic, not necessarily anything sexual. As you feel sexual sensations in your body, this energy will be transmitted, even if you only offer a cup of tea. On the other hand, if you are not feeling excitement and desire, you are not likely to spark it in your partner. Don't wait until you are having sex to get in the mood.
- Find a way to get turned on in your own body before you approach. Fantasize of times when sex was good with your partner. Let yourself feel the associated excitement aroused in your body by the fantasy, but don't try to make something happen.
- Let desire and grow and build. Start out by expressing your loving while keeping the sexual energy contained in your body. Don't rush the approach. Play with extending the time you feel turned on. Let yourself enjoy the charge in your body; express it in the way you breathe and move. Bear in mind that too much mental activity will take you away from your physical feelings of desire.
- Take time with your partner away from children, friends, and work. Make time together without distractions, even if you only take a bath or shower together.
- If you have high desire, don't say anything at first. Notice if your partner moves away or becomes distant when your desire is high, even though you haven't mentioned it. Or, if your lover's desire is high, notice if *you* become more distant. Keep in mind that your partner's desire and love can trigger typical character style distancing behaviors.
- Prolong the time that you spend in the desire phase with your partner. Take your desire out to dinner with you. Extend desire throughout the day by expressing your feelings with a love song or a poem.
- Keep the charge of desire very high in your body by increasing your breathing before you approach. Keep it high while you take a walk, hold hands, dance, swim, take a bath or shower.
- If your partner expresses desire and that turns you on, say so. When anything he or she says or does pleases you, let it be known. Express what that makes you feel in your body and where you feel it. Be receptive to your partner's approach. No matter how sexy your partner is, remember, only *you* can turn *you* on.

The Approach Phase of Sexual Lovemaking

- Get present for yourself. Open your eyes, look at colors, savor smells, sounds, tastes. Allow your senses to come alive. Set everything else aside and enter the realm of erotic, sensuous joining.
- Pay attention to your emotions. Show what you are feeling. If you feel love, convey the *energy* of love. If you feel sexual, convey the *energy* of sexuality. Don't be stingy.
- Before you approach your partner, remember a time when you were both loved and beloved. Feel it in your body before you impart the energy of sex and love. In monogamy, love can open the pelvis more than anything else.
- You don't always have to feel sexual to ask for or agree to have sex, you only need to feel loving and a desire to be close. But if you don't wish to have sex, even if you are loving, request skin time instead. But keep in mind, if skin time is all you ever want, there is something wrong.
- If your answer is, "No, not right now," be relational. Let your partner know when you *will* be available. Don't leave your partner hanging. For instance, you can say, "How about in the morning, later today, or at eight o'clock?" Remember, sometimes saying "no" allows you then to say "yes." You can change your mind as your body becomes aroused.
- Character style can activate a struggle in approach more than the other arenas. Do you consistently ask for sex in a way that angers your partner and wins you a refusal? This a sure sign of your character style asserting itself. Do you consistently find an excuse: "It is not the right time," or, "You asked in the wrong way," etc.? If your partner has a high abandonment-inundation style, there may never be a time in which you can do it right.
- You may not have difficulty turning yourself and even your partner on, but if you have a high abandonment-inundation style, your automatic "no" may come along and stop you

from following through, making you seem like a tease. This behavior is abusive to a sexual relationship.

- It helps to be direct when you wish to approach for sex, to eliminate confusion. "I want to sleep with you," may get you a nap together with hurt feelings and no sex. "I want to make love with you," may be too direct for some people, but you must find an agreed-upon communication that turns neither partner away. This is a subject best discussed when you are *not* approaching for sex.
- If your partner is not as sexually aroused or as interested as you are, start where he or she is, slowly. Think about love-making in terms of both people moving toward the center of many concentric circles.
  - If your partner is at the outer circle and you go for the center, you will miss each other entirely and not feel much mutuality.
  - Be friendly and give your partner room for volition and room to move toward you also.
  - Take turns being in charge; be the leader. Then be the best follower your lover has ever seen.
  - *Respond with enthusiasm if you say yes.* Take responsibility for finding out what you have to do to have a good experience for yourself. Going along and saying, "Okay, use me," or, "Do me," is worse than saying no.
- As with intimacy and desire, approach can be extended over a long period of time. Seduction is glorious in monogamy and heightens charge very effectively. Start with breakfast in bed, kissing. Move to a shower together in the morning, perhaps even a quickie in the shower. Keep the charge alive. Keep breathing and stay present throughout the day. Stay turned on. Then have longer sex in the afternoon or evening. If you have to go to work or otherwise be apart, phone your partner and remind her or him of your love and that you are looking forward to being together once again.
- If you find yourself feeling turned on and then you stop yourself with a thought that turns you off, it's probably your character style. Whether you have disparaging thoughts about yourself, your partner, or about something upsetting or unfinished at work, it is most important to remember that these interruptions are just figments of your character style trying to erect a barrier between you and your partner or you and your sexuality.
- Encourage your partner's approach by being as available as you can without losing your volition. Consistent refusal leads to hurt, anger, withdrawal, or all three. The one who never approaches will eventually feel used, treated like an object; the one who always does the approaching will never feel wanted or desired. Remember, each partner must approach 50 percent of the time.

The Charge-Containment Phase of Sexual Lovemaking
- Pay attention to your own body. Do you feel any tension? Don't say anything to your partner—just turn inward and let go.
- As you begin to build a charge, practice shuttling back and forth between an interior and exterior focus—from within your body to your partner's body and back again.

- Send love through both touch and energy. Send and receive love through your mouth and lips.
- Be generous: Do what your partner wants. Give a little. Put aside any feelings of, "Why do I always have to be the one who…."
- Make sounds with your breathing that show you are enjoying what your lover is doing. Voice your appreciation out loud, "I love the way you look," or, "I love your… (body, eyes, ears, nose, sounds, smell, taste, or anything else that's true)," or, "You are so… (handsome or beautiful or delicious)." If it carries the sound of truth, it speaks directly to the body when you have a high charge. If you can't find something positive to say, then something is wrong—probably your character style.
- Breathe for your own aliveness—don't worry about your partner's charge or what he or she thinks. Don't split off. If your partner doesn't want to have a charge, build one for yourself. Don't fall for the "help me, fix me, turn me on, do me," routine.
- Pay attention to speed limits at these higher charges. Are you comfortable with having a high charge with your partner present? Are you comfortable with your partner's charge? Play with increasing or decreasing your charge to fit your lover. This can bring a feeling of attunement. If your partner has a low speed limit, meet his or her limit and then slowly raise your charges together. This will give your partner the support to move to a higher charge.
- Touch or kiss; send love and energy through the pressure points. They are like direct openings to the fixed body patterns.
- Pay attention to the segment in which your partner is holding. Help bring body awareness by placing your hand over the held area just as you did in chapter 10.
- Stroke your partner lovingly. Use body-release techniques learned in chapter 10. Don't hurry. You have set time aside for this, now enjoy it.
- If there is a big a difference between your charge levels, the partner with the lower charge can try the fish position in chapter 7 and take 50 breaths to raise the charge rapidly. Or just enjoy your partner's pace and continue on with yours. You don't have to charge the same or climax at the same time.
- Open your partner's segments with gentle strokes, massaging, and kissing. Move away from manual stimulation of genitals. Help your partner spread out the charge rather than push for release.
- Have intercourse in very slow motion and notice what you are feeling. Stop your movement. Keep breathing. Stay joined with your genitals, contract your PC muscle, and look at your partner. Do the Eye-alogue presence exercise (chapter 9). Feel the exchange of sexual as well as loving energy.
- While you are having intercourse, imagine that you can't tell who has the penis and who has the vagina, or who is entering, who is being entered. In your imagination, pretend that you are the one who is receiving, then the one who is entering.
- Experiment with sending love with your genitals and with your eyes.

- Men, don't worry about your erection. Your penis is really not as important to your partner as it is to you. Lead with your heart, your genitals will follow. You may find that with loving, your penis might get soft for a while. It's not a crisis. Your erection will come back.

- Experiment with super-charging. Begin to build your charge by breathing. Do ten sets of five. Stop after each set to let energy flow through your bodies. Then add more. Remember the symptoms of overcharge and go slow enough so they don't appear. There will be little chance of this because of your movement. After 50 breaths, just stay joined and looking at each other. Keep your charge high with your breath.

- Some couples find the longer they wait for intromission (vaginal entry), the more exciting the event becomes. Others enter for a few minutes, then uncouple and go to oral sex, then back to intercourse again with higher charges. Sequence doesn't matter. There are no rules except to enjoy, to be loving and kind, and to stay present. And keep a high charge.

- Remember, this is containment, not a race to orgasm. Now is the time to try all the positions (check the five freedoms), all the techniques, pressure points, or gymnastics you wish. Enjoy. Keep breathing. Keep your charge up. Keep moving your pelvis and everything else will follow. Change sexual position to one your partner especially likes.

The Orgastic Phase of Sexual Lovemaking

- Don't change your sexual position if you feel you're at a point of no return (orgastic inevitability). It may lower your charge and cause you to miss your orgasm. If everything is working, don't fix it.

- Enjoy your partner's orgasm. Assist her or him with release. Don't take charge of it. It's not yours, nor is it for you. Try not having an orgasm yourself when your partner does.

- Let your partner participate in your enjoyment as you have an orgasm. Don't hide or suppress your excitement. Allow sound and movement.

- Don't perform for your partner. Don't try to look good. Allow your vulnerability to show. Performance is a trap that can lower your charge and release.

- Take pleasure in the changing colors, the intense energy, the release, the ecstasy.

- You can't make someone have an orgasm if they can't or don't want to have one. Don't take your partner's volition and satisfaction away by claiming his or her orgasm. "Was it good for you?" is an agency plea for approval and a turnoff.

- Some people scream at the moment of release, but excess screaming can lower your charge and lessen your ability for heightened release.

The Satisfaction and Intimacy Phase of Sexual Lovemaking

- Don't talk for a while; just hold each other in silence. Be close. Take long, deep breaths together. Stay quiet.

- If you have to urinate or get a drink or smoke, hold off for a while, or do so and hurry back for the silence and skin time.

- Allow yourself to feel your satisfaction and well-being. Don't give it away to your partner. Don't give your partner all the credit for your orgasm—he or she couldn't have done it without you. Feel what the two of you have experienced, but don't compare the two orgasms.

- If you fall asleep after a while, stay in each other's arms, breathing in each other's energy, deepening satisfaction. When you awake you may find that you can still feel a charge in your body. If so, with a second or third round of lovemaking you will find it only gets better.

- Make love, not sex. Kiss, stroke, nuzzle, lightly massage. Express your loving in touch and words.

- Notice where your partner's body is still letting go and where it is still holding.

- Shuttle back and forth between the emotions and sensations of well-being in your body and the pleasure of being with your partner, fully engaging in your partner's pleasure.

- As lovers, shuttle inside to feel your sense of well-being and satisfaction. Bring this energy up through your body, send it out through your eyes, for a core experience of joining.

Living with Abandonment Anxiety

Because your emotions, longings, and fears are on the surface, you may look as though you are in more emotional trouble than the inundation and abandonment-indundation styles. This is not true. Stop apologizing for your abandonment anxiety and at the same time, learn to how to lower it. Don't forget that your emotional pain did not originate in the present or with your partner. It is your abandonment anxiety and only you can attenuate it. When it is difficult to contain your abundant feelings and thoughts, write them in your journal rather than spilling them out on others in an attempt to soothe your discomfort. In this way your journal can hold them for examination so they can deepen or dissolve with clarity.

Abandonment Anxiety Signals: To become familiar with your abandonment anxiety, turn inward rather than examining how you are treated by others. Discover your unique body signals of abandonment. You must remember that if you carry a large load of abandonment into a relationship, it takes only the tiniest injury to make your load become unbearable. Some of the following body signals may help you identify your body clues more clearly. You may feel an arousal of:

- longings in your chest; a calling to love, embrace, or reach out. Paradoxically, the outpouring of longings may cause a sinking, closing feeling in your chest from the effect of cutting off these painfully strong desires;

- oral habits, desires, or obsessions; smoking, drinking, biting fingernails, eating (especially chocolate). Sexualized longings create a desire to suck or kiss, particularly for oral sex;

- eyes that search restlessly from face to face, object to object, eyes that seek but do not really see. Vision and other senses that are fuzzy or dull;

- holding on to a conversation after delivering the message, a reluctance to hang up the telephone, or a need to reveal more about yourself than anyone wants to know, telling the same stories to many people or too many times;

- colds, sore throats, stomach upsets, headaches, and other

physical symptoms. These inadvertently allow you to nurture yourself;

- breathing shallowly or holding your breath, then desperately sucking air in, sighing or muttering expressions of sadness, "oh dear, my god, oh brother, what will I do?"
- rapid heart rate accompanied by anxiety, jittery feelings of panic in your body;
- tears for no reason, lump in the throat, cracking of the voice, feelings of loneliness;
- thoughts and dreams about death.

Make every effort to detect abandonment signals early while it is easiest to restore your sense of well-being. Abandonment anxiety is cumulative, and the longer symptoms linger in your body-psyche, the more opportunity for everyday slights to be compounded into a fragmentation and all the problems that this state brings about.

Reduce Abandonments: These are practical suggestions for keeping your abandonment anxiety at a lower level. Building consistency in your life is one of the most important themes.

- Create a routine. Eat, exercise, etc. at the same time of day. Shop at the same stores, use the same checkout person. Use an appointment book. Schedule regular activities as well as pleasant social occasions. This will keep you from feeling adrift. In relationships, schedule certain routine times for skin time, for sex, and for conversation and nonproductive playtime.
- Develop friends you can count on and see them regularly.
- Develop consistency, order, a sense of well-being, and prevent feelings of isolation through hobbies, reading, writing poetry, etc.
- Memorize the Good Mother Messages and keep the list handy to remind yourself you are okay.
- Become an avid journal writer. It can become a trusted friend.
- Pets keep you connected to something alive. Gardening does too, and is also grounding. Share your harvest with neighbors.
- When you travel, always plan where and what you are going to do. Stay in familiar hotels. To feel more included, participate in the planning. Carry pictures of loved ones wherever you go.
- Learn to meditate. It will deepen your connection to a spiritual source in yourself. Do the Sustaining Integration exercises on page 116. Then focus on the "I am" sense of well-being that you establish in your body. See how long you can sustain this feeling during and after meditation.
- Try to have jobs where you work with others on a regular schedule. Don't work with unreliable people. People who show up late or not at all will upset you more than you can tolerate. Be choosy as each disappointment will increase a sense of abandonment.
- Change your residence as little as possible. When you must move, make your new home as comfortable and homey as you can, and do so quickly.
- Shop with a friend. You'll be less likely to long for things you can't have or to feel abandoned by salespeople.

- Never spend holidays alone. Plan ahead to spend them with people you want to be with.
- Exercise regularly, with a partner or trainer, if possible. Team sports are ideal. The exercises in this book are superb. Exercise helps you gain a sense of well-being, strength, and consistency in your body.

Living with Inundation Anxiety

If, in your fear of inundation, you are still acting as if you are protecting yourself against excessively controlling or powerful parents, this may be causing you to be nonrelational in intimate relationships. You probably inundate yourself by your own body holding patterns and exaggerated response to people's attempts to be close.

Inundating Situations: Keep in mind that you are not a vulnerable child and *no one can control you*. Common situations that may increase your sense of inundation:

- crowds, confined spaces like airplanes and elevators;
- events of duty such as graduations, weddings, funerals, holidays. These may trigger overwhelming emotions from the past and present and may add pressure on you to live up to the expectations of others;
- a relationship with someone who doesn't have good boundaries or respect for yours;
- work with or for someone who constantly checks up on you or criticizes your work.

Reduce Inundation: These are practical suggestions for keeping your inundation anxiety level low. Creating breathing room is most important. You are not bad for needing more.

- Keep your body relaxed and flexible. A tight body limits internal breathing room and makes any encroachment seem like suffocation. Balance weight training with stretching, yoga, and the exercises in this book. Receive a massage. Have regular sexual releases.
- Put your own inundating thoughts onto paper before they overwhelm you. Notice how much pressure you apply to yourself.
- Create space for yourself; open your collar, loosen a tight belt or brassiere.
- Take a breather when things begin to feel oppressive. Provide your own transportation when you can, so that you can escape when you have had enough.
- Don't say yes when you mean no.
- Remember that you have a right to be alone and to set boundaries, to shut the bathroom door, and to display your belongings and your taste somewhere in the house. You have a right to make reasonable demands for punctuality, cleanliness, neatness, quiet, and other things that are important to you.
- You needn't divulge your innermost secrets nor be as close as your partner wants.

As with abandonment fears, the feelings of inundation are more often imagined than real. Early detection, plus physically changing something can do wonders. Remember, too, that if you are always protecting against inundation, your unguarded backside, abandonment, will be your Achilles' heel.

Anand, Margo. *The Art of Sexual Ecstasy*. California: Jeremy Tarcher, 1989.

Assagioli, Roberto. *The Act of Will*. London: Wildwood House, 1974.

Assagioli, Roberto. *Psychosynthesis*. New York: Hobbs, Dorman & Company, 1965.

Beck, Charolotte. *Nothing Special, Living Zen*. San Francisco: Harper, 1993.

Berman, Morris. *Coming to Our Senses*. New York: Simon & Schuster, 1989.

Bulfinch, Thomas. *Myths of Greece and Rome*. New York: Penguin Books, 1981.

Campbell, Joseph. *Creative Mythology*. New York: Penguin Books, 1968.

Campbell, Joseph. *The Hero with a Thousand Faces*. New Jersey: Princeton University Press, 1949.

Chopra, Deepak. *Ageless Body, Timeless Mind*. New York: Harmony Books, 1993.

Exley, Helen. *Love: A Celebration*. Great Britain: Exley, 1981.

Gage, Suzann. *A New View of a Woman's Body*. New York: Simon & Schuster, 1991.

Govinda, Lama Anagarika. *The Way of the White Clouds*. London: Rider & Company, 1966.

Gunther, Bernard. *Neo Tantra*. New York: Harper & Row, 1980.

Hamill, Sam. *The Erotic Spirit*. Boston: Shambhala, 1996.

Hooper, Anne. *The Ultimate Sex Book*. New York: Dorling Kindersley, 1992.

Johnson, Robert. *She*. New York: Perennial Library, 1979.

Kaplan, Louise. *Oneness & Separateness: From Infant to Individual*. New York: Simon & Schuster, 1978.

Keleman, Stanley. *Your Body Speaks Its Mind*. New York: Simon & Schuster, 1975.

Kopp, Sheldon. *If You Meet the Buddha on the Road, Kill Him*. California: Science and Behavior Books, 1972.

Ladas, A., B. Whipple, and J. Perry. *The G Spot*. New York: Dell Publishing, 1983.

LeShan, Lawrence. *You Can Fight for Your Life*. New York: M. Evans & Company, 1977.

Liebert, Daniel. *Fragments, Ecstasies*. New Mexico: Source Books, 1981.

Michael, R., J. Gagnon, E. Laumann, and G. Kolata. *Sex in America*. Boston: Little, Brown & Company, 1994.

Miller, Alice. *The Drama of the Gifted Child*. New York: Basic Books, 1981.

Money, John. *Sex Research*. New York: Holt, Rinehart and Winston, 1965.

Mookerjee, A., and M. Khanna. *The Tantric Way*. Boston, Massachusetts: Little, Brown & Company, 1977.

Panger, Daniel. *Thoughts and Meditations*. New Mexico: First Unitarian Church of Albuquerque, 1978.

Rahula, Walpola. *What the Buddha Taught*. New York: Grove Press, 1959.

Rajneesh, Osho. *More Gold Nuggets*. Germany: The Rebel, 1989.

Reich, Wilhelm. *Character Analysis*. New York: Noonday Press, 1968.

Rinpoche, Sogyal. *The Tibetan Book of Living and Dying*. San Francisco: Harper, 1992.

Rosenberg, Jack. *Total Orgasm*. New York: Random House, 1973.

Rosenberg, J., M. Rand, and D. Assay. *Body, Self & Soul*. Atlanta: Humanics Limited, 1985.

Sannella, Lee. *Kundalini*. California: H. S. Dakin Company, 1976.

Schnarch, David M. *Constructing the Sexual Crucible*. New York: W. W. Norton & Company, 1991.

Shawn, W., and A. Gregory. *My Dinner with Andre*. New York: Grove Press, 1981.

Stern, Daniel. *The Interpersonal World of the Infant*. New York: Basic Books, 1985.

Stopped, Myriad. *The Magic of Sex*. New York: Dorling Kindersley, 1991.

Tarnas, Richard. *The Passion of the Western Mind*. New York: Harmony Books, 1991.

Welwood, John. *Love and Awakening*. New York: Harper Collins, 1996.

Wilber, Ken. *Grace and Grit*. Boston: Shambhala, 1993.

Wilber, Ken. *Sex, Ecology, Spirituality*. Boston: Shambhala, 1995.

Wolf, Franklin. *Pathways Through Space*. New York: Julian Press, 1973.

Zukov, Gary. *The Seat of The Soul*. New York: Simon & Schuster, 1990.